Comorbidity of Mental and Physical Disorders

Key Issues in Mental Health

Vol. 179

Series Editors

Anita Riecher-Rössler Basel
Norman Sartorius Geneva

Comorbidity of Mental and Physical Disorders

Volume Editors

Norman Sartorius Geneva
Richard I.G. Holt Southampton
Mario Maj Naples

12 figures and 20 tables, 2015

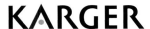

Basel · Freiburg · Paris · London · New York · Chennai · New Delhi ·
Bangkok · Beijing · Shanghai · Tokyo · Kuala Lumpur · Singapore · Sydney

Key Issues in Mental Health

Formerly published as 'Bibliotheca Psychiatrica' (founded 1917)

Professor Norman Sartorius, MA, MD, PhD, FRCPsych
Association for the Improvement of Mental Health Programmes
Geneva, Switzerland

Professor Mario Maj, MD, PhD
Department of Psychiatry
University of Naples
Naples, Italy

Professor Richard I.G. Holt, MA, MB, BChir, PhD, FRCP, FHEA
Human Development and Health Academic Unit
Faculty of Medicine, University of Southampton
University Hospital Southampton NHS Foundation Trust
Southampton, UK

Library of Congress Cataloging-in-Publication Data

Comorbidity of mental and physical disorders / volume editors, Norman Sartorius, Richard I.G. Holt, Mario Maj.
  p. ; cm. -- (Key issues in mental health ; vol. 179)
  Includes bibliographical references and indexes.
  ISBN 978-3-318-02603-0 (hard cover : alk. paper) -- ISBN 978-3-318-02604-7 (electronic version)
  I. Sartorius, N., editor. II. Holt, Richard I. G., editor. III. Maj, Mario, 1953- , editor.
IV. Series: Key issues in mental health ; v. 179.
1662-4874
  [DNLM: 1. Comorbidity. 2. Mental Disorders--etiology. 3. Disease--psychology.
4. Disease Management. 5. Syndrome. W1 BI429 v.179 2015 / WM 140]
  RC454.4
  616.89--dc23
                                                                        2014034031

Bibliographic Indices. This publication is listed in bibliographic services.

© Copyright 2015 by S. Karger AG, P.O. Box, CH-4009 Basel (Switzerland)
www.karger.com
Printed in Germany on acid-free and non-aging paper (ISO 9706) by Kraft Druck GmbH, Ettlingen
ISSN 1662–4874
e-ISSN 1662–4882
ISBN 978–3–318–02603–0
e-ISBN 978–3–318–02604–7

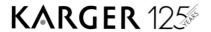

Contents

Foreword

The editors are to be congratulated in having obtained contributions from experts on a wide range of physical disorders in order to throw light on those physical disorders which have a higher rate of psychological disorders associated with them. Recognition and treatment of these disorders have been shown to improve the patient's quality of life, and also collaboration with the treatment regimes for their physical illness.

Of course, the shoe can be fitted to the other foot, and one can ask to what extent do particular psychological disorders have higher rates of expected physical disorders. Both of these are valid questions, but while the second is of great scientific interest, the first is more important from the viewpoint of patient care.

In probing the reasons for these higher than expected comorbidities, it is often found that there is no single way in which one form of morbidity influences the other: each one exacerbates the other, and good clinical care must not be blind to the psychological disorders with which a particular physical disease is associated. This book provides examples of the various ways in which such vicious circles establish themselves.

In addition to the possible factors mentioned by the editors in their preface that may account for the high comorbidity between psychological disorders and physical illnesses, there are a number of other possible relationships. First, the number of different pains caused by the physical illnesses increases the probability of depression: in one primary care study, patients with a single pain were no more likely to be depressed than those without pain, but with two different pains the probability of depression was double, and with three or more pains the probability of depression was five times higher [1]. Secondly, chronic physical illness carries with it the risk of disability, which can be very depressing for an adult who has previously been healthy. For example, Prince et al. [2] showed that the attributable fraction of disability or handicap for the prediction of onset of depression among the elderly was no less than 0.69, and Ormel et al. [3] showed similar findings in Holland. Thirdly, there are physical changes in some diseases which may underlie the development of depression, such as changes in the allostatic load. Allostasis refers to the ability of the body to adapt to stressful conditions. It is a dynamic, adaptive process. Tissue damage, degenerative disease (like arthritis) and life stress all increase allostatic load and can induce inflammatory changes which produce substances such as bradykinin, prostaglandins, cytokines and chemokines. These substances mediate tissue repair and healing, but also act as irritants that result in peripheral sensitisation of sensory neurons, which in turn activate central pain pathways [4]. These are all ways in which a physical disorder can produce higher than expected rates of psychological disorders.

There are also psychological disorders that antedate episodes of physical disorder, such as a depressive illness. Systematic reviews of 11 prospective cohort studies in healthy populations show that depression predicts later development of coronary heart disease in all of them [5, 6]. The occurrence of a depressive episode before an episode of myocardial infarction has been reported by Nielsen et al. [7]. Three prospective studies have also shown that depression is an independent risk factor in stroke [8–10]. In prospective population-based cohort studies, depression has been shown to predict the later development of colorectal cancer [11], back pain [12], irritable bowel syndrome [13] and multiple sclerosis [14], and there is some evidence that depression may precede the onset of type 2 diabetes. Prince et al. [15] argue that there is consistent evidence for depression leading to physical ill-health in coronary heart disease and stroke, as well as depression in pregnancy potentially leading to infant stunting and infant mortality.

It has been hypothesised [16] that increases in pro-inflammatory cytokines in depression and increased adrenocortical reactivity may also lead to atherosclerosis, and with it increased risk for both stroke and coronary artery disease. In the latter, autonomic changes in depression may also cause ECG changes which favour development of coronary disease. Changes in natural killer cells and T-lymphocytes in depression may lead to lowered resistance to AIDS in HIV infections. Menkes and McDonald [17] have argued that exogenous interferons may cause both depression and increased pain sensitivity in susceptible individuals by suppressing tryptophan availability and therefore serotonin synthesis. More prosaic explanations include reduced physical activity in people suffering from depression [18].

It is clear that relationships between the two forms of morbidity are complex and that causal relationships that may be true for one physical disorder may not apply to another disorder. The chapters of this book bring together in one place a comprehensive account of these comorbidities, and an important step has therefore been taken in a field in which there is still much to learn in the future.

Sir David Goldberg, Institute of Psychiatry, King's College, London

References

1 Dworkin S, Vonkorff M, Le Resche L: Multiple pains, psychiatric and social disturbance: an epidemiologic investigation. Arch Gen Psychiatry 1990;47:239–245.

2 Prince MJ, Harwood RH, Blizard RA, et al: Impairment, disability and handicap as risk factors for late life depression. Psychol Med 1998;27:311–321.

3 Ormel J, Kempen GI, Penninx BW, et al: Chronic medical conditions and mental health in old people. Psychol Med 1997;27:1065–1067.

4 Rittner HL, Brack A, Stein C: Pro-algesic and analgesic actions of immune cells. Curr Opin Anaesthesiol 2003;16:527–533.

5 Hemingway H, Marmot M: Evidence based cardiology: psychosocial factors in the aetiology and prognosis of coronary heart disease: systematic review of prospective cohort studies. BMJ 1999;318:1460–1467.

6 Nicholson A, Kuper H, Hemingway H: Depression as an aetiologic and prognostic factor in coronary heart disease: a meta-analysis of 6,362 events among 146,538 participants in 54 observational studies. Eur Heart J 2006;318:1460–1467.

7 Nielsen E, Brown GW, Marmot M: Myocardial infarction; in Brown GW, Harris T (eds): Life Events and Illness. London, Unwin Hyman, 1989, pp 313–342.

8 Everson SA, Roberts RE, Goldberg DE, et al: Depressive symptoms and increased risk of stroke mortality in a 29-year period. Arch Intern Med 1998;158:1133–1138.

9 Ohira T, Iso H, Satoh H, et al: Prospective study of stroke among Japanese. Stroke 2001;32:903–908.

10 Larson SL, Owens PL, Ford D, et al: Depressive disorder, dysthymic disorder and risk of stroke: thirteen-year follow up from Baltimore Epidemiologic Catchment Area study. Stroke 2001;32:1979–1983.

11 Kroenke CH, Bennett GG, Fuchs C, et al: Depressive symptoms and prospective incidence of colorectal cancer in women. Am J Epidemiol 2005;162:839–848.

12 Larson SL, Clark MR, Eaton WW: Depressive disorder as a long-term antecedent risk factor for incident back pain: a 13-year follow-up study from the Baltimore Epidemiological Catchment Area sample. Psychol Med 2004;34:211–219.

13 Ruigómez A, García Rodríguez LA, Panés J: Risk of irritable bowel syndrome after an episode of bacterial gastroenteritis in general practice: influence of comorbidities. Clin Gastroenterol Hepatol 2007;5:465–469.

14 Grant I, Brown GW, Harris T, et al: Severely threatening events and marked life difficulties preceding onset or exacerbation of multiple sclerosis. J Neurol Neurosurg Psychiatry 1989;52:8–13.

15 Prince M, Patel V, Saxena S, et al: No health without mental health. Lancet 2007;370:859–877.

16 Wichers M, Maes M: The psychoneuro-immuno-pathophysiology of cytokine-induced depression in humans. Int J Neuropsychopharmacol 2002;5:375–388.

17 Menkes DB, McDonald JA: Interferons, serotonin and neurotoxicity. Psychol Med 2000;30:259–268.

18 Whooley MA, de Jonge P, Vittinghoff E, et al: Depressive symptoms, health behaviors, and risk of cardiovascular events in patients with coronary heart disease. JAMA 2008;300:2379–2388.

Preface

There is little doubt about the fact that comorbidity – the simultaneous presence of two or more diseases – is a major challenge for health services. The prevalence of comorbidity has increased rapidly and continues to grow for several reasons, mainly the increase in life expectancy following successes in medicine and socioeconomic development. However, also playing a role are environmental factors (such as air pollution), changes in lifestyle, rapid urbanization and medical factors including iatrogenic disease and the fragmentation of medical services which often result in the late recognition of comorbid diseases and the consequent failure to treat them.

An area of particular neglect is the comorbidity between mental and physical disorders. One of the main reasons for this development is the long-standing separation of psychiatry from other branches of medicine. The geographic separation of mental health institutions from the hospitals and departments dealing with other physical diseases is a material expression of the perception that psychiatric disorders are not diseases like others, and a consequence of this perception is the growing distance and separation between psychiatry and the rest of medicine. In practice, this has led to many psychiatrists failing to recognize the presence of physical illness in their patients and being reluctant to provide treatment for the physical disorder when a diagnosis is made. The same is true for specialists in other branches of medicine who pay insufficient attention to the presence and treatment of mental disorders in their patients.

The neglect of comorbidity of mental and physical illness is also linked to the fact that its prevalence has been, for a long time, severely underestimated. This was due in part to the lack of recognition described above; however, it also reflects the fact that the stigma of mental illness makes patients reluctant to speak about their mental health problems to nonpsychiatric physicians. Comorbidity of mental and physical illnesses often leads to a tacit collusion with patients and healthcare professionals agreeing to deal with the physical illness as if the mental disorder did not exist. The fact that people with mental illness are often poor and less well educated may have also contributed to lesser utilization of health services that might have recorded the number and frequency of comorbidity of mental and physical illness.

The scant attention given to the comorbidity of mental and physical disorders is of major public health concern. The simultaneous presence of mental and physical diseases worsens the prognosis of both types of disorders and increases the personal and social cost of dealing with them. Complications of the comorbid diseases become more probable and their treatment is more complex. What is particularly worrisome is that comorbidity of mental and physical disorders is becoming more frequent at a time when medicine is becoming increasingly fragmented into super-specialties and when the numbers of general practitioners who can follow the rapid development of knowledge in the many disciplines of medicine is diminishing.

The reasons for the high prevalence of mental and physical illness are only partially clear. To an extent this may occur because some people with mental illness do not pay sufficient attention to their bodies and do not follow elementary rules of healthy lifestyle, hygiene and disease prevention. That many people with mental illness live in conditions of poverty and deprivation where they may be exposed to the considerable dangers of violence and abuse might also be a part of the explanation. People with mental illness often abuse alcohol and other drugs which expose them to the health consequences of substance misuse such as hepatitis and HIV infections. Although these reasons are important, they do not explain all of the excess comorbidity. A number of biological changes seen in mental illness may also predispose to physical ill health, including enhanced inflammation or endocrine dysfunction, but genetic factors are also important. We are still lacking longitudinal studies of comorbidity that could offer insights into the mechanisms. The recent findings on the effects of early childhood abuse on the prevalence of cardiovascular diseases and on the prevalence of depression are good examples of the gains that might result from long-term and life-perspective studies.

Our main goal for this book was to assemble and present material that will help in efforts to raise awareness of the magnitude and nefarious consequences of comorbidity of mental and physical illnesses while stimulating relevant research as well as the application of knowledge that is already available. We invited leading experts in the field of comorbidity to participate in the production of this volume. We have tried to exemplify issues that arise in three main areas of concern. The first of these are the public health aspects of comorbidity focusing on the ways in which comorbidity can be conceptualized, on the cost that comorbidity presents to society and on the interaction of comorbidity with factors stemming from the context of socioeconomic development. In the second group of chapters we assembled reviews of evidence that illustrate the two main approaches to the understanding of evidence about comorbidity. For the first approach, the chapters look at specific issues that arise in relation to comorbidity of mental disorders with disease groups of major public health importance, such as cardiovascular illness, cancer and infectious diseases. For the second approach we examined physical comorbidity in relation to a range of mental and behavioral disorders, including substance abuse, eating disorders and anxiety. The message imbedded in this way of presenting evidence – using one of the two approaches – is that both are necessary: taking a position of looking at comorbidity from only one side may hide important issues and clues. The last group of chapters includes contributions that deal with the elements of the response to the problems arising from comorbidity – the organization of health services (especially the role of the general practitioners), the training of different categories of health personnel and the multisectoral engagement necessary to prevent comorbidity.

Norman Sartorius, Geneva
Richard I.G. Holt, Southampton
Mario Maj, Naples

Sartorius N, Holt RIG, Maj M (eds): Comorbidity of Mental and Physical Disorders.
Key Issues Ment Health. Basel, Karger, 2015, vol 179, pp 1–14 (DOI: 10.1159/000365522)

Conceptual Perspectives on the Co-Occurrence of Mental and Physical Disease: Diabetes and Depression as a Model

Edwin B. Fisher[a, b] · Juliana C.N. Chan[c] · Sarah Kowitt[a, b] · Hairong Nan[d] · Norman Sartorius[e] · Brian Oldenburg[f]

[a]Peers for Progress, American Academy of Family Physicians Foundation, Leawood, Kans., and [b]Department of Health Behavior, Gillings School of Global Public Health, University of North Carolina, Chapel Hill, N.C., USA; [c]Department of Medicine and Therapeutics, Hong Kong Institute of Diabetes and Obesity, Chinese University of Hong Kong and Prince of Wales Hospital, and [d]Faculty of Health and Social Sciences, The Hong Kong Polytechnic University, Hong Kong, SAR, P.R. China; [e]Association for the Improvement of Mental Health Programmes, Geneva, Switzerland; [f]School of Population and Global Health, The University of Melbourne, Melbourne, Vic., Australia

Abstract

Diabetes and depression provide a model for understanding the comorbidity of mental and physical disorders, as each influences the other while sharing a broad range of biological, psychological, socioeconomic and cultural determinants. Diabetes and depression may be viewed as: (1) categories or dimensions, (2) single problems or parts of broader categories, e.g. metabolic/cardiovascular abnormalities or negative emotions, (3) separate comorbidities or integrated so that depression is seen as part of the comprehensive, normal clinical picture of diabetes, and (4) expressions of a shared, complex biosocial propensity to chronic disease and psychological distress. Interventions should reflect the commonalities among chronic mental and physical disorders and should include integrated clinical care and self-management programs along with population approaches to prevention and management. Among these, peer support, self-management and problem solving, and programs for whole communities are promising approaches. Self-management and problem solving may also provide a coherent framework for integrating the diverse management of tasks and objectives of those affected by diabetes and depression and as a model for prevalent multimorbidity.

© 2015 S. Karger AG, Basel

Amidst growing evidence of the bidirectional relationship between diabetes and depression at the pathophysiological, clinical, behavioral, and social levels [e.g. 1], their co-occurrence also provides a window on a broader range of comorbidities among mental health, psychological distress, and diverse chronic diseases and health condi-

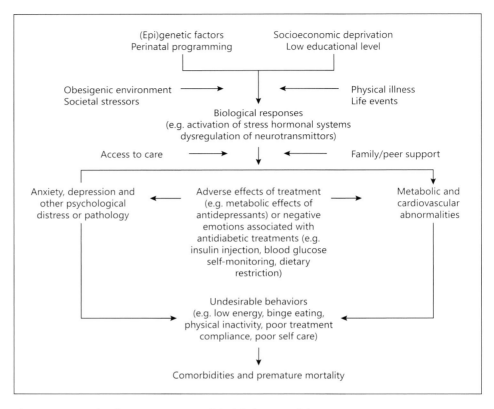

Fig. 1. An example of an integrative model of diabetes and depression.

tions. Diabetes itself is an excellent model of chronic disease in general, and depression, with its broad range of influences, severity and intervention strategies provides an excellent model for understanding psychological distress and mental health problems as they interact with other aspects of health and well-being.

Biological, Psychological and Socioeconomic Influences in Diabetes and Depression

How social and psychological factors 'get under the skin' to influence biological processes is central to understanding the complexity of relationships between mental health and chronic disease [e.g. 2]. Figure 1 provides a useful model in diabe-

tes and depression that recognizes how depression and stressful life events can lead to the activation of the hypothalamic-pituitary-adrenal axis and complex hormonal interactions in the pathogenesis of metabolic disorders. These complex hormonal interactions can give rise to a wide range of metabolic and cardiovascular abnormalities which characterize diabetes and are increasingly observed in people with depression, thus threatening an increasing cycle of psychological and physical ill health [3].

Starting with epigenetic effects of early maternal care, a variety of social, psychological and biological influences may interact in the etiology and course of both depression and diabetes, and accelerate the psychological and metabolic abnormalities of each [1]. As symptoms and complications of diabetes increase, associated psychosocial stress and reduced coping ability may contribute to depression. Additionally, the psychological burdens of diabetes treatments, such as insulin injection or blood glucose self-monitoring, can increase negative emotions and maladaptive behaviors and lead to a loss of interest, low energy, abnormal eating patterns, sleep disturbance, poor treatment compliance and poor concentration. As diabetes may exacerbate depression, likewise evidence indicates deleterious effects of coexisting depression on clinical status, subsequent complications, mortality and increased healthcare expenditures [4].

Following the model in figure 1, broad social and economic contexts of family and social relationships as well as organizational, economic and cultural factors influence depression, diabetes and other mental and physical disorders. Examples of these are detailed in a report available at http://sph.unc.edu/profiles/edwin-b-fisher-phd/.

The Breadth of Environmental Influence: Neighborhood Design and Social Isolation

Illustrating the broad range of potential influences on mental and physical disorders, the next paragraphs provide examples of how neighborhood and architectural design may influence social relationships and health status.

One study on housing involving older adults showed that architectural features such as porches and stoops encouraged greater person-to-person contact and were positively associated with perceived social support. These in turn were associated with less self-reported depression and anxiety [5]. Other architectural features, such as windows, allowed for broader observation of the surrounding area, but removed individuals from close person-to-person contact and were associated with lower levels of perceived social support and greater psychological distress [5].

Research has also documented associations between neighborhood characteristics and diabetes prevalence and management. In a natural experiment in the mid-1990s, the Department of Housing and Urban Development randomly assigned approximately 4,500 women with children living in public housing in high-poverty urban areas to one of three conditions: housing vouchers to move to low-poverty areas and receive counseling, unrestricted vouchers and no counseling, and control – no vouchers. In follow-up data (2008–2010), those who had been offered vouchers for low-poverty neighborhoods were less likely than controls to have BMI ≥35 or ≥40, and less likely to have a glycated hemoglobin ≥6.5% (48 mmol/mol). Those receiving the unrestricted vouchers did not differ from controls [6].

A study in Quebec, Canada sheds light on specific neighborhood features that may be especially important. Individuals who reported their neighborhoods as having worse physical and social order (i.e. deteriorated buildings, graffiti, noise, trash, crime and vandalism), less social cohesion, and less access to services and resources had greater diabetes distress including emotional burden, dissatisfaction with medical care, difficulty with treatment regimen, interpersonal impacts and support for diabetes management. Even after controlling for confounders, such as income, education and race, these relationships remained significant [7].

The complex interweaving of multiple levels of influence results in sharp social and economic stratification of both diabetes and depression. Failure to recognize the influence of contextual factors may have at least three deleterious consequences. First, interventions may be less powerful than they might be. Second, benefits of medical or psychological interventions delivered to individuals may be *underestimated* if important contextual moderators of their effects are not accounted for in analyses. Third, individuals may be viewed as responsible for problems in a manner that constitutes a kind of 'victim blaming'.

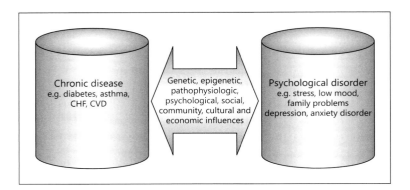

Fig. 2. Simple model of comorbidity.

What Are We Preventing, Treating, and Managing? Key Definitional and Conceptual Issues

In order to develop comprehensive approaches to the effective prevention and/or management of diabetes and depression, it is necessary to clarify just how the problems and their interrelationships are to be approached. The term 'comorbidity' connotes two well-defined and distinct clinical entities, occurring simultaneously and each tending to occur more frequently in the presence of the other, as simply illustrated in figure 2. However, the interrelationships between diabetes and depression may be viewed in other ways as well.

A Dimensional versus Categorical View of Each of Diabetes and Depression

Both depression and diabetes are commonly defined categorically with specific criteria used to classify individuals as having either depression or diabetes. However, an alternative to this categorical definition of depression has been a dimensional characterization of mood or dysphoria, often using standardized instruments such as the popular Beck Depression Inventory which was originally developed and validated as a measure of depressed mood, not of categorical depression. As an example of the dimensional perspective in diabetes, the success of preventing incident diabetes in high-risk subjects has led to the identifi-

cation of a dimension of dysglycemia including varying degrees of insulin resistance and deficiency that underlie manifest abnormalities in glucose metabolism. Supporting the dimensional perspective, 'graded relationships' between depression and both myocardial infarction and all-cause mortality suggest that depression 'is best viewed as a continuous variable that represents a chronic psychological characteristic rather than a discrete and episodic psychiatric condition' [8].

With both depression and diabetes, categorical definitions may be superimposed on the dimensional by defining the diagnostic category according to a convention of some criterion score as in common – and changing [9] – definitions of hypertension. Additionally, the International Classification of Diseases distinguishes three categories – mild, moderate and severe depression – that also reflect the practical usefulness of the dimensional approach.

Single Problem versus Group of Problems

In addition to the difference between viewing problems as distinct categories or as dimensions, diabetes and depression may each be categorized as part of a broader class of problems: cardiometabolic abnormalities for diabetes and negative emotions for depression. For example, studies of depression in various groups indicate high co-occurrence of depression, anxiety and other varieties of psychological distress [10]. Similarly, studies in cardiovascular risk indicate the utility of grouping together a set of negative emotions that includes depression, anxiety, hostility and stress, and their complex interactions in pathways related to cardiovascular pathogenesis [11]. Recent work in diabetes has also indicated that general measures of diabetes distress may be more closely related to poor metabolic control than measures of depressed mood alone [12]. Parallel to the overlap among measures of psychological disorder and distress, hyperlipidemia, central adiposity and hypertension often co-occur with 'prediabetes' or diabetes, leading some to refer to the group as comprising a 'metabolic syndrome' [13].

Whether depression and diabetes are best viewed as distinct or as members of broader categories is controversial. For example, some argue that, however much they may co-occur, one needs to treat the individual cardiovascular and metabolic problems encompassed by the term 'metabolic syndrome' with appropriate medications for diabetes, hypertension and hyperlipidemia [14]. Similarly, one may argue that beyond the co-occurrence with anxiety, hostility and stress, depressed mood alone has a specific and distinctive role with both diabetes and cardiovascular disease, requiring specific treatment rather than a more generalized approach.

Whether diabetes or depression are best viewed as distinct entities or as parts of broader syndromes may depend on the purpose of the viewing. For example, Valderas et al. [15] noted that the value of different models of comorbidity would vary according to the perspective taken by specialist, primary care, public health or health services. From the perspective of clinical care of individuals, differentiating among specific problems – depression, anxiety and hostility on the one hand and diabetes, hypertension and hyperlipidemia on the other – makes great sense. Whether with psychotherapy or psychopharmacology, management of depressed mood differs from treatment of hostility or anxiety, just as medication for diabetes differs from that for hy-pertension or hypercholesterolemia. At the population level, however, co-prevalent problems may share common treatment and prevention targets, such as healthy diet, physical activity, weight management and communities that encourage them [e.g. 6] for diabetes and cardiovascular disease, or, for negative emotions, socioeconomic well-being and communities and families that encourage cooperation and satisfying relationships among neighbors [5]. Thus, the broader categories of cardiometabolic abnormalities and negative emotions may help guide population-wide prevention and treatment campaigns. At the same time, their individual components are duly the focus of clinical intervention.

Separate 'Comorbidities' or Depression as Part of Normal Clinical Picture of Diabetes

Viewing diabetes and depression as part of broader groupings or syndromes may also make sense *across* the categories of mental health and medical illness. Research such as from the Diabetes Prevention Program [16] raises the possibility that depression is an early sign or precursor of diabetes. Thus, as we think of the comorbidity of diabetes and depression, we might consider whether they are best viewed as distinct clinical entities that occasionally exist together, or as components of a broader syndrome encompassing both psychological and physical problems. The consideration of depression as part of such a broader syndrome would not necessarily include depressive disorders with specific symptoms, courses and outcomes such as severe depressive disorders with psychotic features (DSM 296.24) or depression in typical bipolar disorders. More generally, the term 'depression' needs to be understood as referring to mood changes that may be combined with a large – probably larger than currently recognized – number of problems and syndromes, rather than as a single entity.

Table 1 depicts options to view diabetes and depression as: (1) distinct but comorbid conditions, (2) closely related conditions with appropriately

Table 1. Conceptualizations of the diabetes-depression relationship and implications for treatment

Conceptualization of relationship between diabetes and depression	Approach to treatment
Depression as a separate clinical problem but one that complicates diabetes management, e.g. 'There's no way these folks can address their diabetes until we treat their depression'	Referral for specialty care
Depression and diabetes as overlapping, e.g. helping patients to set and reach goals for increasing physical activity is good for *both* diabetes and depression	Develop resources for psychological and psychiatric services that are closely linked to diabetes care team; include attention to emotional issues in self-management programs
Integration: depression is part of the normal scope of diabetes and *vice versa*	Attention to psychosocial and emotional issues is a routine part of diabetes care; clinical depression as part of a range of emotional problems in diabetes Reflecting the bidirectional nature of these relationships, obesity, metabolic syndromes, diabetes and related problems are considered as part of the management of depression

coordinated care and (3) clinical problems that normally and commonly co-occur, requiring integrated care. In an integrated approach, the treatment of depression becomes a routine part of diabetes care, just as foot care and yearly retinal checks. So, too, the psychological or medical treatment of depression may be expanded to address its routine metabolic and cardiovascular dimensions. Consider, for example, physical activity, which is often included in diabetes self-management and increasingly recognized as helpful in reducing depression. When promoting physical activity in diabetes self-management, one should routinely consider reticence to engage in exercise as potentially linked to mood problems. Additionally, one should structure goal setting and monitoring to maximize the possible benefits not only of physical activity itself, but also of the mood-elevating effects of achieving a personal goal [17]. At the same time, promoting physical activity as part of depression treatment may draw added emphasis from the recognition of its value not only in increasing mood, but also in reducing cardiovascular risks to which those with depression are prone.

Biosocial Propensity to Chronic Disease and Psychological Distress

Bringing together a number of the points illustrated so far in this chapter, figure 3 outlines a biosocial complex of determinants of chronic disease ranging from genetic and epigenetic effects (including those of maternal nurturance during early childhood) to community design. Given sufficient deficiencies in this complex, some kind of chronic disease (diabetes, asthma, etc.) is very likely as is some variety of appreciable psychological distress or psychopathology. The particular *expression* of this biosocial complex in one or another chronic disease and one or another type of psychological problem may be hard to predict, but the likelihood of at least one of each – chronic disease and psychological distress – is highly likely. In a casual survey of practicing primary care clinicians, the common response is 'That's half of my waiting room.'

Figure 3 raises an important point, 'What is fundamental that requires attention?' In the simpler terms of figure 2, that fundamental may be, for example, diagnosed diabetes and diagnosed

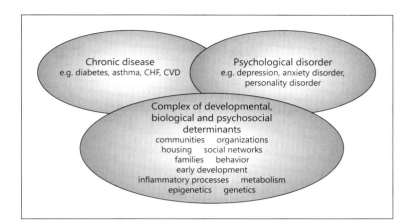

Fig. 3. Chronic disease and psychological disorders as expressions of a biosocial complex of influences.

depression co-occurring in a particular individual. In the more developmental, genetic terms of figure 3, what is fundamental is the biosocial complex of events that make expression in diabetes and depression or some other varieties of medical and psychological morbidity highly likely. The particular choice of expressions may be almost accidental or perhaps guided by some specific factors, but the likelihood of such expressions is almost assured.

Treatment: Integrative Clinical and Comprehensive Population Approaches

A range of pharmacologic and psychological [18] interventions have been found to be useful for comorbid diabetes and depression. Here we highlight those that reflect the integrative, social and community perspectives suggested in the preceding pages.

Integrative Chronic Disease Care and Self-Management

Recent reports [19, 20] have documented improved clinical outcomes in diabetes through integrative care that includes team care, evidence-based guidelines, procedures for coordinating care, and registry-based monitoring and prioriti-

zation of cases and strategies. Self-management interventions are key components of integrative approaches to clinical care. They teach and promote skills for doing the things in day-to-day life that are necessary to enhance clinical status and well-being [21]. Diabetes self-management interventions have been well documented as effective in improving metabolic control [22]. Notable within the context of the present review, reports of diabetes self-management and education programs have included benefits in quality of life [23].

Integrative models have also emerged in mental health. Assertive community treatment focuses on treating individuals with severe mental illness (schizophrenia, depression, bipolar disorder) within the community through a team of professionals from psychiatry, nursing and social work. Rather than providing support within hospital or clinical settings, community care is provided 24 h a day, 7 days a week. Research has documented the effectiveness of assertive community treatment in reducing hospitalization days, inpatient psychiatric services and emergency room visits, especially among high utilizers of healthcare services [24]. Especially pertinent to the present volume, integrated assertive community treatment models have also been used to provide care for co-occurring physical and mental health problems [25].

Integrating such approaches to both mental and physical disorders, Katon and colleagues [26] developed 'collaborative care' models that combined pharmacotherapy, psychotherapy, general counseling, problem solving and support provided by a depression care manager. They included those with depression as well as either diabetes and/or elevated cardiovascular risk, and found that collaborative care improved treatment (as indicated by medication adjustments), clinical risk measures (glycemic control, lipids, blood pressure), quality of life and social role disability [26]. A 2012 meta-analysis of 69 studies of collaborative care [27] documented substantial improvements on a variety of indicators, including adherence to depression treatment (OR = 2.22) and recovery from symptoms (OR = 1.75). Such findings have also been replicated with low-income ethnic minority patients in the USA [28].

Social Influences: Peer Support

Peer supporters, also known as 'community health workers', 'lay health advisors', 'promotores' and a number of other terms, can assist individuals in self-management of diabetes and prevention and management of other diseases [e.g. 29]. They may also provide emotional support and encourage problem solving to address depression and other emotional distress. Both the social isolation or lack of a confidant that often accompany psychopathology and distress [29] and the importance of simple social contact and emotional support suggest that simple, frequent, affirming and pleasant contact from a supporter may be especially helpful to those with emotional distress.

In a striking cluster randomized evaluation in Pakistan, 'Lady Health Workers' implemented a cognitive-behavioral, problem-solving intervention for women who met criteria for major depression during the third trimester of their pregnancies. Relative to controls, the intervention substantially reduced depression 12 months postpartum (OR = 0.23, p < 0.0001) [30]. In India,

peer support for depression, anxiety and other mental health problems included education about psychological problems and ways of coping with them (e.g. deep breathing for anxiety symptoms) as well as interpersonal therapy, and was delivered by lay health counselors with back-up by primary care and monthly consultations from psychiatrists. Results included a 30% decrease in the prevalence of depression and other common mental disorders among those with these problems at baseline, 36% reduction in suicide attempts or plans, and an average of 4.43 fewer days with no or reduced work in the previous 30 days [31], resulting in the intervention being both cost saving as well as cost-effective [32].

A population-based study in the USA evaluated Medicaid enrollees who had made a claim for both community mental health and peer support services. A comparison group who had made only claims for community mental health services was matched by gender, race, age, urban/rural residence and principle diagnosis. Those who had received peer support were less likely to be hospitalized (OR = 0.766) and more likely to achieve crisis stabilization (OR = 1.345) [33].

An important impact of psychological distress in chronic disease is its role in complicating efforts to reach and engage patients in recommended care. Peer support may be an especially effective strategy for reaching the 'hardly reached' [34]. Asthma coaches pursuing a nondirective, flexible, stage-based approach were able to engage 89.7% of mothers of Medicaid-covered children hospitalized for asthma. The coaches sustained that engagement, averaging 21.1 contacts per parent over a 2-year intervention. Of those randomized to an asthma coach, 36.5% were rehospitalized over the 2 years compared to 59.1% receiving usual care (p < 0.01) [35].

In a successful peer support intervention for diabetes management among patients of safety net clinics in San Francisco, participants were categorized as low, medium or high medication adherence at baseline. The peer support led to greater reductions in glycated hemoglobin than in controls across all groups, but the differential impact of peer support was greatest among those initially in the low adherence group [36]. In a dyadic support intervention among veterans with diabetes, improvements in blood glucose measures were substantially more pronounced among those with low initial levels of diabetes support (p for interaction <0.001) and those with low health literacy (p for interaction <0.05) [37].

Comprehensive Population Approaches to Interventions for Depression and Diabetes
Community-wide health promotion programs focus on populations affected or at risk. The major community programs aiming to prevent cardiovascular disease [38] and encourage non-smoking [39] may provide lessons for comprehensive approaches to management of physical and mental disorders. The North Karelia project in Finland addressed heightened cardiovascular disease through a broad range of interventions. In comparison to other parts of the country, North Karelia showed impressive reductions in cardiovascular risk factors and mortality, as well as reductions of cancer risk factors [38].

Several characteristics appear important in the North Karelia program. Its wide range of initiatives included development of new treatment guidelines for hypertension and care following myocardial infarction and other clinical preventive approaches, community-based health education and social marketing of preventive practices, and diverse engagement of community organizations, mass media and key businesses such as dairies, sausage factories, and food merchandising groups and grocery stores to improve the availability of healthy foods [40]. Across all interventions, great attention was given to collaborative planning and implementation with local organizations.

Similar lessons may be drawn from successful campaigns to encourage prevention and cessation of smoking in the USA [41]. Most notably, declines in per capita cigarette consumption and closely associated declines in cardiovascular mortality in California were attributable to a statewide campaign supported by taxes on cigarettes that included prevention programs for youth, cessation programs for adults, aggressive counteradvertising campaigns, and community-based program coordination and planning [42].

Illustrating community approaches to mental health, the German city of Nuremberg implemented a multilevel 2-year community intervention to treat depression and suicide [43]. Using community facilitators, the program intervened with three sectors of society: primary care physicians to provide training and awareness about depression, the general public to raise awareness and knowledge of services, and depressed patients to provide support. After 2 years, the program found significant reductions in suicide acts and depressive symptoms, and the program was expanded to other regions of Europe under the name 'The European Alliance against Depression' [43].

How such community approaches might be extended to multimorbidity of physical and mental disorders is unclear. One might begin with behaviors that community health promotion programs have been able to improve and that are also pertinent to diabetes and depression, such as healthy diet, regular physical activity, medication adherence, and regular clinical care, and in successful approaches to hypertension, such as strategically directed screening. In addition to broad involvement of community organizations, business and local government, intervention strategies might include:

(1) Attention to the built environment and design of neighborhoods and housing to promote physical activity as well as enhance psychological adjustment and well-being
(2) Engaging worksites to recognize two roles they may play: useful and socially influential

sites for implementation of programs, and identifying ways in which personnel policies and procedures might be improved to facilitate daily management of diabetes (e.g. blood glucose monitoring, healthy diet) and to reduce stress and enhance emotional as well as physical health

(3) Community organization and social marketing to build social capital and promote the kinds of community values, social interactions and approaches to conflict resolution that may also enhance emotional and physical health

(4) Recruiting members of key audiences as peer supporters to build links between programs and those audiences as well as providing emotional and tangible support to those most in need

New Media of Intervention: e-Learning, Telehealth, Web-Based Interventions

Promising results from Web-based and telehealth interventions have spurred interest in new modalities for intervening with people experiencing depression and diabetes [44]. A recent systematic review of Internet support groups for individuals with depressive symptoms provides evidence for the role of e-health in managing depression [45]. Of the 16 studies reviewed, a majority (62.5%) reported a positive effect of Internet support on depressive symptoms. Although only 20% of the studies used a control group, other randomized control trials of Internet interventions have demonstrated statistically significant reductions in depression compared to control groups [46]. Telephone-delivered cognitive-behavioral programs have also been successfully used with Veterans Administration patients in the USA to reduce depressive symptoms and improve quality of life and functioning [17]. For patients who have been 'hardly reached' by the traditional medical care system, these new modalities offer a model for enhanced patient outreach and care.

Discussion

Articulation of the roles of social and economic factors is sometimes perceived as being in opposition to the articulation of individual-level factors or clinical treatment. The intent of the broad ecological perspective taken here is an integration rather than opposition of multiple levels of explanation. Recognition of the range of influences on mental health and chronic disease will best illuminate the relationships between them. Understanding the utilities of different perspectives on those relationships will best guide selection of perspectives that serve specific purposes. Furthermore, integrating clinical, social and community approaches to prevention and management will best meet the global burden of multimorbidities.

Clinical Implications

There is often a tendency to see the world of clinical care as separate and distinct from that of prevention and population health; however, these are overlapping. Healthy communities may enable patient adherence to diabetes management and treatment of depression. At the same time, the availability of quality clinical care may provide both a channel for reaching populations as well as a resource for promoting healthy lifestyles [47].

As discussed above, peer support may be an especially promising strategy for integrating clinical and preventive as well as individual and population approaches. Peer supporters can help sustain the behaviors that comprise diabetes and depression management [29] and provide emotional support and encourage problem solving to address depression and other emotional distress [30] while engaging those who otherwise fail to receive appropriate care [35, 48]. All of these can assist in identifying and recruiting into treatment those with mental and physical disorders and in helping them take full advantage of the available resources.

A simple consideration that is too often unrecognized cuts across all the approaches to intervention outlined here. The emotional aspect is an important part of chronic disease care. Attention to depression, emotional well-being and healthy relationships is not a secondary consideration in chronic disease care, but – based on the evidence [e.g. 1] – of central importance. In diabetes and cardiovascular disease, for example, the recognition and treatment of depression may be as important as biological treatment targets. Further, knowledge gained by a comprehensive approach to diabetes and depression may be highly relevant to the care of other chronic diseases. Attention to depression, anxiety and stress disorders is likely to have impacts on health and healthcare costs far greater than currently appreciated.

Integrative Role of Self-Management in Diabetes and Depression

Self-management programs in chronic disease may provide important models for approaches to mental health problems in general as well as those which co-occur with physical disorders. Surely the core elements of chronic disease self-management – healthy diet, physical activity, adherence to medication regimens, stress management, problem solving, and cultivating family and friend support – would all seem equally pertinent to the management of depression. It should also be noted that meta-analysis of interventions for depression and diabetes has implicated diabetes self-management education in the metabolic benefits associated with cognitive behavioral interventions [18].

Within self-management, problem solving may have a special role in integration of care for depression and diabetes. Problem solving is central to almost all models of self-management in diabetes and chronic disease. At the same time, problem solving has emerged as a prominent approach to psychotherapy for depression and other problems [49]. Indeed, recent research indicates that the benefits of cognitive behavior therapy for depression rest largely on the more behavioral, skill-oriented components of problem solving and 'behavioral activation' within cognitive behavior therapy [50]. Thus, problem solving can address the management of both mental and physical disorders. For example, helping individuals set objectives for increasing physical activity, take steps to accomplish those objectives, and reflect on the pleasure of reaching them may advance both diabetes self-management as well as self-management of depression.

In addition to its effectiveness in both domains, an emphasis on problem solving may also provide a useful framework for providing coherence to the individual's tasks in management of mental and physical disorders. Organizing overall care as problem solving or self-management to achieve a healthy diet, physical activity, adherence to medications, stress management, and maintenance of satisfying social and community engagements may provide patients a coherent framework for accommodating the changes that emerge inevitably in the natural history of chronic disease. It may also avoid concerns about stigma surrounding depression, other forms of emotional distress or chronic diseases in many cultures.

Self-management procedures emerged largely out of research on self-control and related processes in psychology, behavior therapy and health psychology. This might lead one to expect great attention to self-management approaches to depression and other mental health problems that psychology has traditionally addressed. Yet, while a search of PubMed (January 13, 2014) for papers with 'self-management' and cognates of 'diabetes' in their titles yielded 762, a parallel search for papers with 'self-management' and cognates of 'depression' in their titles yielded only 36. When expanded to include mention in abstracts, results were 2,390 for 'self-management' with cognates of 'diabetes' and 567 with cognates of 'depression'. Further, many of those mentioning depression were focused on self-management of other diseases and simply included a measure of depression, not the focus of the self-management program. It should be noted that mental health researchers may use other terms like 'psychotherapy', 'supportive therapy', and 'bibliotherapy' to refer to similar services as 'self-management'. Nevertheless, it appears that the *combination* of proactive medical treatment and self-management which constitutes the state-of-the-art in diabetes has not been fully recognized in mental health.

Experience teaches that paradigm or conceptual shifts do not follow from rational argument as often as they emerge in response to events. The growing burden of diabetes, depression and other multimorbidities may compel medicine, public health and mental health to move forward with improved and comprehensive interventions. Closely related to this, the pressure of healthcare costs has led (e.g. US Affordable Care Act) to increased emphasis on primary care and integration of chronic disease management and behavioral health.

The perspectives here have substantial implications for training professionals. Beyond covering chronic diseases and the behavioral health issues that so often accompany them, training needs to inculcate an understanding of the integration of these, as they are experienced by patients and as they need to be treated by clinicians. Moving down the problem list from diabetes, to joint problem, down to depression is not an approach to organizing clinical care that reflects the ways in which these problems emerge and function. One might argue that such an approach is, indeed, bad medicine. Beyond the pitfalls of polypharmacy that it engenders, it fails to recognize the interconnected nature of behavioral health and biological problems and to bring to bear evidence-based models for addressing them.

Whether through mental health, primary care, specialty care or community-based programs, individuals should receive services that reflect the co-occurrence of diabetes and other chronic diseases with depression and other emotional distress and that provide integration and continuity of services for these. Integrating the clinical with social, organizational and community approaches as advocated here may offer a strong model not only for the global burdens of diabetes, depression and other mental and physical health problems, but also for more general prevention and healthcare in an era of aging populations, growing prevalence and burden of noncommunicable diseases, and *normative multimorbidity*.

Disclosure Statement

Dr. Fisher and Ms. Kowitt are supported by the American Academy of Family Physicians Foundation through its program, Peers for Progress, which is supported by the Eli Lilly and Company Foundation, the Bristol-Myers Squibb Foundation and Sanofi US.

The Association for the Improvement of Mental Health Programmes, directed by Dr. Sartorius, received a grant from Eli Lilly and Company to assist in the development of the Dialogue on Diabetes and Depression from deliberations of which the present manuscript developed. With the exception of support for travel to meetings provided through the Dialogue on Diabetes and Depression, and the support of Dr. Fisher and Ms. Kowitt by Peers for Progress of the American Academy of Family Physicians Foundation, the authors have collaborated in the development of this paper without any support for the work.

References

1 Holt RI, de Groot M, Lucki I, Hunter CM, Sartorius N, Golden SH: NIDDK international conference report on diabetes and depression: current understanding and future directions. Diabetes Care 2014;37:2067–2077.

2 Uchino BN: Social support and health: a review of physiological processes potentially underlying links to disease outcomes. J Behav Med 2006;29:377–387.

3 Ma RC, Kong AP, Chan N, Tong PC, Chan JC: Drug-induced endocrine and metabolic disorders. Drug Saf 2007;30:215–245.

4 Katon WJ, Rutter C, Simon G, Lin EH, Ludman E, Ciechanowski P, Kinder L, Young B, Von Korff M: The association of comorbid depression with mortality in patients with type 2 diabetes. Diabetes Care 2005;28:2668–2672.

5 Brown SC, Mason CA, Lombard JL, Martinez F, Plater-Zyberk E, Spokane AR, Newman FL, Pantin H, Szapocznik J: The relationship of built environment to perceived social support and psychological distress in Hispanic elders: the role of 'eyes on the street'. J Gerontol B Psychol Sci Soc Sci 2009;64:234–246.

6 Ludwig J, Sanbonmatsu L, Gennetian L, Adam E, Duncan GJ, Katz LF, Kessler RC, Kling JR, Lindau ST, Whitaker RC, McDade TW: Neighborhoods, obesity, and diabetes – a randomized social experiment. N Engl J Med 2011;365:1509–1519.

7 Gariepy G, Smith KJ, Schmitz N: Diabetes distress and neighborhood characteristics in people with type 2 diabetes. J Psychosom Res 2013;75:147–152.

8 Barefoot JC, Schroll M: Symptoms of depression, acute myocardial infarction, and total mortality in a community sample. Circulation 1996;93:1976–1980.

9 James PA, Oparil S, Carter BL, Cushman WC, Dennison-Himmelfarb C, Handler J, Lackland DT, Lefevre ML, Mackenzie TD, Ogedegbe O, Smith SC Jr, Svetkey LP, Taler SJ, Townsend RR, Wright JT Jr, Narva AS, Ortiz E: 2014 evidence-based guideline for the management of high blood pressure in adults: report from the panel members appointed to the Eighth Joint National Committee (JNC 8). JAMA 2014;311:507–520.

10 Hjerl K, Andersen EW, Keiding N, Mortensen PB, Jorgensen T: Increased incidence of affective disorders, anxiety disorders, and non-natural mortality in women after breast cancer diagnosis: a nation-wide cohort study in Denmark. Acta Psychiatr Scand 2002;105:258–264.

11 Brummett BH, Boyle SH, Ortel TL, Becker RC, Siegler IC, Williams RB: Associations of depressive symptoms, trait hostility, and gender with C-reactive protein and interleukin-6 response after emotion recall. Psychosom Med 2010; 72:333–339.

12 Fisher L, Mullan JT, Arean P, Glasgow RE, Hessler D, Masharani U: Diabetes distress but not clinical depression or depressive symptoms is associated with glycemic control in both cross-sectional and longitudinal analyses. Diabetes Care 2010;33:23–28.

13 Eckel RH, Grundy SM, Zimmet PZ: The metabolic syndrome. Lancet 2005;365: 1415–1428.

14 Kahn R: Metabolic syndrome – what is the clinical usefulness? Lancet 2008;371: 1892–1893.

15 Valderas JM, Starfield B, Sibbald B, Salisbury C, Roland M: Defining comorbidity: implications for understanding health and health services. Ann Fam Med 2009;7:357–363.

16 Rubin RR, Ma Y, Marrero DG, Peyrot M, Barrett-Connor EL, Kahn SE, Haffner SM, Price DW, Knowler WC: Elevated depression symptoms, antidepressant medicine use, and risk of developing diabetes during the diabetes prevention program. Diabetes Care 2008;31:420–426.

17 Piette JD, Richardson C, Himle J, Duffy S, Torres T, Vogel M, Barber K, Valenstein M: A randomized trial of telephonic counseling plus walking for depressed diabetes patients. Med Care 2011;49: 641–648.

18 van der Feltz-Cornelis CM, Nuyen J, Stoop C, Chan J, Jacobson AM, Katon W, Snoek F, Sartorius N: Effect of interventions for major depressive disorder and significant depressive symptoms in patients with diabetes mellitus: a systematic review and meta-analysis. Gen Hosp Psychiatry 2010;32:380–395.

19 Chan JC, So WY, Yeung CY, Ko GT, Lau IT, Tsang MW, Lau KP, Siu SC, Li JK, Yeung VT, Leung WY, Tong PC; SURE Study Group: Effects of structured versus usual care on renal endpoint in type 2 diabetes: the SURE study: a randomized multicenter translational study. Diabetes Care 2009;32:977–982.

20 Daniel DM, Norman J, Davis C, Lee H, Hindmarsh MF, McCulloch DK, Wagner EH, Sugarman JR: A state-level application of the chronic illness breakthrough series: results from two collaboratives on diabetes in Washington State. Jt Comm J Qual Saf 2004;30:69–79.

21 Fisher EB, Brownson CA, O'Toole ML, Shetty G, Anwuri VV, Glasgow RE: Ecologic approaches to self-management: the case of diabetes. Am J Public Health 2005;95:1523–1535.

22 Norris SL, Lau J, Smith SJ, Schmid CH, Engelgau MM: Self-management education for adults with type 2 diabetes: a meta-analysis of the effect on glycemic control. Diabetes Care 2002;25:1159–1171.

23 Thorpe CT, Fahey LE, Johnson H, Deshpande M, Thorpe JM, Fisher EB: Facilitating healthy coping in patients with diabetes: a systematic review. Diabetes Educ 2013;39:33–52.

24 Morrissey JP, Domino ME, Cuddeback GS: Assessing the effectiveness of recovery-oriented act in reducing state psychiatric hospital use. Psychiatr Serv 2013;64:303–311.

25 Shattell MM, Donnelly N, Scheyett A, Cuddeback GS: Assertive community treatment and the physical health needs of persons with severe mental illness: issues around integration of mental health and physical health. J Am Psychiatr Nurses Assoc 2011;17:57–63.

26 Von Korff M, Katon WJ, Lin EH, Ciechanowski P, Peterson D, Ludman EJ, Young B, Rutter CM: Functional outcomes of multi-condition collaborative care and successful ageing: results of randomised trial. BMJ 2011;343:d6612.

27 Thota AB, Sipe TA, Byard GJ, Zometa CS, Hahn RA, McKnight-Eily LR, Chapman DP, Abraido-Lanza AF, Pearson JL, Anderson CW, Gelenberg AJ, Hennessy KD, Duffy FF, Vernon-Smiley ME, Nease DE Jr, Williams SP: Collaborative care to improve the management of depressive disorders: a community guide systematic review and meta-analysis. Am J Prev Med 2012;42:525–538.

28 Ell K, Katon W, Xie B, Lee PJ, Kapetanovic S, Guterman J, Chou CP: Collaborative care management of major depression among low-income, predominantly Hispanic subjects with diabetes: a randomized controlled trial. Diabetes Care 2010;33:706–713.

29 Fisher EB, Boothroyd RI, Coufal MM, Baumann LC, Mbanya JC, Rotheram-Borus MJ, Sanguanprasit B, Tanasugarn C: Peer support for self-management of diabetes improved outcomes in international settings. Health Aff (Millwood) 2012;31:130–139.

30 Rahman A, Malik A, Sikander S, Roberts C, Creed F: Cognitive behaviour therapy-based intervention by community health workers for mothers with depression and their infants in rural Pakistan: a cluster-randomised controlled trial. Lancet 2008;372:902–909.

31 Patel V, Weiss HA, Chowdhary N, Naik S, Pednekar S, Chatterjee S, Bhat B, Araya R, King M, Simon G, Verdeli H, Kirkwood BR: Lay health worker led intervention for depressive and anxiety disorders in India: impact on clinical and disability outcomes over 12 months. Br J Psychiatry 2011;199:459–466.

32 Buttorff C, Hock RS, Weiss HA, Naik S, Araya R, Kirkwood BR, Chisholm D, Patel V: Economic evaluation of a task-shifting intervention for common mental disorders in India. Bull World Health Organ 2012;90:813–821.

33 Landers GM, Zhou M: An analysis of relationships among peer support, psychiatric hospitalization, and crisis stabilization. Community Ment Health J 2011;47:106–112.

34 Fisher EB, Coufal MM, Parada H, Robinette JB, Tang P, Urlaub D, Castillo C, Filossof YR, Guzman-Corrales LM, Hino S, Hunter J, Katz AW, Worley HP, Xui C: Peer support in health care and prevention: cultural, organizational and dissemination issues; in Fielding J, Brownson RC, Green L (eds): Annual Review of Public Health. Palo Alto, Annual Reviews, 2014, vol 35.

35 Fisher EB, Strunk RC, Highstein GR, Kelley-Sykes R, Tarr KL, Trinkaus K, Musick J: A randomized controlled evaluation of the effect of community health workers on hospitalization for asthma: the asthma coach. Arch Pediatr Adolesc Med 2009;163:225–232.

36 Moskowitz D, Thom DH, Hessler D, Ghorob A, Bodenheimer T: Peer coaching to improve diabetes self-management: which patients benefit most? J Gen Intern Med 2013;28:938–942.

37 Piette JD, Resnicow K, Choi H, Heisler M: A diabetes peer support intervention that improved glycemic control: mediators and moderators of intervention effectiveness. Chronic Illn 2013;9:258–267.

38 Puska P, Vartiainen E, Tuomilehto J, Salomaa V, Nissinen A: Changes in premature deaths in Finland: successful long-term prevention of cardiovascular diseases. Bull World Health Organ 1998; 76:419–425.

39 Fisher EB, Brownson RC, Luke DA, Sumner WI, Heath AC: Cigarette smoking; in Raczynski J, Bradley L, Leviton L (eds): Health Behavior Handbook. Washington, American Psychological Association, 2004, vol II.

40 Puska P, Nissinen A, Tuomilehto J, Salonen JT, Koskela K, McAlister A, Kottke TE, Maccoby N, Farquhar JW: The community-based strategy to prevent coronary heart disease: conclusions from the ten years of the North Karelia project. Annu Rev Public Health 1985;6: 147–193.

41 Cole HM, Fiore MC: The war against tobacco: 50 years and counting. JAMA 2014;311:131–132.

42 Fichtenberg CM, Glantz SA: Association of the California tobacco control program with declines in cigarette consumption and mortality from heart disease. N Engl J Med 2000;343:1772–1777.

43 Hegerl U, Rummel-Kluge C, Varnik A, Arensman E, Koburger N: Alliances against depression – a community based approach to target depression and to prevent suicidal behaviour. Neurosci Biobehav Rev 2013;37:2404–2409.

44 Williams ED, Bird D, Forbes AW, Russell A, Ash S, Friedman R, Scuffham PA, Oldenburg B: Randomised controlled trial of an automated, interactive telephone intervention (TLC diabetes) to improve type 2 diabetes management: baseline findings and six-month outcomes. BMC Public Health 2012;12:602.

45 Griffiths KM, Calear AL, Banfield M: Systematic review on internet support groups (ISGs) and depression (1): do ISGs reduce depressive symptoms? J Med Internet Res 2009;11:e40.

46 Glozier N, Christensen H, Naismith S, Cockayne N, Donkin L, Neal B, Mackinnon A, Hickie I: Internet-delivered cognitive behavioural therapy for adults with mild to moderate depression and high cardiovascular disease risks: a randomised attention-controlled trial. PLoS One 2013;8:e59139.

47 Plescia M, Groblewski M: A community-oriented primary care demonstration project: refining interventions for cardiovascular disease and diabetes. Ann Fam Med 2004;2:103–109.

48 Boothroyd RI, Fisher EB: Peers for progress: promoting peer support for health around the world. Fam Pract 2010; 27(suppl 1):i62–i68.

49 D'Zurilla TJ, Nezu AM: Problem-Solving Therapy, ed 2. New York, Springer, 1999.

50 Cuijpers P, van Straten A, Warmerdam L: Behavioral activation treatments of depression: a meta-analysis. Clin Psychol Rev 2007;27:318–326.

Edwin B. Fisher, PhD
Department of Health Behavior
Gillings School of Global Public Health
University of North Carolina
Box 7440
Chapel Hill, NC 27599-7440 (USA)
E-Mail edfisher@unc.edu

Background

Sartorius N, Holt RIG, Maj M (eds): Comorbidity of Mental and Physical Disorders.
Key Issues Ment Health. Basel, Karger, 2015, vol 179, pp 15–22 (DOI: 10.1159/000365524)

Public Health Perspectives on the Co-Occurrence of Non-Communicable Diseases and Common Mental Disorders

Brian Oldenburg[a] · Adrienne O'Neil[b] · Fiona Cocker[a]

[a]School of Population and Global Health, The University of Melbourne, and [b]IMPACT Strategic Research Centre, Deakin University, Melbourne, Vic., Australia

Abstract

This chapter uses a public health perspective to provide an overview of the key determinants and shared pathways for the causes of non-communicable diseases and common mental disorders and their outcomes. Current understandings about their co-occurrence, prevention and control will be discussed, as well as the implications of emerging frameworks that target modifiable risk factors. We will conclude by outlining some of the issues and challenges associated with wide-scale implementation and scale-up of public health interventions that target the prevention and control of these conditions when they co-occur in different community settings.

© 2015 S. Karger AG, Basel

Current Views on the Prevention and Control of Non-Communicable Diseases and Common Mental Disorders

Cardiovascular disease, type 2 diabetes mellitus, cancer and chronic respiratory disease are often referred to as 'the big four' non-communicable diseases. The World Health Organization (WHO) reports that these conditions account for almost 90% of all deaths due to non-communicable disease, globally. However, in recent times, growing support has emerged for the need for common mental disorders, such as major depression and anxiety, to also be recognised as non-communicable diseases [1]. Indeed, it is now *very* well established that these common mental disorders contribute significantly to the global burden of disability-adjusted life years. In fact, when considering disability-adjusted life years, rather than just cause of death, the so-called 'big four' account for only half (54%) of non-communicable disease-related disability-adjusted life years, with major depression the second leading cause of disability. In response, the WHO Global Action Plan (2013–2016), developed to reduce the global burden of non-communicable diseases and preventable mortality, now incorporates targets and strategies related to mental health prevention and control [2]. A shift towards a model that incorporates mental *and* physical disorders into the same constellation of conditions also has important implications for conceptualising their prevention and management, both as independent conditions, but even more importantly, when they co-occur. Before further discussing the implications of such a model for approaches to their prevention and control, the key determinants and pathways that link high prevalence non-communicable diseases to common mental disorders will be discussed. We shall particularly focus on the inter-relationships and co-occurrence among cardiovascular disease, type 2 diabetes and depression.

Shared Determinants for Non-Communicable Diseases and Common Mental Disorders

When identifying population-wide prevention and control strategies for non-communicable diseases, the WHO has emphasised the role of the lifestyle determinants of these conditions. Traditionally, common mental disorders have received relatively little attention from this perspective, and treatment options that target the modifiable lifestyle factors known to ameliorate non-communicable diseases have been seldom applied to common mental disorders. Jacka et al. [1] have argued that while contextual factors including social inequity and networks, child maltreatment, and neglect clearly contribute to depression risk, it is important that prevention and control efforts focus much more on those determinants with the 'greatest plasticity and reach'. The authors describe a growing evidence base that identifies lifestyle factors (e.g. physical inactivity, smoking and diet quality) as important determinants for the development of common mental disorders such as depression, i.e. the same lifestyle determinants already known to be important determinants of non-communicable diseases. This evidence suggests an opportunity exists to prevent and control mental and physical disorders that occur comorbidly by using a consolidated framework in which several overlapping, modifiable risk factors, such as tobacco use, unhealthy alcohol use, physical inactivity and unhealthy diet are targeted with the potential to reduce both non-communicable dis-

eases *and* common mental disorders. Before reviewing such a framework, the shared pathways that link the common mental disorders to non-communicable diseases will be described.

Shared Pathways for Non-Communicable Diseases and Common Mental Disorders

It may seem intuitive that the occurrence of depression or anxiety in those with a chronic physical condition exacerbates the risk of poor clinical outcomes. For example, after the occurrence of a life-threatening event such as acute coronary syndrome (heart attack), or symptoms and potential complications of type 2 diabetes, the associated worry and distress impair functioning, recovery and/or coping ability, and the overall burden of self-management may exacerbate symptoms of depression [3]. For example, some estimates suggest 25–46% of people with type 2 diabetes mellitus [4] or cardiac disease [5] experience symptoms indicative of depression. However, these symptoms are not just a common clinical outcome of these conditions. Major depression has emerged as a powerful and robust risk factor for both conditions in recent years [6]. While the pathways implicating depression in the pathogenesis and outcomes of cardiovascular disease and/or diabetes remain unclear, they are clearly multifaceted. Psychophysiological, biobehavioural and social influences interact to elevate the risk of cardiovascular disease and/or type 2 diabetes in those with depression (both in its genesis and clinical course), accelerating the psychological and cardiometabolic abnormalities of each [3]. For example, of the former, depression and psychosocial stressors can lead to hypothalamic-pituitary-adrenal axis activation and complex hormonal and (auto)immuno-inflammatory interactions in the pathogenesis of cardiometabolic disorders. Such a response can elicit a host of metabolic and cardiovascular abnormalities which characterise the cardiovascular disease and diabetes over-represented in people with depression. This response can perpetuate a cycle of psychological and physical ill health [3].

Another explanation for this relationship is biobehavioural; the presence of shared risk factors like smoking, obesity, poor diet or physical inactivity can lead to systemic inflammation, which is common in the development of both depression [7, 8] and these systemic disorders [9]. Further, environmental and contextual factors commonly linking mental and physical disorders, including socio-economic status and social isolation, have also been shown to increase the risk of all of these disorders [7, 10, 11]. Fisher et al. [3] argues that these up- and downstream determinants are complex in that they are interwoven at multiple levels. Failure to consider the role of such factors has potentially deleterious consequences with respect to the delivery and effectiveness of public health interventions. While these consequences will be discussed further in a following section, we will define what is meant by 'public health' interventions before looking at those that exist for the prevention and control of comorbid mental and physical health disorders.

Defining Public Health Interventions

The term 'public health interventions' can have different meanings, in part because the term 'public health' is used in different ways. First, the term 'public health', particularly 'public health research', is often used as a general and very broad term to be inclusive of all epidemiologic, intervention and health services research. Second, it can be used to imply a primary focus on the health of the public and whole populations, rather than being concerned with just the health and well-being of single individuals; often this focus also includes a particular interest in the situation as it pertains to disadvantaged individuals or groups, and/or an emphasis on this issue globally. Third, 'public health' is often taken to mean an emphasis on pre-

vention rather than a focus on treatment services and management of a clinical problem. With these theoretical differences in mind, we will now consider the evidence in relation to the prevention and control of comorbid non-communicable diseases and common mental disorders.

Prevention and Control of Comorbid Physical and Mental Disorders

To date, the evidence base for the effectiveness and feasibility of real-world public health interventions for the prevention and management of common comorbid non-communicable diseases and common mental disorders is stronger for people with existing conditions than for primary prevention or secondary prevention in those at 'high risk'; we shall consider both of these.

Prevention of Comorbid Non-Communicable Diseases and Common Mental Disorders

As outlined in previous sections, there is sound evidence that similar lifestyle factors shown to precipitate the 'big four' non-communicable diseases are also important contributors in the development of common mental disorders. Notwithstanding the complexity of factors contributing to the pathophysiology and trajectory of common mental disorders like depression and anxiety, this evidence suggests that modification of lifestyle behaviours as risk factors may have the potential to ameliorate some of the risk of common mental disorders. This rationale has underpinned recent calls for a population-based approach that integrates such 'plastic' lifestyle factors for the universal prevention of common mental disorders [1]. Recent research in this field suggests whilst the potential contribution of modifiable factors such as social inequality, social networks, and child, drug and alcohol abuse to depression risk should not be underestimated or ignored, preventive efforts should also aim to address individuals' health-related lifestyle behaviours.

Lifestyle is a term that encompasses behaviours related to diet, physical activity and smoking, amongst other behaviours, known to increase the risk of disease and poor health. There is increasing evidence which identifies physical inactivity as a risk factor for common mental disorders [12, 13], with exercise shown to be effective in treatment studies [14]. Further, some evidence exists linking smoking to an increased risk of developing common mental disorders [15, 16]. Diet quality has also received much attention in recent times in the lifestyle-mental health research field [17, 18]. For example, one notable study, the PREDIMED trial, identified a link between adherence to the Mediterranean diet, the hallmark of which is the abundant use of olive oil [19], which is rich in monounsaturated fatty acids, and reduced depression risk [20]. Results revealed a significant 40% reduction in depression risk for individuals with type 2 diabetes who adhered to the Mediterranean diet when compared with the control group.

Despite these encouraging findings, evidence is somewhat scarce and moreover limited by underpowered sample sizes or inadequate study designs. However, the primary prevention of common mental disorders remains a burgeoning area in public health that has garnered support in recent years in light of data suggesting that, for the majority of people (75%), common mental disorders manifest before the age of 24 years [21]. Moreover, lifestyle-based strategies that target the primary prevention of common mental disorders could play an important role in the subsequent prevention of the 'big four' non-communicable diseases. The beneficial effects of targeting lifestyle factors are likely to extend beyond that of psychological well-being to ameliorate the risk of non-communicable diseases, potentially producing a 'double hit' by delaying or preventing chronic disease later in the lifespan. From a well-being, health and economic perspective, the (in)direct 'flow-on' effects resulting from investment in the primary prevention of common mental disorders

using this approach become apparent. We shall discuss the issues related to economic responsibility in the following section.

Control and Management of Comorbid Non-Communicable Diseases and Common Mental Disorders in 'High-Risk' Populations

Traditionally, non-communicable diseases and common mental disorders have been treated uniquely and independently within the public health sphere. From a systematic perspective, many healthcare systems are not designed to incorporate the multidisciplinary approach required to manage patients with co-occurring physical and mental disorders adequately. This is largely due to increasingly specialised and fragmented structures. Additionally, a range of downstream determinants are likely to impede the cohesive management of these comorbidities, including a lack of recognition around their high prevalence, poor awareness on behalf of the patient, practitioner or both, and deficits in physician training.

If we use the specific example of diabetes, a lack of continuity of care has been shown to translate to poorer clinical outcomes and suboptimal care provision. For example, Mitchell et al. [22] provide evidence that despite greater service use, those with a mental illness are less likely to be screened for diabetes, associated eye or foot complications, receive statins or diabetes education, or be offered HbA1c and cholesterol screening.

The converse is also true. Using the example of heart disease, people who have been admitted to hospital for a coronary event are unlikely to be screened for depression. Stewart et al. [23] report that only 3% of clinicians in Australia perform routine screening for depression. In order to address these deficiencies within healthcare systems, models of the clinical management for comorbid mental and physical disorders have been developed. Perhaps the most well-known is the IMPACT model developed by Katon et al. [24], which draws on evidence-based medical models such as those described by Wagner et al. [25] (chronic care model in primary care settings) and Lorig et al. [26] (self-management models in community-based settings). The model of care by Katon et al. was one of the first to consider the concurrent management of depression, heart disease and type 2 diabetes using a collaborative care approach, and has been shown to be more effective for chronic disease management than standard medical care [27]. Collaborative care models emphasise the 'up-skilling' of practice nurses as case managers who aim to provide continuity of care. This includes [24]:

- Encouraging support and effective communication to patients from clinicians
- Utilising evidence-based guidelines to promote patient self-management
- Monitoring risk factors
- Scheduling visits
- Providing audit information

Algorithms provide guidance on the direction of care based on severity of symptoms, often using a stepped-care approach with various healthcare professionals based on patient need. Perhaps the most important characteristic underpinning this model is its operation within existing structures of the healthcare setting, rather than amending the healthcare structure itself. It is designed to capitalise on existing workforce and financial infrastructures by refocussing the roles of the existing members and organisational structures of the setting.

Collaborative care models have now been extrapolated to a range of other comorbidities, such as depression and coronary artery bypass grafting [28], where they have demonstrated efficacy and feasibility, and have been shown to reduce cardiovascular risk in elderly people with depression [29]. However, such models have been subject to criticism. For example, it has been argued that they have limited generalisability, require a cultural shift in norms and roles, are too resource intensive to implement and there may be unnecessary overlap with other related programs [30].

These models also depend largely on local culture, health systems, workforce and many other contextual factors and influences.

Considerations for Implementation and Scale-Up of Prevention and Control of Comorbid Non-Communicable Diseases and Common Mental Disorders

Context

With the development and adaptation of any public health intervention – much less one that targets both mental and physical disorders – one needs to consider particular contexts and settings. Fisher et al. [3] maintains that failure to consider contextual factors can result in a number of potentially deleterious outcomes. First, efficacy and/or effectiveness of specific interventions may be diluted. Second, the benefits of interventions may be further underestimated should contextual moderators remain unaccounted for in analyses. Third, individuals participating in these interventions could be perceived as responsible for their condition resulting in a type of 'victim blaming' [3]. To this end, future opportunities exist to explore and evaluate different approaches to increase awareness and understanding of these issues in both health professionals and patient populations.

Cost and Responsibility

There remains a need to shift the balance towards greater investment in not only population-based prevention strategies in public health, but those which incorporate attention being given to either the increased risk *or* the co-occurrence of non-communicable diseases and common mental disorders. The broader issue of responsibility must be considered, as with the primary prevention of any condition. Indeed, cost remains a barrier. A WHO report suggests a key factor underscoring the traditional focus on, and preference for, curative strategies are the short-term, tangible benefits as opposed to the longer pay-off periods required to see the effects of prevention [31]. This is particularly evident as the cost of healthcare increases globally, thereby increasing competition for resources [31]. Because more than 80% of the world's population lives in developing regions of the world [32] – particularly, very populous countries, such as India, China and Indonesia, where non-communicable disease risk factors continue to increase [33] – focus on the management of these comorbidities in so-called 'low and middle income' countries is of particular importance.

Economic Impact of the Co-Occurrence of Non-Communicable Diseases and Common Mental Disorders: A Focus on the Workforce

The economic impact of non-communicable diseases and common mental disorders when they occur alone is significant. However, the associated costs, largely attributed to increased healthcare use and expenditure (e.g. specialist care, hospital care and medication) and lost productive time, are substantially increased when non-communicable diseases and common mental disorders co-occur. In most developed countries, the majority of people with non-communicable diseases are able to keep working, with the latest estimates of workforce participation among Australian adults with non-communicable diseases being 79% for men and 63% for women [34]. As a result, a substantial economic burden from non-communicable diseases is borne by workplaces, in particular, lost productivity resulting from absenteeism and presenteeism (working while ill) [34]. Additionally, a sizeable minority of employed people with non-communicable diseases, an estimated 18% amongst Australian employees, will be managing another major health conditions such as heart disease, arthritis, depression, asthma, diabetes and stroke [34], and these multimorbid disease combinations commonly also include depression [35]. With an ageing workforce globally, a greater understanding of how to promote the health and productivity of workers with multiple chronic illnesses is a priority, as the impact of comorbid and multimorbid mental and physical disorders is not restricted to older adults outside the workforce.

Absenteeism from work is a major issue for governments across the world as it not only decreases productivity resulting in loss of financial growth, but also costs governments a significant amount of money annually to treat ill individuals, giving absenteeism a twofold economic effect [36]. Aside from the economic impact of absenteeism, there are also social benefits for adults who participate in paid employment such as financial independence, a higher standard of living, and the potential for personal satisfaction and social acceptance [37]. Data reveal absenteeism is higher amongst people with one or more chronic illnesses and that employees with a chronic illness have higher rates of long-term work disability than the general population [37]. Interestingly, one study revealed that for absenteeism attributed to a physical illness, psychological factors played a greater part in the decision to take a sickness absence than the physical illness itself [37].

Most of the research to date on multimorbidity and health and social outcomes has focused on quality of life [38], use of medical services [39], and hospitalisation and mortality [40], and has been in clinical or primary care populations [35, 41], or selected older adult populations [41]. However, given that many chronic diseases affect healthier, working age adults [34], this focus on clinical populations and clinical outcomes provides an insufficient evidence base for a public health approach to the health of the workforce [35, 42]. Further, one recent Australian study demonstrated that comorbid psychological distress causes an increased risk of productivity loss, from both absenteeism and presenteeism, for a range of health conditions. Therefore, in terms of population health approaches to managing comorbid non-communicable diseases and common mental disorders, an increased focus needs to be on developing evidence-based guidance to inform a reduction of the burden of common chronic diseases and comorbid depression among working age adults. Specifically, this includes the prevention of long-term work absences and the associated costs, generally poor outcomes of return-to-work programmes, and the development of decision aids for individuals and their clinicians to help guide management of work demands and resources for employers on how best to manage work attendance in employees with comorbid non-communicable diseases and common mental disorders.

Future Efforts in Public Health

There is a need to close the gap between the epidemic growth of common mental disorders, like depression, and non-communicable diseases, such as type 2 diabetes and cardiovascular diseases, and the provision of appropriate healthcare and public health programs that address the shared determinants and pathways of these disorders. Whilst some public health interventions have proven effective, there remains a range of contextual and economic factors to consider for wide-scale implementation in different settings. Specific considerations include the responsibility of investment and cost recovery, and a lack of awareness and action concerning comorbidity by public health and medical authorities. Where there is not sufficient evidence for either testing and/or implementing programs for prevention or control, there is still an important need for research that is more focused on understanding the epidemiology and determinants of comorbid mental and physical conditions in different cultures and population groups within and between countries and different regions of the world.

Acknowledgment

A.O. is supported by the National Health and Medical Research Council (1052865).

References

1 Jacka F, Mykletun A, Berk M: Moving towards a population health approach to the primary prevention of common mental disorders. BMC Med 2012;10: 149.
2 World Health Organization: WHO Global NCD Action Plan 2013–2020. Geneva, WHO, 2013.
3 Fisher EB, Chan JC, Nan H, Sartorius N, Oldenburg B: Co-occurrence of diabetes and depression: conceptual considerations for an emerging global health challenge. J Affective Disorders 2012; 142(suppl):S56–S66.
4 Speight J, Browne JL, Holmes-Truscott E, et al: Diabetes MILES – Australia 2011 Survey Report. Canberra, Diabetes Australia, 2011.
5 Cheok F, Schrader G, Banham D, Marker J, Hordacre AL: Identification, course, and treatment of depression after admission for a cardiac condition: rationale and patient characteristics for the identifying depression as a comorbid condition (IDACC) project. Am Heart J 2003;146:978–984.
6 Van der Kooy K, van Hout H, Marwijk H, Marten H, Stehouwer C, Beekman A: Depression and the risk for cardiovascular diseases: systematic review and meta analysis. Int J Geriatr Psychiatry 2007; 22:613–626.
7 Jacka FN, Pasco JA, Mykletun A, Williams LJ, Hodge A, O'Reilly SL, et al: Association of Western and traditional diets with depression and anxiety in women. Am J Psychiatry 2010;167:305–311.
8 Pasco JA, Kotowicz MA, Henry MJ, Nicholson GC, Spilsbury HJ, Box JD, et al: High-sensitivity C-reactive protein and fracture risk in elderly women. JAMA 2006;296:1353–1355.
9 Chiu C, Wray L, Beverly E, Dominic O: The role of health behaviors in mediating the relationship between depressive symptoms and glycemic control in type 2 diabetes: a structural equation modeling approach. Soc Psychiatry Psychiatr Epidemiol 2010;45:67–76.
10 Pasco JA, Williams LJ, Jacka FN, Henry MJ, Coulson CE, Brennan SL, et al: Habitual physical activity and the risk for depressive and anxiety disorders among older men and women. Int Psychogeriatr 2011;2:292–298.
11 Pasco JA, Williams LJ, Jacka FN, Ng F, Henry MJ, Nicholson GC, et al: Tobacco smoking as a risk factor for major depressive disorder: population-based study. Br J Psychiatry 2008;193:322–326.

12 Lucas M, Mekary R, Pan A, Mirzaei F, O'Reilly ÉJ, Willett WC, et al: Relation between clinical depression risk and physical activity and time spent watching television in older women: a 10-year prospective follow-up study. Am J Epidemiol 2011;174:1017–1027.

13 Pasco JA, Williams LJ, Jacka FN, Henry MJ, Coulson CE, Brennan SL, et al: Habitual physical activity and the risk for depressive and anxiety disorders among older men and women. Int Psychogeriatr 2011;23:292–298.

14 Stathopoulou G, Powers MB, Berry AC, Smits JA, Otto MW: Exercise interventions for mental health: a quantitative and qualitative review. Clin Psychol Sci Pract 2006;13:179–193.

15 Mykletun A, Overland S, Aarø LE, Liabø H-M, Stewart R: Smoking in relation to anxiety and depression: evidence from a large population survey: the HUNT study. Eur Psychiatry 2008;23:77–84.

16 Pasco JA, Williams LJ, Jacka FN, Ng F, Henry MJ, Nicholson GC, et al: Tobacco smoking as a risk factor for major depressive disorder: population-based study. Br J Psychiatry 2008;193:322–326.

17 Murakami K, Sasaki S: Dietary intake and depressive symptoms: a systematic review of observational studies. Mol Nutr Food Res 2010;54:471–488.

18 Jacka FN, Pasco JA, Mykletun A, Williams LJ, Nicholson GC, Kotowicz MA, et al: Diet quality in bipolar disorder in a population-based sample of women. J Affect Disorder 2011;129:332–337.

19 Sánchez-Villegas A, Delgado-Rodríguez M, Alonso A, et al: Association of the Mediterranean dietary pattern with the incidence of depression: the Seguimiento Universidad de Navarra/University of Navarra follow-up (SUN) cohort. Arch Gen Psychiatry 2009;66:1090–1098.

20 Sanchez-Villegas A, Martinez-Gonzalez M, Estruch R, Salas-Salvado J, Corella D, Covas M, et al: Mediterranean dietary pattern and depression: the PREDIMED randomized trial. BMC Med 2013;11:208.

21 Kessler R, Bergland P, Demler O, Jin R, Walters E: Lifetime prevalence and age-of-onset distributions of DSM-IV disorders in the National Comorbidity Survey Replication. Arch Gen Psychiatry 2005;62:593–602.

22 Mitchell AJ, Malone D, Doebbeling CC: Quality of medical care for people with and without comorbid mental illness and substance misuse: systematic review of comparative studies. Br J Psychiatry 2009;194:491–499.

23 Stewart AJ, Driscoll A, Hare DL: National survey of Australian cardiologists' beliefs and practice regarding screening, diagnosis and management of depression. Heart Lung Circ 2009;18:S5.

24 Katon W, Korff MV, Lin E: Collaborative management to achieve treatment guidelines. Impact on depression in primary care. JAMA 1995;273:1026–1031.

25 Wagner EH, Glasgow RE, Davis C, et al: Quality improvement in chronic illness care: a collaborative approach. Jt Comm J Qual Improv 2001;27:63–80.

26 Lorig KR, Sobel DS, Stewart AL, Brown BW Jr, Bandura A, Ritter P, et al: Evidence suggesting that a chronic disease self-management program can improve health status while reducing hospitalization: a randomized trial. Med Care 1999;37:5–14.

27 Gilbody S, Bower P, Fletcher J, et al: Collaborative care for depression: a cumulative meta-analysis and review of longer-term outcomes. Arch Intern Med 2006;166:2314–2321.

28 Rollman BL, Belnap BH: The Bypassing the Blues trial: collaborative care for post-CABG depression and implications for future research. Cleve Clin J Med 2011;78(suppl 1):S4–S12.

29 Stewart JC, Perkins AJ, Callahan CM: Effect of collaborative care for depression on risk of cardiovascular events: data from the IMPACT randomized controlled trial. Psychosom Med 2014;76:29–37.

30 Tully PJ: Telephone-delivered collaborative care for post-CABG depression is more effective than usual care for improving mental-health-related quality of life. Evid Based Med 2010;15:57–58.

31 Prevention of Mental Disorders: Effective Interventions and Policy Options: Summary Report. A Report of the World Health Organization, Department of Mental Health and Substance Abuse, Prevention Research Centre of the Universities of Nijmegen and Maastricht. Geneva, WHO, 1994.

32 United Nations Development Program. New York, United Nations Develop Program, 2007.

33 Global Status Report on Non-Communicable Diseases. Geneva, World Health Organization, 2010.

34 Australian Institute of Health and Welfare: Chronic Disease and Participation in Work. Cat. No. PHE 109. Canberra, AIHW, 2009.

35 Britt HC, Harrison CM, Miller GC, Knox SA: Prevalence and patterns of multimorbidity in Australia. Med J Aust 2008;189:72–77.

36 AIHW: Chronic Disease and Participation in Work. Canberra, AIHW, 2009.

37 Boot C, Koppes L, can den Bossche S, Anema J, can der Beek A: Relation between perceived health and sick leave in employees with a chronic illness. J Occup Rehabil 2011;21:211–219.

38 Fortin M, Bravo G, Hudon C, Lapointe L, Almirall J, Dubois MF, et al: Relationship between multimorbidity and health-related quality of life of patients in primary care. Qual Life Res 2006;15:83–91.

39 Starfield B, Lemke KW, Herbert R, Pavlovich WD, Anderson G: Comorbidity and the use of primary care and specialist care in the elderly. Ann Fam Med 2005;3:215–222.

40 Lee TA, Shields AE, Vogeli C, Gibson TB, Woong-Sohn M, Marder WD, et al: Mortality rate in veterans with multiple chronic conditions. J Gen Intern Med 2007;22:403–407.

41 van den Akker M, Buntinx F, Metsemakers JF, Roos S, Knottnerus JA: Multimorbidity in general practice: prevalence, incidence, and determinants of co-occurring chronic and recurrent diseases. J Clin Epidemiol 1998;51:367–375.

42 Holden L, Scuffham PA, Hilton MF, Muspratt A, Ng SK, Whiteford HA: Patterns of multimorbidity in working Australians. Popul Health Metr 2011;9:15.

Brian Oldenburg, PhD
School of Population and Global Health
The University of Melbourne
207 Bouverie Street, Parkville, VIC 3010 (Australia)
E-Mail brian.oldenburg@unimelb.edu.au

Background

Sartorius N, Holt RIG, Maj M (eds): Comorbidity of Mental and Physical Disorders.
Key Issues Ment Health. Basel, Karger, 2015, vol 179, pp 23–32 (DOI: 10.1159/000365941)

Counting All the Costs: The Economic Impact of Comorbidity

David McDaid[a, b] · A-La Park[a]

[a]Personal Social Services Research Unit and [b]European Observatory on Health Systems and Policies,
London School of Economics and Political Science, London, UK

Abstract

This chapter provides an overview on what is known about the economic impacts of comorbid physical and mental disorders. The chapter begins by briefly describing the concept of economic cost, before going on to look at different examples of the costs of comorbidity. There is an increasing, albeit still small, number of studies that have looked at the economic impacts of comorbid physical and mental health problems. The majority of these examples are from a US context and thought must be given on how they translate to other contexts. Nonetheless, these studies illustrate potentially substantial costs to healthcare systems and society as a whole, which might be avoided through early identification of potential risk factors and early intervention to mitigate the effects of comorbidity. The chapter ends by examining how information on the costs of comorbidity can be used to inform economic arguments for investment in actions to prevent or alleviate some of these morbidities, and how this evidence base may be strengthened further.

© 2015 S. Karger AG, Basel

This chapter provides an overview on what is known about the economic impacts of comorbid physical and mental disorders. As later chapters discuss, illnesses such as psychoses, bipolar disorder and major depression can increase the risk of many physical health problems, including obesity, diabetes, cardiovascular disease, chronic obstructive pulmonary disorder and some infectious diseases. Poor physical health, for instance related to cancer or musculoskeletal health problems, may also increase the risk of developing mental health problems such as depression and anxiety-related disorders. As a result, there is likely to be a considerable overlap in those living with long-term physical and mental health problems. In England, for example, it has been estimated that up to 46% of all those with mental health problems also have some chronic physical health problem, while 30% of those with long-term physical conditions also have a mental health problem [1].

All of these comorbidities will have economic consequences that impact right across society. Some of these costs may potentially be avoidable. Thus, there is a growing interest from policy makers, particularly in countries where health and social care spending is under great strain, about the potential importance of actions that can effectively prevent and/or reduce the impacts of comorbidity.

This chapter therefore begins by briefly describing the concept of economic cost, before going on to look at different examples of the costs of comorbidity. It ends by examining how better information on the costs of comorbidity can be used to inform economic arguments for investment in actions to prevent and alleviate some of these morbidities, and how this evidence base may be strengthened further.

What Is Meant by Economic Cost?

Before going further, it is worth briefly explaining what economists mean by cost, as this is about much more than simple monetary cost. In fact economists often talk about three different components of cost. There may be increased direct costs to the healthcare systems associated with the management of multiple health problems, for instance if mental disorders exacerbate the risk of adverse events and complications in chronic physical health problems or if recovery times are prolonged. This could include the salary costs of healthcare staff, the cost of medicines and the use of diagnostic procedures. In England it has been estimated that as much as GBP 1 in every GBP 8 spent on chronic long-term conditions is due to adverse outcomes arising from poor mental health [1]. There may also be direct costs for the provision of services that fall on other sectors such as social care services. In some cases there might be additional costs falling on other sectors, such as for home modifications due to physical disabilities.

There are also 'indirect' costs, which focus on the lost opportunity to contribute to economic productivity, such as when individuals are absent from the labour market due to poor health or premature death. Productivity costs for many mental disorders already account for more than 60% of all costs because of the low rate of participation in employment [2]. A major reason for these costs is the much higher rate of mortality due to poor physical health. For instance, one study of men and women with severe mental disorders in Denmark, Finland and Sweden reported that they lived between 20 and 15 years less than the general population [3].

Other forms of productivity loss also occur. Comorbid health problems may reduce participation in school or university, potentially impacting on career possibilities. In fact, the long-term adverse costs to the economy due to children with mental health problems not obtaining employment in adulthood has been one key reason for substantial policy interest in measures to help support the health and well-being of children from a very young age [4]. Family members may also give up some of their time from employment or other activities because of the need to provide care and support to a loved one.

The third cost category is known as 'intangible' because it refers to impacts that are often difficult to quantify and value. Examples include the stigma associated with mental illness, communicable disease or physical disabilities, as well as the grief experienced by families as a result of an unexpected death.

What Do We Already Know about the Economic Impacts of Comorbidity on Healthcare Systems?

Remarkably, health economists have not focused much of their energies on assessing the economic impact of comorbidity in any area of health, let alone looking at the issue of mental and physical

Table 1. Selected examples of impact of physical comorbidity on annual healthcare costs of adults with mental disorders

Study	Mental disorder	Comorbid physical disorder	Relative increase in costs of comorbidity (mental disorder alone = 1)[a]
Chwastiak et al. [5]	schizophrenia	obesity	1.3:1
McDonald et al. [6]	schizophrenia	diabetes	1.9:1
McDonald et al. [6]	schizophrenia	dyslipidaemia	1.8:1
McDonald et al. [6]	schizophrenia	hypertension	2.1:1
McDonald et al. [6]	schizophrenia	heart disease	1.7:1
Centorrino et al. [8]	bipolar disorder	metabolic disorders	2.3:1
Welch et al. [10]	depression	congestive heart failure	2.0:1
Welch et al. [10]	depression	coronary artery disease	2.1:1
Welch et al. [10]	depression	diabetes	2.0:1

All of the studies were from the USA. [a] All differences statistically significant $p < 0.05$.

comorbidity. This may be due to the difficulties in attributing healthcare costs to any specific comorbidity, as well as the separation of the way in which mental and physical health services are organised in many countries. There is, however, an increasing, albeit still small number of studies, which have looked at the economic impacts of comorbid physical and mental health problems. The majority of these examples are from a US context and thought must be given on how they translate to other contexts. Nonetheless, they illustrate potentially substantial costs to healthcare systems and society as a whole that might be avoided through early identification of potential risk factors and early intervention to mitigate the effects of comorbidity. The next sections provide an overview of some of these economic analyses, looking at economic impacts within and beyond healthcare systems.

Impacts on Healthcare Systems

Comorbidities between physical and mental health problems provide major challenges to healthcare systems; they can worsen health out-

comes, prolong recovery time and thus exacerbate costs to healthcare systems. Some, as shown in table 1, look at the additional excess costs to the healthcare system of a comorbid physical health problem compared to having a mental health problem alone, while others, as illustrated in table 2, focus on the additional excess costs of a comorbid mental health problem to having a physical health problem alone. Much of this evidence is from the USA, but it provides valuable insights on the extra costs of comorbidities in other countries, suggesting that there is the potential to avoid substantial costs to healthcare systems through early identification and intervention.

Several studies focus on schizophrenia and physical health problems. Analysis of healthcare costs for more than 1,400 individuals with schizophrenia who participated in the 18-month CATIE trial (Clinical Antipsychotic Trials of Intervention Effectiveness) in the USA reported statistically significant 25% higher costs for those who were obese [5]. Data from the US Medical Expenditure Panel Survey of more than 571,000 individuals in 2001 and 2002 found annual healthcare costs for people living with schizophrenia alone of USD 5,990, compared with USD 11,611, 10,803,

Table 2. Selected examples of impact of mental comorbidity on annual healthcare costs of adults with mental disorders

Author and country	Physical disorder	Comorbid mental disorder	Relative increase in costs of comorbidity (physical disorder alone = 1)[a]
Richardson et al. [25], USA	asthma	depression	1.5:1
Hochlehnert et al. [23], Germany	cardiovascular disease	depression and/or anxiety	1.5:1
Atlantis et al. [14], Australia	diabetes	depression	1.5:1
Le et al. [13], USA	diabetes	depression	1.7:1
Simon et al. [15], USA	diabetes	depression	1.8:1

[a] All differences statistically significant $p < 0.05$.

12,292 and 10,415 for those with comorbid diabetes, dyslipidaemia, hypertension or heart disease, respectively [6].

The healthcare costs of more than 31,000 older people with and without schizophrenia were analysed for the 10-year period from 1998 to 2008. Mean healthcare costs were significantly higher in the schizophrenia group; a key driver of greater healthcare costs was the significantly higher rate of physical health problems, including congestive heart failure (45.1 vs. 38.8%), chronic obstructive pulmonary disease (52.7 vs. 41.4%), hypothyroidism (36.7 vs. 26.7%) and dementia (64.5 vs. 32.1%) [7].

Turning to bipolar disorder, in the USA the medical records (spanning 1 year) of more than 28,000 people with bipolar disorder were compared with matched controls without any mental health problems [8]. Those with bipolar disorder had a significantly higher prevalence of metabolic comorbidities than the general population (37 vs. 30%). Annual healthcare costs for metabolic conditions were twice those of controls (USD 531 vs. 233). The bipolar cohort also had significantly higher overall medical service and prescription drug costs than those of the control cohort (USD 12,764 vs. 3,140). Prescription medication costs for metabolic conditions were also higher, with bipolar cohort per-patient costs of USD 571 ver-

sus 301 for the control cohort. Analysis of data on 67,000 members of a health insurance fund in seven US states also suggests that 67% of total healthcare costs of bipolar disorder were related to the treatment of comorbid physical health conditions [9].

Comorbid depression or anxiety disorders and physical health problems have also been associated with higher levels of cost to healthcare systems. One US study reported that the costs of 11 chronic health problems are significantly greater when an individual has comorbid depression. Costs related to diabetes, coronary artery disease and congestive heart failure were approximately twice the costs of individuals without depression [10].

Two reviews, one with 27 [11] and the other with 41 largely US-set studies [12], looked at the impact on healthcare resource utilisation of comorbid diabetes and depression. Both reviews consistently showed increased healthcare resource use to manage diabetes in people with depression. For example, in one study of more than 400,000 adults with diabetes in the USA, the costs of depression increased mean annual healthcare costs from USD 11,000 to 19,000 [13], while in Australia, health service use by people with comorbid diabetes and depression was 49% higher compared to those with diabetes alone [14]. In another US study, the healthcare costs of managing diabetes over a 6-month period were found to be between 50 and 75% higher in people with major depression than in people with diabetes alone [15]. Furthermore, this study observed a significant difference in the costs of managing one or more complications of diabetes in people with major depression compared to those with subclinical thresholds of depression. Other studies also point to higher costs of managing complications. In the USA, the costs of managing complications of diabetes, such as diabetic neuropathy, in people with comorbid depression have also been shown to be significantly greater than in those without depression [16].

Another US study looked at the healthcare costs of more than 14,000 people with depression, congestive heart failure, or both [17]. People who also had depression had significantly higher total annual healthcare costs than those without: USD 20,046 versus 11,956. Costs increased with the severity of comorbidity, but mental healthcare costs accounted for less than 1% of total healthcare costs.

Outside of the USA, significantly increased costs to healthcare systems have also been observed when comorbidity involved depression. English data from more than 86,000 patients in the General Practice Research Database were used to assess whether comorbidity increases the costs of managing patients in primary care [18]. The study found that 20% of all patients had more than one chronic health problem and that all instances of comorbidity increased the costs of primary healthcare compared to the costs of managing these conditions separately. Depression was found to be the most important cost-increasing condition, significantly increasing costs in adult patients of all ages when comorbid with a wide range of conditions. For instance, the costs of managing comorbid depression and asthma or diabetes were greater for patients of all ages, whilst depression and comorbid cancer were associated with significant-

ly higher costs in people aged 40–59 years. Depression and comorbid obesity, heart failure or epilepsy were associated with significantly higher primary care costs in patients aged over 60 years. Increases in cost ranged from GBP 269 for people aged 40–59 years with depression and cancer to GBP 2,817 in people with comorbid depression and obesity aged 40–59 years. In younger adults, mean additional costs related to asthma and comorbid depression were GBP 1,257, while comorbid diabetes and depression increased costs by GBP 2,133 in people aged over 60 years.

Other examples of additional costs from around the world can be identified. In Singapore, adults attending a specialist diabetes centre over a 1-year period who also had depression had a 30% chance of hospitalisation compared to 10% in the diabetes-alone group. They were four times more likely to be hospitalised for non-psychiatric conditions and three times more likely to be hospitalised for complications of diabetes [19].

In Hungary, a survey of more than 12,000 people looking at their use of health services over a 12-month period found that those with comorbid diabetes and depression had a 2.6 times greater risk of a lengthy period of hospitalisation and had almost double the risk of multiple hospital admissions compared to people with diabetes alone [20]. Another study looked at the impacts of physical comorbidity on healthcare costs for 65,000 people receiving primary care in Spain in 2004. Individuals with a depressive disorder had a significantly greater number of comorbid conditions or risk factors, including obesity, dyslipidaemia and smoking per year compared to other primary care service users (7.4 conditions vs. 4.3). Overall the annual costs of care were EUR 1,084 and 684 per patient in the comorbid and control populations, respectively [21]. In the UK, the economic impacts of smoking in people with mental disorders have been estimated to cost primary and secondary care service providers GBP 720 million per annum in treating smoking-related disease. The study also estimated that about a third of all cigarettes smoked in England are smoked by people with a mental disorder. This could mean that there are 2.6 million avoidable hospital admissions, 3.1 million avoidable primary care consultations and 18.8 million prescriptions that can be avoided each year [22].

In Germany, analysis at one teaching hospital over a 2-year period again reported that the average total costs of hospitalisation for people with cardiovascular disease alone compared to those with psychiatric comorbidity (largely depression and anxiety disorders) differed significantly (EUR 5,142 vs. 7,663). The average length of stay for patients with comorbidity was 13.2 days compared to 8.9 for patients with cardiovascular disease only [23]. Furthermore, this paper highlighted that the funding system in that hospital did not fully cover the costs of comorbidity, which means that patients might not receive appropriate levels of care.

There is also some limited information looking at the association between healthcare costs and comorbid asthma and mental disorders. One systematic review found 20 studies, largely focused on depression or anxiety disorders and asthma. It reported increased rates of hospitalisation, emergency department visits and visits to primary care practitioners in people with asthma and a mental disorder [24]. In the USA, a telephone survey of adolescents (aged 11–17 years) with asthma found that those assessed to have depressive disorders as well had on average 51% higher healthcare costs [25]. Most of these additional costs were related to non-asthma and non-mental health-related healthcare costs.

Impacts beyond Healthcare Systems

There appear to be fewer estimates of the impacts of comorbidity beyond the healthcare system. Published estimates concentrate on indirect costs – mainly productivity losses from employment due to absenteeism, with much less discussion of poor performance at work (presenteeism); there does not appear to be much information on the intangible costs of comorbidity. One review looked at the impact on participation in employment of people with coronary artery disease and mental disorders [26]. Only 13 studies were identified, 10 of which focused on comorbid depression. The review concluded that people with comorbid depression had a reduced likelihood of returning to work following the onset of illness (odds ratio 0.37) compared to people with coronary artery disease alone. A systematic review on comorbid diabetes and depression identified 11 studies that looked at the impacts on productivity, but only two of these studies assigned a monetary value to productivity losses and none included losses from premature mortality or informal care [12].

Data from a cross-sectional survey of 78,000 workers in Australia [27] show higher relative risks of both absenteeism and poor functioning while at work in individuals with comorbid psychological distress and physical health problems compared to those with physical health problems only. For instance, compared to people with no health problems, the risk of absenteeism from work was 33% higher for people who were experiencing psychological distress alongside obesity, and 27% higher for those who had high levels of cholesterol. Rates of presenteeism were between 2.5 and 5 times greater in populations with comorbid asthma, obesity, arthritis, diabetes and high cholesterol compared with the reference population.

Data from the 2007 Australian National Survey of Mental Health and Wellbeing (n = 8,841) have also been used to compare work functioning and absenteeism rates in people with depression, cardiovascular disease, or both conditions, with a disease-free population [28]. As table 3 shows, compared to a population with neither condition, and adjusted for various social and demographic

Table 3. Work participation, work functioning and disease group in Australia [28]

Disease group	Full- or part-time employment in the workforce (adjusted odds ratio)	Amount of difficulty in day to day work (full-time workers) (adjusted odds ratio)	Number of days unable to work (full-time workers) (adjusted odds ratio)
Neither MDD or CVD	1.0	1.0	1.0
MDD only	0.8*	4.0*	1.7*
CVD only	0.8*	0.9	0.9
Comorbid CVD and MDD	0.4*	10.6*	3.0*

MDD = Major depressive disorder; CVD = cardiovascular disease. * p < 0.05.

characteristics, the odds ratio for people with co-morbid depression and cardiovascular disease participating in work was significantly lower at just 0.4. This compared with odds ratios for work participation of 0.8 for depression or cardiovascular disease only. The comorbid group were also 10 times more likely to experience poor work functioning compared to the healthy workforce, 9 times greater than for people with cardiovascular disease alone and 2.5 times greater than for people with depression alone. Rates of absenteeism were also significantly higher for the comorbid group.

Data from a large Canadian survey of more than 130,000 people found (even after adjusting for socio-demographic characteristics, alcohol dependence and chronic physical illness burden), that the presence of comorbid major depressive disorders was associated with twice the likelihood of healthcare utilisation, and increased functional disability and work absence compared to the presence of a chronic physical illness without comorbid depression [29]. Significant increases in resource use and productivity losses have also been reported in a population survey of more than 12,000 adults in Hungary [20]. People with comorbid diabetes and depression were more than twice as likely to have lengthier stays in hospital (>20 days) and to have more hospital admissions. They were also more than 3 times as likely

to have a prolonged absence (>10 days) from paid work and to be unemployed.

In Finland, analysis of certified sickness absence in 33,000 public sector employees reported that non-cardiovascular comorbid conditions for employees with diabetes, including depression, accounted for over 50% of excess risk of sickness absence [30]. A US study of a manufacturing company with 15,000 employees reported 13.5 sick days per annum on average due to depression and physical comorbidity (diabetes, heart disease, hypertension or back problems) compared to 6.6 and 8.8 days for those with a physical condition or depression alone. Total mean costs, including healthcare and disability, per employee with comorbidity were USD 7,906. This is conservative as the costs of poor performance (presenteeism) at work were not included [31].

Data from the UK Psychiatric Morbidity Survey also indicate that over a year individuals with diabetes and depression were 7.7 and 5.3 times more likely to take sick days and have their work and other activities impaired by poor health compared to people with diabetes alone [32]. The number of working days lost was also found to be significantly higher in people with comorbid diabetes and depression compared to diabetes alone in Singapore – 1.9 versus 1.4 working days lost over a 3-month period [19].

Strengthening the Case for Tackling Comorbid Mental and Physical Health Problems

This chapter has illustrated that there are substantial economic costs associated with comorbidity. These costs fall both within and beyond healthcare systems. It is not, however, enough to identify these costs. Given that healthcare budget holders have to make difficult choices on how to allocate scarce resources to mental health and other services, it is critical is to identify cost-effective ways of reducing the risks or consequences of comorbidity.

Potentially, given the high additional costs of comorbidity, even modest success in reducing its prevalence may have economic payoffs. Policy makers will want to know whether early intervention and investment in actions to protect the physical health of people with mental health problems are a cost-effective use of resources, generating benefits not only to healthcare systems, but also more widely, perhaps reducing rates of absenteeism from work or the need for informal family care. They may also want to know whether a greater focus on managing the mental health of people with chronic physical health problems is a cost-effective way of improving outcomes.

There is a need to strengthen the evidence base, and in particular to look more at the cost-effectiveness of interventions outside of a US context. To date, the evidence on cost-effective approaches to manage comorbidity is modest, although it supports investment, suggesting that a number of cost-effective interventions are available. For instance, empirical work and modelling studies focusing on comorbid diabetes and depression includes several studies that have highlighted the cost-effectiveness of better integration between psychological and diabetes care [33–35]. Only a handful of studies have considered the economic, as well as the clinical impact, of interventions to promote and protect the physical health of people with mental disorders [36].

One way of strengthening the evidence base in the short-term is to make use of economic modelling techniques to take existing data on the effectiveness of different actions to tackle comorbidity and model plausible costs and benefits under different scenarios in different country contexts and over different time periods [37]. One recent example of a modelling approach suggests that it may be cost-effective to invest in group-based actions to promote better weight management in people with schizophrenia and diabetes [38]. In the mid to longer term it would be helpful to embed economic analysis, collecting data on resource use, costs and economic consequences, into evaluations of interventions to tackle comorbidity. This can facilitate better comparability across different interventions and help policymakers prioritise the way in which they allocate resources.

Where mental health services are largely separate from physical health services, the provision of seamless care for both physical and mental health problems becomes more difficult to achieve. Therefore, another important step may be to evaluate the cost-effectiveness of different incentives and organisational structures to encourage a more collaborative approach to the detection and management of comorbidity; there are often substantive silos in both the financing and organisation of mental health and general health services [39].

This chapter has illustrated that economics can help provide powerful arguments to support a case for tackling comorbidity. It has shown that there are substantial impacts both within and beyond health systems linked to comorbidity. For too long, much of these costs remained hidden; this is now changing and in the future more information will be available on these additional costs as well. This hopefully will provide more impetus for actions to address an issue which leads not only to some avoidable costs to health and society, but also has profound personal human consequences.

References

1 Naylor C, Parsonage M, McDaid D, Knapp M, Fossey M, Galea A: Long-Term Conditions and Mental Health. The Costs of Co-Morbidities. London, The King's Fund, 2012.

2 Wittchen HU, Jacobi F, Rehm J, Gustavsson A, Svensson M, Jonsson B, et al: The size and burden of mental disorders and other disorders of the brain in Europe 2010. Eur Neuropsychopharmacol 2011;21:655–679.

3 Wahlbeck K, Westman J, Nordentoft M, Gissler M, Laursen TM: Outcomes of Nordic mental health systems: life expectancy of patients with mental disorders. Br J Psychiatry 2011;199:453–458.

4 McDaid D, Park A-L, Currie C, Zanotti C: Investing in the wellbeing of young people: making the economic case; in McDaid D, Cooper CL (eds): Wellbeing: A Complete Reference Guide. The Economics of Wellbeing. Oxford, John Wiley, 2014, vol 5.

5 Chwastiak LA, Rosenheck RA, McEvoy JP, Stroup TS, Swartz MS, Davis SM, et al: The impact of obesity on health care costs among persons with schizophrenia. Gen Hosp Psychiatry 2009;31:1–7.

6 McDonald M, Hertz RP, Lustik MB, Unger AN: Healthcare spending among community-dwelling adults with schizophrenia. Am J Manag Care 2005; 11(8 suppl):S242–S247.

7 Hendrie HC, Tu W, Tabbey R, Purnell CE, Ambuehl RJ, Callahan CM: Health outcomes and cost of care among older adults with schizophrenia: a 10-year study using medical records across the continuum of care. Am J Geriatr Psychiatry 2014;22:427–436.

8 Centorrino F, Mark TL, Talamo A, Oh K, Chang J: Health and economic burden of metabolic comorbidity among individuals with bipolar disorder. J Clin Psychopharmacol 2009;29:595–600.

9 Guo JJ, Keck PE Jr, Li H, Jang R, Kelton CM: Treatment costs and health care utilization for patients with bipolar disorder in a large managed care population. Value Health 2008;11:416–423.

10 Welch CA, Czerwinski D, Ghimire B, Bertsimas D: Depression and costs of health care. Psychosomatics 2009;50: 392–401.

11 Hutter N, Schnurr A, Baumeister H: Healthcare costs in patients with diabetes mellitus and comorbid mental disorders – a systematic review. Diabetologia 2010;53:2470–2479.

12 Molosankwe I, Patel A, Jose Gagliardino J, Knapp M, McDaid D: Economic aspects of the association between diabetes and depression: a systematic review. J Affect Disord 2012;142(suppl):S42–S55.

13 Le TK, Curtis B, Kahle-Wrobleski K, Johnston J, Haldane D, Melfi C: Treatment patterns and resource use among patients with comorbid diabetes mellitus and major depressive disorder. J Med Econ 2011;14:440–447.

14 Atlantis E, Goldney RD, Eckert KA, Taylor AW, Phillips P: Trends in health-related quality of life and health service use associated with comorbid diabetes and major depression in South Australia, 1998–2008. Soc Psychiatry Psychiatr Epidemiol 2012;47:871–877.

15 Simon GE, Katon WJ, Lin EH, Ludman E, VonKorff M, Ciechanowski P, et al: Diabetes complications and depression as predictors of health service costs. Gen Hosp Psychiatry 2005;27:344–351.

16 Boulanger L, Zhao Y, Foster TS, Fraser K, Bledsoe SL, Russell MW: Impact of comorbid depression or anxiety on patterns of treatment and economic outcomes among patients with diabetic peripheral neuropathic pain. Curr Med Res Opin 2009;25:1763–1773.

17 Unutzer J, Schoenbaum M, Katon WJ, Fan MY, Pincus HA, Hogan D, et al: Healthcare costs associated with depression in medically Ill fee-for-service Medicare participants. J Am Geriatr Soc 2009;57:506–510.

18 Brilleman SL, Purdy S, Salisbury C, Windmeijer F, Gravelle H, Hollinghurst S: Implications of comorbidity for primary care costs in the UK: a retrospective observational study. Br J Gen Pract 2013;63:e274–e282.

19 Subramaniam M, Sum CF, Pek E, Stahl D, Verma S, Liow PH, et al: Comorbid depression and increased health care utilisation in individuals with diabetes. Gen Hosp Psychiatry 2009;31:220–224.

20 Vamos EP, Mucsi I, Keszei A, Kopp MS, Novak M: Comorbid depression is associated with increased healthcare utilization and lost productivity in persons with diabetes: a large nationally representative Hungarian population survey. Psychosom Med 2009;71:501–507.

21 Sicras Mainar A, Rejas Gutierrez J, Navarro Artieda R, Serrat Tarres J, Blanca Tamayo M, Diaz Cerezo S: Patterns of health services use and costs in patients with mental disorders in primary care (in Spanish). Gac Sanit 2007;21:306–313.

22 Royal College of Physicians, Royal College of Psychiatrists: Smoking and Mental Health. London, Royal College of Physicians, 2013.

23 Hochlehnert A, Niehoff D, Wild B, Jünger J, Herzog W, Löwe B: Psychiatric comorbidity in cardiovascular inpatients: costs, net gain, and length of hospitalization. J Psychosom Res 2011;70: 135–139.

24 Hutter N, Knecht A, Baumeister H: Health care costs in persons with asthma and comorbid mental disorders: a systematic review. Gen Hosp Psychiatry 2011;33:443–453.

25 Richardson LP, Russo JE, Lozano P, McCauley E, Katon W: The effect of comorbid anxiety and depressive disorders on health care utilization and costs among adolescents with asthma. Gen Hosp Psychiatry 2008;30:398–406.

26 Haschke A, Hutter N, Baumeister H: Indirect costs in patients with coronary artery disease and mental disorders: a systematic review and meta-analysis. Int J Occup Med Environ Health 2012;25: 319–329.

27 Holden L, Scuffham PA, Hilton MF, Ware RS, Vecchio N, Whiteford HA: Health-related productivity losses increase when the health condition is comorbid with psychological distress: findings from a large cross-sectional sample of working Australians. BMC Public Health 2011;11:417.

28 O'Neil A, Williams ED, Stevenson CE, Oldenburg B, Sanderson K: Co-morbid depression is associated with poor work outcomes in persons with cardiovascular disease (CVD): a large, nationally representative survey in the Australian population. BMC Public Health 2012;12: 47.

29 Stein MB, Cox BJ, Afifi TO, Belik SL, Sareen J: Does co-morbid depressive illness magnify the impact of chronic physical illness? A population-based perspective. Psychol Med 2006;36:587–596.

30 Kivimäki M, Vahtera J, Pentti J, Virtanen M, Elovainio M, Hemingway H: Increased sickness absence in diabetic employees: what is the role of co-morbid conditions? Diabet Med 2007;24:1043–1048.

31 Druss BG, Rosenheck RA, Sledge WH: Health and disability costs of depressive illness in a major U.S. corporation. Am J Psychiatry 2000;157:1274–1278.

32 Das-Munshi J, Stewart R, Ismail K, Bebbington PE, Jenkins R, Prince MJ: Diabetes, common mental disorders, and disability: findings from the UK National Psychiatric Morbidity Survey. Psychosom Med 2007;69:543–550.

33 Katon W, Russo J, Lin EH, Schmittdiel J, Ciechanowski P, Ludman E, et al: Cost-effectiveness of a multicondition collaborative care intervention: a randomized controlled trial. Arch Gen Psychiatry 2012;69:506–514.

34 Hay J, Katon W, Ell K, Lee PJ, Guterman J: Cost-effectiveness analysis of collaborative care management of major depression among low income, predominantly Hispanics with diabetes. Value Health 2012;15:249–254.

35 King D, Molosankwe I, McDaid D: Collaborative care for depression in individuals with type II diabetes; in Knapp M, McDaid D, Parsonage M (eds): Mental Health Promotion and Mental Illness Prevention: The Economic Case. London, Department of Health, 2011.

36 Park AL, McDaid D, Weiser P, Von Gottberg C, Becker T, Kilian R: Examining the cost effectiveness of interventions to promote the physical health of people with mental health problems: a systematic review. BMC Public Health 2013;13:787.

37 McDaid D: Economic modelling for global mental health; in Thornicroft G, Patel V (eds): Global Mental Health Trials. Oxford, Oxford University Press, 2014.

38 Park AL: Exploring the economic implications of a group-based lifestyle intervention for middle-aged adults with chronic schizophrenia and co-morbid type 2 diabetes. J Diabetes Metab 2014; 5:366.

39 Knapp M, McDaid D, Amaddeo F, Constantopoulos A, Oliveira MD, Salvador-Carulla L, et al: Financing mental health care in Europe. J Ment Health 2007;16: 167–180.

David McDaid, MSc, BSc
Personal Social Services Research Unit, London School of Economics and Political Science
Houghton Street
London WC2A 2AE (UK)
E-Mail d.mcdaid@lse.ac.uk

Background

Sartorius N, Holt RIG, Maj M (eds): Comorbidity of Mental and Physical Disorders.
Key Issues Ment Health. Basel, Karger, 2015, vol 179, pp 33–41 (DOI: 10.1159/000365545)

Difficulties Facing the Provision of Care for Multimorbidity in Low-Income Countries

David Beran

Division of Tropical and Humanitarian Medicine, Geneva University Hospitals and University of Geneva, Geneva, Switzerland

Abstract

Low-income countries face a double burden of noncommunicable and communicable diseases, which further strains their limited resources. In response, the global community has prioritized four chronic noncommunicable diseases and four risk factors, not including neuropsychiatric disorders. Health systems play a key role in addressing the challenges of noncommunicable diseases, mental health and multimorbidity, but have failed to tackle this effectively. Noncommunicable disease as well as noncommunicable/communicable disease multimorbidity cannot be managed from only a biomedical perspective, but needs to include consideration of inequality and poverty. The health systems in low-income countries are currently failing in their management of individuals with single noncommunicable diseases; therefore, when a person is exposed to multiple risk factors and/or has multiple conditions, the health system cannot cope, leading to poor outcomes for individuals. Eleven elements were found to be necessary for diabetes care in low-income settings, and since diabetes makes a good tracer condition, these elements are presented for the issue of multimorbidity. They include organization of the health system, data collection, prevention, diagnostic tools and infrastructure, medicine procurement and supply, accessibility and affordability of medicines and care, healthcare workers, adherence issues, patient education and empowerment, community involvement and positive policy environment. Primary healthcare has been proposed as a solution, but there are numerous barriers to implementing this. Given health system constraints, there is a need to shift care back to the individual and their family for managing both the medical (self-care) and social aspects (e.g. stigma) of their conditions for better outcomes.

© 2015 S. Karger AG, Basel

Low-income countries are defined by the World Bank as countries where income per capita is USD 1,035 or less [1]. This grouping includes 28 countries from sub-Saharan Africa, 5 from Asia, 3 from Central Asia and 1 in the Caribbean. Because of their low income, these countries spend on average only USD 22 per person per year on health [2]. While traditionally it was thought that the burden of disease in these countries was predominantly from communicable diseases, noncommunicable diseases represent 80% of deaths in low- and middle-income countries [3]. Noncommunicable diseases and poverty have a symbiotic relationship, with poverty increasing exposure to noncommunicable disease risk factors and actual noncommunicable diseases forcing individuals and households into poverty as the burden of the cost of care falls on the individual in these countries [3]. Noncommunicable diseases also impact health systems, economies and countries as a whole, as every 10% increase in noncommunicable diseases is associated with a 0.5% decrease in economic growth.

In September 2011, the United Nations held its second health-related general assembly on noncommunicable diseases after its 2001 meeting on HIV/AIDS. Four diseases were prioritized by the World Health Organization, namely cardiovascular diseases, cancer, chronic respiratory diseases and diabetes, which were chosen since they contribute the largest amount to morbidity and mortality [4]. In 2013, the World Health Organization's noncommunicable disease global action plan was endorsed and aims to provide a guide to attain nine voluntary global targets, including the overall goal of a 25% relative reduction in premature mortality from cardiovascular disease, cancer, diabetes and chronic respiratory disease by 2025 [4]. Although neuropsychiatric disorders contribute an estimated 13% of the global burden of disease [5], they are not formally included in the World Health Organization's global noncommunicable diseases action plan. Mental health is mentioned in the context of comprehensive care for noncommunicable diseases needing to include 'primary prevention, early detection or screening, treatment, secondary prevention, rehabilitation and palliative care and attention to improving mental health' [4].

Health systems play a key role in addressing the challenges of noncommunicable diseases, mental health and multimorbidity. The management of these requires care be provided over a long period of time, which needs the input from a multidisciplinary team of healthcare workers, access to medicines and diagnostic tools, patient empowerment, and coordination of different elements of the health system [6].

Multimorbidity in a Low-Income Context

With the number of people aged 65 years or above projected to increase from approximately 524 million in 2010 to about 1.5 billion in 2050, with the highest increase in developing countries, the issue of multimorbidity needs to be addressed. It is estimated that 1 in 4 adults suffer from multimorbidity, with most evidence coming from high-income countries [7]. Studies from low-income countries have found that 53.7% of people aged above 60 years had two or more chronic conditions in Bangladesh [8], 66.7% of people with diabetes also had hypertension in Cameroon [9] and in a nationally representative sample in South Africa it was found that 29.6% had two or more of the following conditions: hypertension, diabetes, asthma, depression, angina, stroke and arthritis [10].

Synergies to address and integrate care for communicable and noncommunicable diseases have not been addressed [11]. The links between the four main noncommunicable diseases are clearly established through their shared risk factors and high rates of comorbidity [8, 9]. In low-income country settings, however, there is not only the existence of comorbidity of noncommunicable diseases, but also comorbidity of noncommunicable diseases with communicable disease [12].

The issue of multimorbidity can be linked to the causal pathways of the diseases [13]. For example, there is a link between a high burden of tuberculosis with smoking and harmful alcohol use [14–16], or mental health with sexual behavior, alcohol and tobacco use [17]. Another way of looking at multimorbidity is that having one condition means the individual is more likely to develop another [13]. For example, diabetes has

Table 1. The interplay of multiple risk factors and diseases

	Noncommunicable disease risk factor	Actual non-communicable disease	Communicable disease	Mental health
Noncommunicable disease risk factor	person who smokes and is obese	person with diabetes who smokes	obese individual with HIV/AIDS	smoking and alcohol consumption
Actual non-communicable disease		person with diabetes and hypertension	person with diabetes and tuberculosis	people with diabetes are more prone to depression
Communicable disease			person with HIV/AIDS and tuberculosis	people with HIV/AIDS more likely to have mental disorders

Underlying issues include, for example, ageing and poverty.

been associated with a threefold incident risk of tuberculosis [18–20], HIV/AIDS causes Kaposi sarcoma and lymphoma [21], and people with HIV/AIDS are more likely to have mental disorders [22].

It is not only the condition that may lead to another condition, but also the treatments for these. One particular example relevant to low-income countries is the link between antiretroviral treatment and the metabolic syndrome [18], increased rate of cardiovascular risk factors [23], diabetes [24], and other cardiac, neurological and musculoskeletal conditions [25].

Finally, the last aspect is that proper management of both conditions is necessary in order to ensure good outcomes from each disease perspective. Good tuberculosis management is necessary for good diabetes management, and good diabetes management helps ensure the success of tuberculosis treatment; however, the medicines used to treat tuberculosis may worsen blood glucose control [19, 20]. Management of depression is also necessary to ensure proper outcomes for noncommunicable diseases [26].

Addressing these situations needs to be done not only from a biomedical perspective, but also from a socioeconomic angle, taking into account inequalities and poverty. Table 1 details these interlinkages as well as the underlying issues of ageing and poverty.

The challenge in low-income countries is that there is a knowledge, treatment and outcome gap for noncommunicable diseases and multimorbidity. In Mozambique the prevalence of hypertension is 33.1%, but only 14.8% of people who have hypertension are aware they have it [27]. Of those aware, 51.9% receive treatment and of those receiving treatment, only 39.9% are controlling their hypertension. That means for every 100 people with hypertension, only 3 know they have the disease, receive treatment and have controlled hypertension. A nationally representative survey in South Africa found that despite the high prevalence of mental disorders and related disability, these conditions, especially depression, were less likely to be treated than physical disorders [28]. Data from the World Health Organization show that between 76 and 85% of people with mental health problems in low- and middle-income countries receive no treatment for their disorder and that resources for mental health are primarily assigned to mental hospitals [29].

The health systems in low-income countries are currently failing in their management of individuals with single conditions. Therefore, when a person has multiple conditions or multiple risk factors for these conditions, the health system is not organized in a manner that can face such a situation, which leads to poor outcomes for individuals.

The Health System Barriers to Care for Multimorbidity in Low-Income Countries

A health system is defined as all the 'activities whose primary purpose is to promote, restore and maintain health' [30]. Health systems have three main objectives: (1) to improve the health of the populations they serve, (2) respond to the population's expectations and (3) provide financial protection against the costs of ill-health [30].

Health systems do not work in isolation of the other sociopolitical elements of a given country, and therefore different models of health systems exist [31, 32]. Certain key factors that health systems need to perform are procurement and supply of medicines, disposables and equipment, healthcare workers in sufficient numbers and with the right skills for the given population and disease burden, and sustainable financing and healthcare costs that do not overburden the poor and have a financial, budgetary and regulatory framework [31, 32]. Research into diabetes in low-income countries [33] found that 11 elements were necessary for diabetes care. Diabetes makes a good tracer condition for health systems, from which the lessons learnt can be applied to other chronic conditions [34–36].

The first element is organization of the health system. Currently, health systems in low-income countries are not organized to manage noncommunicable disease, let alone individuals with multiple conditions, and are more focused on infectious diseases [37]. Many health system responses in low-income countries for HIV/AIDS and tuberculosis have focused on vertical programs only addressing these specific conditions and not tackling all the challenges faced by individuals in the health system [38]. Although these have shown some success, they fail to take a person-centered focus and do not manage all the conditions the individual may have, but only the one that is being funded, leading to fragmentation of healthcare [39]. This fragmentation also exists because care in urban areas is hospital based whereas in rural areas health services focus on a specific disease (e.g. HIV/AIDS) or selective services (e.g. maternal health) [39]. In parallel, the use of traditional medicine is widespread, with 80% of the population in Sub-Saharan Africa relying on this as their primary source of care [13], which has as of yet not been integrated for the management of noncommunicable diseases.

Although primary healthcare has been promoted in low-income countries, it has not been able to address the challenge of noncommunicable disease or play a role in prevention and health promotion [13, 37]. Noncommunicable disease care is still the remit of specialists in specialist centers; for example, mental health in low-income countries is still predominantly focused on hospital care [40]. As these specialist centers are limited, this also causes problems for referrals and counterreferrals. Specifically for the issue of multimorbidity, the degree of overspecialization may mean multiple referrals, if feasible, are made to different specialists for the individual's multiple conditions.

When providing care for a person both over a long period of time and with multiple conditions, another element the health system needs to provide is data collection. Data are needed at all levels of the health system in order to inform policies, medicine procurement, and staffing and individual care. However, there is a general lack of quality health information systems in many low-income countries [37]. At the level of the individual, poor use of patient records means that previous consultations or other conditions are not taken into account, thus leading to an unstructured monitoring of clinical care [37]. There is also a lack of a recall system to ensure continuity of care [38]. In terms of studies, very few have looked at the issue of multimorbidity in low-income countries except for the issue of HIV/AIDS and tuberculosis.

Another area where studies are lacking from low-income countries and which is important for the issue of multimorbidity is prevention. As mentioned previously, primary healthcare in low-income countries does not fulfill its role in terms of prevention and health promotion [33]. This is linked to lack of training, human resources and culturally appropriate materials to ensure wider knowledge of noncommunicable disease and their risk factors in these settings. For example, asthma and chronic respiratory disease are underrecognized, underdiagnosed, undertreated and insufficiently prevented. With one of the main risk factors in low-income countries being the use of biomass fuel, local healthcare workers need the knowledge about these conditions in their specific context to enable them to play a preventive role and not only provide care [41]. The World Health Organization has also developed 'best buys' for noncommunicable diseases for the four common risk factors (tobacco use, harmful use of alcohol, unhealthy diets and physical inactivity) and for cardiovascular disease, diabetes and cancer [42]. However, many low-income countries lack the capability of implementing, enforcing and sustaining these.

As prevention also includes screening measures, diagnostic tools and infrastructure are needed. However, health infrastructure is poor at all levels of the health system with, for example, 19 and 39% of primary healthcare facilities in Tanzania and Senegal, respectively, having access to electricity, water and sanitation [13]. In addition, basic equipment is lacking in these facilities and access to diagnostic tools for diabetes has been seen to be poor in low-income countries [43]. There are also financial constraints for the individual if they need to pay for the test as well as budget limits that impact a prescribers' ability to ask for certain tests [38].

Besides diagnostic tools and infrastructure, health systems need to be able to procure and supply medicines to manage multimorbidity. Looking at the issue of insulin in low-income countries, a variety of factors impact its procurement and supply, such as budget allocation for medicines, adequate buying procedures, quantifi-

cation of needs, efficient procurement, efficient distribution, rational prescription and proper compliance [43].

Mental health is an example highlighting the challenge of medicine procurement and supply with such issues as prescription regulations, availability and use of certain treatments, and limited expenditure (low-income countries spend 10 times less than lower-middle and 1,547 less than high-income countries, respectively) [40]. Ultimately, all of these factors impact the affordability and accessibility of medicines. Accessibility is linked not only to distribution, but also to where the individual lives, with urban areas having better access than rural areas. In terms of affordability, government policies will impact this; for example, insulin is free in Nicaragua, while individuals have to pay for this in Mali because of the government policy of cost recovery [43]. Generic medicines to treat noncommunicable disease were found to be less available than medicines for communicable conditions in both the public (36.0 vs. 53.5%) and private sectors (54.7 vs. 66.2%) [44]. Specifically, antiasthmatic inhalers were available to 30.1% in the public sector and to 43.1% in the private sector. In terms of affordability, it has been found that 1 month of treatment for coronary heart disease costs 18.4 days' wages in Malawi while for insulin in Mali the annual cost represented 38% of per capita gross domestic product [43, 45]. These conditions also place a huge financial burden on countries, with diabetes care representing 5% of the total budget for the Ministry of Health in Nicaragua and insulin representing 10% of the total medicines budget in Mozambique [43].

An essential element of the health system is healthcare workers. Issues of availability, rational use and training need to be addressed [46]. Low-income countries face a severe shortage of healthcare workers and the human resources present are inequitably distributed [13]. Specifically for mental health in the Africa region of the World Health Organization, there is significant variation in the number of psychiatrists, ranging from more than 10 per 100,000 to fewer than 1 per 100,000 [47]. There is also a low focus of these human resources on community care [40]. Overall, this problem is linked to an internal and external 'brain drain' with doctors preferring the private over public sector, urban over rural areas, and tertiary levels of care versus primary care [48]. In addition, this internal brain drain to nongovernmental organizations specifically in the area of HIV/AIDS has impacted the availability of health professionals, e.g. 50% of medical graduates in Uganda were found to be working for an HIV-related nongovernmental organization [49].

It is important to define the role of different cadres of healthcare workers in managing noncommunicable disease and the role of specialists, such as in the initiation of treatment versus follow-up and continuation of treatment and how this is linked to treatment guidelines that are adapted to the local context or include the best clinical evidence. Another issue is actual training and how this training currently focuses on clinical management of certain diseases and not the issue of multimorbidity. Current training of health professionals, especially doctors, does not include the preventive role they can play.

Patient education is lacking both as health professionals are not trained in this area, have very little time for this, and also lack the materials and the means to deliver this. In addition, the view of certain diseases may impact how health professionals educate and empower their patients. For example, in some settings people with mental health problems are shackled and beaten because of traditional beliefs about the causes of these conditions [47]. Therefore, issues of stigma also need to be addressed not only for individuals with these conditions, but also in the wider community. There is also the issue of using Western concepts of disease. For example, Patel et al. [50] while studying depression in Zimbabwe found a variety of presentations and

descriptions for this condition including supernatural causes. The health system may provide the majority of aspects that a person with a noncommunicable disease requires; however, the burden of care falls on the individual and their family as the majority of the time spent managing a noncommunicable disease is done outside of the health system [51].

Adherence is impacted by education about the condition and the financial burden of care. In low-income countries, patient education is lacking for noncommunicable disease and there is still a large financial burden of care. In a systematic review of adherence to cardiovascular medications in resource-limited settings, Bowry et al. [52] found that poor adherence was due to these factors as well as negative perceptions about medicines and their side effects.

Community involvement and patient associations can play a role in patient education and empowerment, thereby impacting adherence, with the proper support from the health system. Many types of patient organizations (e.g. diabetes associations) exist, with varying roles, such as advocacy, training for patients and healthcare workers, and acting as a support group for patients and families, as well as being a provider of care [53]. The 2011 *Mental Health Atlas* [40] found that 39% of low-income countries had associations compared with 80% of high-income countries. It is not only the number of these organizations that is important, but also that many of them focus on specific diseases, such as cancer societies, diabetes associations, etc.

Overall, the health system elements described above need to be present and supported by a positive policy environment. In low-income countries, there is a large reliance on external funding for specific disease programs [13]. Due to this it was found that 30% of countries do not have a specified budget for mental health [47]. In parallel, in order to address the issue of noncommunicable disease properly, a multisectorial approach is needed that not only includes the health sector, but also education, trade and agriculture [33]. For mental health there is also a need to include police and judicial systems. Although many low-income countries have started to develop national non-communicable disease plans, these fail to recognize the true issue of multimorbidity and include mental health [54]. In low-income countries, only 48.7% of countries have a mental health policy in comparison to 77.1% of high-income countries [40].

Conclusion

There is both the need to address prevention and the wider determinants of noncommunicable disease as well as ensuring access to affordable care [37]. Primary healthcare has been proposed as a solution to address this challenge as it enables a shift in focus to managing the individual and not the specific condition; however, there are numerous barriers to delivery of noncommunicable disease interventions and not all noncommunicable disease interventions, due to their complexity, can be integrated in primary healthcare. This is even more relevant for multimorbidity whereby the complexity of the individual may mean that primary healthcare does not have the human and resource capacity to manage this.

Each level of the health system has a role to play in multimorbidity prevention and management, and thus needs certain materials and human resources to be available. Also, a certain level of organization and coordination between different levels of the health system and different sectors within the same institution (inpatient and outpatient services, pharmacy, laboratory, etc.) need to be in place for patient management and referral. Guidelines need to be developed and used as well as data to ensure efficient and effective care and help define referral pathways from different levels of the health system to avoid overuse of hospital care and ensure prompt referral to specialists only when needed.

An innovative approach to addressing the issue of noncommunicable diseases in low-income countries was a Twinning project between Diabetes UK (UK-based diabetes association) and Mozambique [55]. This project showed that by taking a systematic approach to developing diabetes care, including activities addressing all 11 elements presented above, it was able to improve healthcare worker knowledge, access to medicines and the government's response not only to diabetes, but also all noncommunicable diseases [56].

In looking at lessons from low-income countries in improving access to psychological treatments, Patel et al. [57] found that the two main barriers were a lack of human resources and the acceptance of the treatments proposed in different sociocultural contexts. The human resource challenge in low-income countries will not be solved quickly, and with the rising burden of noncommunicable disease and multimorbidity, solutions need to be found. Specifically looking at mental health, Petersen et al. [58] propose task-shifting to nonspecialists. These nonspecialists need to shift the power back to the individual and their family, and have informed and active individuals in their own care who are able to have a partnership with their healthcare providers [59].

One lesson from HIV/AIDS that may be useful for multimorbidity is to involve local communities actively [60]. As chronic diseases are mainly managed outside the formal health system, individuals need the skills to be able to care for themselves. Parallel to the ageing population, community-based care is necessary. This will of course require trained healthcare workers to be involved, but by involving civil society, traditional healers and other groups, the issues of knowledge and stigma can effectively be addressed, ensuring better management, medically and socially, and therefore better outcomes for people with multiple conditions.

References

1 Country and Lending Groups. Washington, The World Bank, 2013.
2 World Health Statistics 2009. Geneva, World Health Organization, 2009.
3 Global Status Report on Noncommunicable Diseases. Geneva, World Health Organization, 2010.
4 Global Action Plan for the Prevention and Control of Noncommunicable Diseases 2013–2020 – Revised Draft (version dated February 11, 2013). Geneva, World Health Organization, 2013.
5 The Global Burden of Disease: 2004 Update. Geneva, World Health Organization, 2004.
6 Nolte E, McKee M: Introduction; in Nolte E, McKee M (eds): Caring for People with Chronic Conditions: A Health System Perspective. Maidenhead, Open University Press, 2008.
7 Alaba O, Chola L: The social determinants of multimorbidity in South Africa. Int J Equity Health 2013;12:63.
8 Khanam MA, Streatfield PK, Kabir ZN, Qiu C, Cornelius C, Wahlin A: Prevalence and patterns of multimorbidity among elderly people in rural Bangladesh: a cross-sectional study. J Health Popul Nutr 2011;29:406–414.
9 Choukem SP, Kengne AP, Dehayem YM, Simo NL, Mbanya JC: Hypertension in people with diabetes in sub-Saharan Africa: revealing the hidden face of the iceberg. Diabetes Res Clin Pract 2007;77: 293–299.
10 Negin J, Martiniuk A, Cumming RG, Naidoo N, Phaswana-Mafuya N, Madurai L, Williams S, Kowal P: Prevalence of HIV and chronic comorbidities among older adults. AIDS 2012;26(suppl 1): S55–S63.
11 Marais BJ, Lonnroth K, Lawn SD, Migliori GB, Mwaba P, Glaziou P, Bates M, Colagiuri R, Zijenah L, Swaminathan S, Memish ZA, Pletschette M, Hoelscher M, Abubakar I, Hasan R, Zafar A, Pantaleo G, Craig G, Kim P, Maeurer M, Schito M, Zumla A: Tuberculosis comorbidity with communicable and non-communicable diseases: integrating health services and control efforts. Lancet Infect Dis 2013;13:436–448.
12 Maher D, Ford N, Unwin N: Priorities for developing countries in the global response to non-communicable diseases. Global Health 2012;8:14.

13 Marquez PV, Farrington JL: The Challenge of Non-Communicable Diseases and Road Traffic Injuries in Sub-Saharan Africa. Washington, The World Bank, 2013.
14 Lonnroth K, Castro KG, Chakaya JM, Chauhan LS, Floyd K, Glaziou P, Raviglione MC: Tuberculosis control and elimination 2010–50: cure, care, and social development. Lancet 2010;375: 1814–1829.
15 Lonnroth K, Jaramillo E, Williams BG, Dye C, Raviglione M: Drivers of tuberculosis epidemics: the role of risk factors and social determinants. Soc Sci Med 2009;68:2240–2246.
16 Brunet L, Pai M, Davids V, Ling D, Paradis G, Lenders L, Meldau R, van Zyl Smit R, Calligaro G, Allwood B, Dawson R, Dheda K: High prevalence of smoking among patients with suspected tuberculosis in South Africa. Eur Respir J 2011; 38:139–146.
17 Lundberg P, Rukundo G, Ashaba S, Thorson A, Allebeck P, Ostergren PO, Cantor-Graae E: Poor mental health and sexual risk behaviours in Uganda: a cross-sectional population-based study. BMC Public Health 2011;11:125.
18 Young F, Critchley JA, Johnstone LK, Unwin NC: A review of co-morbidity between infectious and chronic disease in sub Saharan Africa: TB and diabetes mellitus, HIV and metabolic syndrome, and the impact of globalization. Global Health 2009;5:9.
19 Dooley KE, Chaisson RE: Tuberculosis and diabetes mellitus: convergence of two epidemics. Lancet Infect Dis 2009;9: 737–746.
20 Dooley KE, Tang T, Golub JE, Dorman SE, Cronin W: Impact of diabetes mellitus on treatment outcomes of patients with active tuberculosis. Am J Trop Med Hyg 2009;80:634–639.
21 Parkin DM: The global health burden of infection-associated cancers in the year 2002. Int J Cancer 2006;118:3030–3044.
22 Freeman M, Patel V, Collins PY, Bertolote J: Integrating mental health in global initiatives for HIV/AIDS. Br J Psychiatry 2005;187:1–3.
23 Muronya W, Sanga E, Talama G, Kumwenda JJ, van Oosterhout JJ: Cardiovascular risk factors in adult Malawians on long-term antiretroviral therapy. Trans R Soc Trop Med Hyg 2011;105:644–649.

24 Rao MN, Mulligan K, Schambelan M: HIV infection and diabetes principles of diabetes mellitus; in Poretsky L (ed): Principles of Diabetes Mellitus, ed 2. New York, Springer, 2010, pp 617–642.
25 Dawson R, Rom WN, Dheda K, Bateman ED: The new epidemic of non-communicable disease in people living with the human immunodeficiency virus. Public Health Action 2013;3:4–6.
26 Moussavi S, Chatterji S, Verdes E, Tandon A, Patel V, Ustun B: Depression, chronic diseases, and decrements in health: results from the World Health Surveys. Lancet 2007;370:851–858.
27 Damasceno A, Azevedo A, Silva-Matos C, Prista A, Diogo D, Lunet N: Hypertension prevalence, awareness, treatment, and control in Mozambique: urban/rural gap during epidemiological transition. Hypertension 2009;54:77–83.
28 Suliman S, Stein DJ, Myer L, Williams DR, Seedat S: Disability and treatment of psychiatric and physical disorders in South Africa. J Nerv Ment Dis 2010;198: 8–15.
29 Draft Comprehensive Mental Health Action Plan 2013–2020. Geneva, World Health Organization, 2013.
30 The World Health Report 2000 – Health Systems: Improving Performance. Geneva, World Health Organization, 2000.
31 Strengthening Health Systems to Improve Health Outcomes: WHO's Framework for Action. Geneva, World Health Organization, 2007.
32 Reich MR, Takemi K, Roberts MJ, Hsiao WC: Global action on health systems: a proposal for the Toyako G8 summit. Lancet 2008;371:865–869.
33 Beran D, Yudkin J: Diabetes care in sub-Saharan Africa. Lancet 2006;368:1689–1695.
34 Kessner D, Carolyn E, Singer J: Assessing health quality: the case for tracers. N Engl J Med 1973;288:189–194.
35 Nolte E, Bain C, McKee M: Diabetes as a tracer condition in international benchmarking of health systems. Diabetes Care 2006;29:1007–1011.
36 Beran D: Health systems and the management of chronic diseases: lessons from type 1 diabetes. Diabetes Manag 2012;2:1–13.

37 Maher D, Harries AD, Zachariah R, Enarson D: A global framework for action to improve the primary care response to chronic non-communicable diseases: a solution to a neglected problem. BMC Public Health 2009;9:355.

38 Levitt NS, Steyn K, Dave J, Bradshaw D: Chronic noncommunicable diseases and HIV-AIDS on a collision course: relevance for health care delivery, particularly in low-resource settings – insights from South Africa. Am J Clin Nutr 2011; 94:1690S–1696S.

39 World Health Report 2008: Primary Health Care – Now More than Ever. Geneva, World Health Organization, 2008.

40 Mental Health Atlas 2011. Geneva, World Health Organization, 2011.

41 van Gemert F, van der Molen T, Jones R, Chavannes N: The impact of asthma and COPD in sub-Saharan Africa. Prim Care Respir J 2011;20:240–248.

42 WHO, WEF: From Burden to 'Best Buys': Reducing the Economic Impact of Non-Communicable Diseases in Low- and Middle-Income Countries. Geneva, World Economic Forum, 2011.

43 Beran D, Yudkin JS: Looking beyond the issue of access to insulin. What is needed for proper diabetes care in resource poor settings. Diabetes Res Clin Pract 2010;88:217–221.

44 Cameron A, Roubos I, Ewen M, Mantel-Teeuwisse AK, Leufkens HG, Laing RO: Differences in the availability of medicines for chronic and acute conditions in the public and private sectors of developing countries. Bull World Health Organ 2011;89:412–421.

45 Mendis S, Fukino K, Cameron A, Laing R, Filipe A Jr, Khatib O, Leowski J, Ewen M: The availability and affordability of selected essential medicines for chronic diseases in six low- and middle-income countries. Bull World Health Organ 2007;85:279–288.

46 Wagner EH, Austin BT, Von Korff M: Organizing care for patients with chronic illness. Milbank Q 1996;74:511–544.

47 WHO Resource Book on Mental Health, Human Rights and Legislation. Geneva, World Health Organization, 2005.

48 Padarath A, Chamberlain C, McCoy D, Ntuli A, Rowson M, Loewenson R: Health personnel in Southern Africa: confronting maldistribution and brain drain. London, Regional Network for Equity in Health in Southern Africa, 2003.

49 Bajunirwe F, Twesigye L, Zhang M, Kerry VB, Bangsberg DR: Influence of the US President's Emergency Plan for AIDS Relief (PEPfAR) on career choices and emigration of health-profession graduates from a Ugandan medical school: a cross-sectional study. BMJ Open 2013;3:pii, e002875.

50 Patel V, Abas M, Broadhead J, Todd C, Reeler A: Depression in developing countries: lessons from Zimbabwe. BMJ 2001;322:482–484.

51 Von Korff M, Glasgow R, Sharpe M: ABC of psychological medicine: organising care for chronic illness. BMJ 2002; 325:92–94.

52 Bowry AD, Shrank WH, Lee JL, Stedman M, Choudhry NK: A systematic review of adherence to cardiovascular medications in resource-limited settings. J Gen Intern Med 2011;26:1479–1491.

53 Diabetes Foundation Report on Insulin-Requiring Diabetes in Sub-Saharan Africa. London, International Insulin Foundation, 2005.

54 Silva-Matos C, Beran D: Non-communicable diseases in Mozambique: risk factors, burden, response and outcomes to date. Global Health 2012;8:37.

55 Yudkin JS, Holt RI, Silva-Matos C, Beran D: Twinning for better diabetes care: a model for improving healthcare for non-communicable diseases in resource-poor countries. Postgrad Med J 2009;85: 1–2.

56 Beran D, Silva Matos C, Yudkin JS: The Diabetes UK mozambique Twinning Programme. Results of improvements in diabetes care in Mozambique: a reassessment 6 years later using the Rapid Assessment Protocol for Insulin Access. Diabet Med 2010;27:855–861.

57 Patel V, Chowdhary N, Rahman A, Verdeli H: Improving access to psychological treatments: lessons from developing countries. Behav Res Ther 2011; 49:523–528.

58 Petersen I, Lund C, Stein DJ: Optimizing mental health services in low-income and middle-income countries. Curr Opin Psychiatry 2011;24:318–323.

59 Bodenheimer T, Lorig K, Holman H, Grumbach K: Patient self-management of chronic disease in primary care. JAMA 2002;288:2469–2475.

60 Narayan KM, Ali MK, del Rio C, Koplan JP, Curran J: Global noncommunicable diseases – lessons from the HIV-AIDS experience. N Engl J Med 2011;365:876–878.

David Beran, MSc, PhD
Division of Tropical and Humanitarian Medicine
Geneva University Hospitals and University of Geneva
Rue Gabrielle-Perret-Gentil 6, CH–1211 Geneva 14 (Switzerland)
E-Mail David.Beran@unige.ch

Sartorius N, Holt RIG, Maj M (eds): Comorbidity of Mental and Physical Disorders.
Key Issues Ment Health. Basel, Karger, 2015, vol 179, pp 42–53 (DOI: 10.1159/000365529)

Depression, Diabetes and Dementia

Joshua D. Rosenblat[a, d] · Rodrigo B. Mansur[a, f, g] · Danielle S. Cha[a, b] ·
Anusha Baskaran[a, e] · Roger S. McIntyre[a–c]

[a]Mood Disorders Psychopharmacology Unit (MDPU), University Health Network, [b]Institute of Medical
Science, and [c]Department of Psychiatry and Pharmacology, University of Toronto, Toronto, Ont., [d]Schulich
School of Medicine and Dentistry, Western University, London, Ont., and [e]Centre for Neuroscience Studies,
Queen's University, Kingston, Ont., Canada; [f]Interdisciplinary Laboratory of Clinical Neuroscience (LINC) and
[g]Program for Recognition and Intervention in Individuals in At-Risk Mental States (PRISMA), Department of
Psychiatry, Federal University of São Paulo, São Paulo, Brazil

Abstract

Depression, diabetes and dementia are three disorders associated with staggering morbidity and mortality worldwide. The association between depression and diabetes has been well established. Furthermore, both depression and diabetes have been shown to increase the incidence of dementia individually and synergistically. The metabolic-brain axis appears to be a key mediator connecting depression, diabetes and dementia. Brain regions important for cognition and emotional regulation may be damaged by the effects of hyperglycemia and insulin resistance. Indeed, insulin resistance and decreased insulin in the central nervous system (CNS) results in decreased intracellular glucose levels in frontal and subcortical regions, neurotoxicity, decreased neuroplasticity, decreased signaling, decreased synaptic connectivity and disturbances in neural circuitry. The aforementioned changes may be attributable to brain bioenergetics wherein there is a bias toward energy conservation. The insulin pathway also has a bidirectional interaction with amyloid-β oligomer formation, one of the hallmarks of Alzheimer's disease. As well, depression may further facilitate neural circuit damage through the inflammatory pathway, hypothalamic-pituitary-adrenal axis dysregulation, monoamine changes and lowering of neurotrophic support to the CNS. Stress and psychosocial determinants of health may also be key mediators in how these systems interact. The involvement of several pathways may present new potential drug targets for the treatment and prevention of dementia using a lifetime approach. Systemic and intranasal insulin, oral diabetic medications, exercise, dietary changes, bariatric surgery and improved screening practices with early treatment of depression and diabetes all show promise in the treatment and prevention of comorbid depression, diabetes and dementia.

© 2015 S. Karger AG, Basel

Depression has been recognized by the World Health Organization (WHO) as one of the leading causes of disability worldwide, affecting an estimated 350 million people globally [1]. Depression has also been identified as a risk factor and poor prognostic indicator for several medical comorbidities including, but not limited to, metabolic disorders such as diabetes, metabolic syndrome and obesity [2]. According to WHO estimates, diabetes, which now affects more than 350 million people globally, will be the seventh leading cause of death by 2030 [3]. Moreover, depression and diabetes have a well-established link as numerous investigators have shown a bidirectional association between these disorders [4]. Both depression and diabetes have been independently associated as risk factors for the development of cognitive impairment and dementia [5, 6]. Furthermore, depression and diabetes have been recognized as having a synergistic effect in increasing the risk for dementia above and beyond the effects that depression or diabetes would have on the risk of developing dementia independently. More specifically, comorbid type 2 diabetes mellitus and major depressive disorder have been documented to increase the incidence of Alzheimer's disease greatly later in life [7].

Alzheimer's disease is the leading cause of dementia, the sixth leading cause of mortality and the third most costly disease in the USA [8–10]. It is progressive in nature and is ultimately fatal [10]. Currently, available treatments are only palliative as there are no agents that have been shown to have disease-modifying properties [11]. Therefore, primary prevention represents a priority research vista for identifying and targeting modifiable risk factors of Alzheimer's disease. Modifiable risk factors that are addressed in this review are type 2 diabetes and major depressive disorder.

The overarching aim of this review is to review the potential pathophysiologic mechanisms which may account for this observed association between Alzheimer's disease, type 2 diabetes and major depressive disorder. There is also a brief discussion about preventative and therapeutic options with particular emphasis on a lifetime approach to dementia. Evidence for the association between diabetes, depression and dementia has been extensively reviewed and can be found elsewhere [7, 12–14].

Mechanisms Linking Depression, Diabetes and Dementia

Evidence from preclinical and clinical studies has suggested several potential mechanisms connecting diabetes, depression and dementia. Essential to this discussion is the recognition that the neural networks implicated in cognitive and emotional function and dysfunction have significant overlap, as shown in figure 1 [15], which is central to the observed interactions between cognition and mood. It has been amply documented that cognitive dysfunction and changes in mood are key symptoms that have been observed to appear together in individuals diagnosed with major depressive disorder [6, 16]. Therefore, the observed symptoms of Alzheimer's disease and major depressive disorder may be associated with a spectrum of structural and functional changes of shared neural circuits of the frontal and subcortical regions [6, 16]. Likewise, the epidemiological observation and proposal of major depressive disorder as a prodrome of Alzheimer's disease may be indicative of progressive damage to these neural circuits with repeated major depressive episodes [6, 13, 16].

In addition, central to the discussion of mechanisms involved in diabetes, depression and dementia is the bidirectional relationship of the body's metabolic milieu and neural circuitry [17]. Pathologic metabolic processes may damage these foregoing neural circuits. Evidence for such damage to neural circuits is shown through impaired cognition and altered brain connectivity in people with diabetes, independent of vascular pathology, as demonstrated through functional imaging techniques, such as electroencephalography, magnetoencephalography and functional magnetic resonance imaging [18, 19]. The damage to frontosubcortical circuits by metabolic pathology, namely diabetes, insulin resistance, and obesity, may thus impair cognition and affect mood [18, 20].

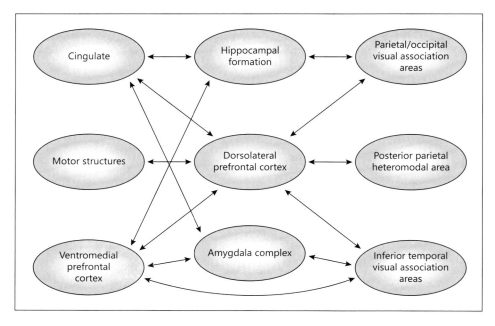

Fig. 1. The neural basis of cognitive and emotional processes. Reprinted with permission from Wood and Grafman [15].

Impaired Central Insulin and Glucose Supply

Insulin, produced by the pancreas, enters the blood stream allowing for its systemic circulation and systemic effects [21]. To enter the central nervous system (CNS), blood-borne insulin is transported across the blood-brain barrier via a saturable, receptor-mediated process [15]. Once in the CNS, insulin may exert a plethora of important effects, including, but not limited to, promoting glucose uptake in specific regions, neurogenesis, neuroplasticity, synaptic strengthening and preventing neurodegeneration [22, 23]. CNS insulin and glucose have also been proposed to be an important modulator of the reward system and appetite [24].

The previous understanding that insulin had no effect on the brain has now been abolished with the discovery of insulin receptors in numerous brain regions [25]. Notably, insulin receptors have been identified in regions involved with cognition and emotion including the hypothalamus,

olfactory bulb, cerebral cortex, substantia nigra, basal ganglia, hippocampus and amygdala [25]. As such, altered insulin levels and signaling, as seen in type 2 diabetes, may have important CNS consequences.

Type 2 diabetes is characterized by hyperglycemia, insulin resistance with compensatory hyperinsulinemia, and subsequent pancreatic decompensation, resulting in hypoinsulinemia at later stages, unless treated [21]. Preliminary evidence indicates that the blood-brain barrier insulin transporters may be downregulated in chronic hyperinsulinemia [15] and that, consequentially, CNS insulin levels may be decreased [26–28]. As previously discussed, CNS insulin is an important signaling molecule in numerous CNS processes. Therefore, in the setting of type 2 diabetes where CNS insulin has been decreased because of blood-brain barrier receptor downregulation, several deleterious effects may ensue [23, 26].

The simplest deleterious effect to conceptualize is a decrease in intracellular glucose, secondary to decreased CNS insulin levels, as certain brain regions, notably the medial temporal lobe and hippocampus, have insulin-dependent glucose uptake [26]. GLUT4 receptors in the hippocampus have been shown to facilitate insulin-dependent glucose uptake [29]. In type 2 diabetes animal models of insulin resistance, there is decreased glucose uptake in the hippocampus [26]. Therefore, metabolically active CNS tissue important for cognition and emotion receive suboptimal levels of glucose and thus may have suboptimal function.

CNS insulin not only increases glucose uptake in particular regions, but also acts as a growth factor through its downstream effects. In brief, in vitro studies and animal models have shown that when insulin binds its receptor, the phosphoinositide-3 kinase pathways are activated, which promotes the production and release of several growth factors including brain-derived neurotrophic factor (BDNF) and vascular endothelial growth factor [30], thereby promoting neuronal survival, synaptogenesis and dendritic arborisation [23]. Similarly, long-term potentiation cascades, important for learning and memory, are promoted by insulin [26]. Indeed, animal models have shown a strong trophic effect of insulin on hippocampus size and benefits in cognition and memory [22, 23, 26, 27, 31]. Furthermore, in animal models, inhibiting the binding of insulin to hippocampal cells has a marked negative effect on hippocampus size and function (as manifested through impaired memory) [26, 31].

Taken together, insulin acts as a growth factor and mediator of glucose uptake in the hippocampus and other areas of emotion and cognition, promoting the health of these neural circuits. Therefore, insulin resistance may lead to decreased CNS insulin levels, leading to decreased hippocampal glucose uptake and decreased growth factor signaling, which may lead to impaired neurogenesis and ultimately hippocampal

atrophy. In keeping with this hypothesis, imaging and postmortem studies have found hippocampal atrophy in type 2 diabetes, major depressive disorder and Alzheimer's disease [32].

Bioenergetics

Numerous energetically 'expensive' processes are continually occurring in the brain. These energetically intensive processes include, but are not limited to, maintenance of an electrochemical gradient in cells, neurogenesis, cellular depolarization and repolarization, synaptogenesis, and release and reuptake of neurotransmitters [33, 34]. In addition, brain topology studies have shown that higher functioning neural circuits have a greater volume and length of connections, and as such, are even more energetically expensive [35].

To support these processes, the brain, while representing only 2% of total body mass, consumes 25% of the body's available glucose [34]. Furthermore, Peters et al. [24] hypothesized that the 'selfish brain' ensures adequate energy for itself through modulating appetite, prioritizing glucose supply to the brain above other organs and decreasing energy demands. In support of this hypothesis, empirical data have shown that carbohydrate intake is increased in humans after a stressful intervention (a model shown to increase brain energy consumption by 10–15%) [36, 37]. In addition to postintervention changes in food consumption, participants had increased blood glucose with a blunted insulin response. Since brain glucose uptake is largely insulin independent, this pattern is indicative of a preferential bias of brain glucose uptake relative to other organs when brain energy demands are increased [37].

Low CNS insulin and intracellular glucose levels, as seen in type 2 diabetes with downregulated blood-brain barrier insulin transport and insulin resistance, may lead to the perception of low energy availability and thus may trigger downstream mechanisms to conserve energy [24, 38]. To conserve energy, neurogenesis is prevented as it requires great consumption of energy [24, 29,

39]. Animal models of type 2 diabetes have reported that N-methyl-D-aspartate (NMDA) signaling for the purpose of long-term potentiation is inhibited as it too is energetically expensive [40].

Ultimately, energy deficits perceived by the brain (e.g. lowered CNS insulin and glucose in the case of type 2 diabetes) may negatively impact neuroplasticity, optimal neural circuitry and thus optimal function [24, 29, 39]. In keeping with this view, when the frontosubcortical regions are forced to reduce energy expenditure by allocating resources to less demanding neural circuits, the domains of mood and cognition may be impaired to conserve energy in times of perceived energy depletion [17, 24, 38]. Furthermore, chronic perceived bioenergetic depletion may lead to chronic and progressive impairment of these circuits [17]. Taken together, comorbid mood and cognitive symptoms, commonly observed and reported in epidemiological studies as the co-occurence of major depressive disorder and Alzheimer's disease, may represent late-stage bioenergetic bias. More specifically, older individuals with type 2 diabetes experience years of brain insults resulting from glycemic dysregulation and aberrant insulin levels, affecting neuroplasticity and neural function, leading to bioenergetic bias towards energy conservation rather than higher functioning [17].

Insulin-Amyloid Pathway
Another mechanism whereby hyperinsulinemia with insulin resistance and low CNS insulin may impact function is through the insulin-amyloid pathway. Amyloid-β protein oligomers have been strongly implicated in the pathoetiology of Alzheimer's disease [41]. What induces amyloid-β oligomer formation is not yet fully understood; however, a strong interaction between amyloid-β and insulin has been identified [41, 42]. Notably, insulin and amyloid-β compete for the same degrading enzyme, namely, insulin degrading enzyme, thereby indirectly affecting each other's systemic and central concentration [43, 44]. Fur-

thermore, insulin degrading enzyme levels are reduced in type 2 diabetes animal models [14, 18]. Moreover, insulin has been shown to modulate amyloid-β removal, reduce amyloid-β load and prevent pathogenic binding of amyloid-β [28, 43].

The interaction between insulin and amyloid-β is bidirectional. More specifically, accumulating amyloid-β can bind to insulin receptors and downregulate insulin signaling, thus impairing neurogenesis and function through the previously discussed mechanisms [45]. The foregoing bidirectional interaction may perpetuate a deleterious positive feedback loop whereby insulin resistance promotes increased amyloid-β and amyloid-β induces further insulin resistance [26]. This loop may provide another reason for the high prevalence of Alzheimer's disease in people with type 2 diabetes [26].

Neuroplasticity, Inflammation, Oxidative Stress and the Hypothalamic-Pituitary-Adrenal Axis
Neuroplasticity is the brain's ability to change in response to environmental stimuli [46]. The inability of the brain to change at a molecular, cellular, structural and ultimately functional level is an important cause of impaired cognition and mood. Diabetes and depression have been shown to impair neuroplasticity through the inflammatory pathway, oxidative stress, depletion of neurotrophic factors and hypothalamic-pituitary-adrenal (HPA) axis derangement, leading to impaired neurogenesis, impaired long-term potentiation and neurotoxicity [47, 48].

A proinflammatory state has been shown to be associated with stress (physical, emotional, psychological), inflammatory medical comorbidities (infection, obesity, diabetes, metabolic syndrome, autoimmune diseases, cardiovascular disease) and psychiatric comorbidities (mood disorders, anxiety disorders, psychotic disorders) [49]. The cytokines produced, most notably TNF-α, IL-6 and IL-1β, in this proinflammatory state have been associated with 'sickness behavior' including depressive symptoms of lethargy, anhedonia and cognitive decline [49]. The downstream effects of the proinflammatory state include derangement of monoamine levels, pathologic microglial cell dysfunction, increased oxidative stress, HPA axis activation and structural changes of the subcortical regions, all of which may lead to decreased neuroplasticity and dysfunctional emotional and cognitive processing [50].

More specifically, proinflammatory cytokines have been shown to cause tryptophan depletion and increased serotonin turnover, both well-known causes of altered mood and cognition [51]. Increased oxidative stress also accompanies the elevated metabolic rate induced by a proinflammatory state, thus increasing cellular damage at the molecular level ultimately leading to neurotoxicity [51].

Also implicated in the inflammatory pathway are microglial cells, the macrophages of the CNS. Microglial cells are important for normal brain function and synaptic pruning; however, in a chronic inflammatory state, microglial cells may induce high levels of neural death through pathologic synaptic pruning leading to impairment of the cognitive and mood neural circuits [52, 53].

The proinflammatory state is also associated with activation of the HPA axis leading to hypercortisolemia as well was impaired HPA negative feedback through decreased glucocorticoid receptor expression, translocation and signaling [54]. Of note, diabetes and depression as well as stress all have the ability to activate the HPA axis, inducing hypercortisolemia [54, 55] which leads to further hyperglycemia and thus to poorer control of diabetes and increased insulin requirements [21]. Chronic exposure to high levels of cortisol can also cause neurotoxicity in the hippocampus, leading to impaired cognition and mood symptoms [56]. This neurotoxic effect is amplified in the presence of insulin resistance [26]. Notably, cortisol has also been implicated in altering metabolism of amyloids and may thus exhibit pro-Alzheimer's disease properties through the amyloid mechanism as well [57].

Brain-Derived Neurotrophic Factor
Low levels of BDNF are commonly observed in people with type 2 diabetes, impaired glucose tolerance, major depressive disorder and Alzheimer's disease [58]. This observation may suggest another common mechanism of pathogenesis of these diseases. For example, during a major depressive episode, hippocampal 5-HT2A receptors are upregulated, which may lead to decreased BDNF and a subsequent decrease in hippocampal volume [59]. Moreover, BDNF is one of the downstream targets of insulin receptor activation [30]. Therefore, in the setting of insulin resistance where signaling is diminished, BDNF levels are also lower [26]. The low levels of BDNF, as seen in both type 2 diabetes and major depressive disorder, may thus increase vulnerability to hippocampal dysfunction and atrophy secondary to inadequate growth factor stimulation [26, 31, 60].

Monoamine Changes
The monoamine pathway has been the primary therapeutic target of major depressive disorder for decades. Causes of monoamine derangement are numerous, including the previously discussed inflammatory pathway [49] and CNS insulin [26]. Monoamines, notably serotonin, norepinephrine and dopamine, are now also being recognized as having significant roles in cognition [61]. For example, serotonin receptors are found abundantly in cognitive regions such as the hippocampus, prefrontal cortex and septum, where they play an important role in cognition, most notably creation of episodic memories as evidenced by tryptophan depletion studies [62]. Norepinephrine plays a significant role in alertness and arousal, thus affecting cognitive function in the domains of working memory, memory consolidation, attention and executive function [61]. Dopamine levels are also salient to cognition, motivation and the reward system [63]. In sum, the monoamine system can be altered by depression and type 2 diabetes and has large effects on both cognition and emotion. Therefore, it may provide another

pathophysiologic nexus to account for the interplay between depression, diabetes and cognitive impairment [61].

Microbiota-Gut-Brain Axis
Many decades ago, the vast and dynamic ecosystem of the gut microbiota was hypothesized to affect mental health; however, only recently has this idea been revisited [64]. Currently, there is only limited evidence for the bidirectional interaction between the gut and the CNS, but interest across the fields of psychiatry, neurology, gastroenterology and endocrinology is increasing [65]. Preclinical evidence suggests that this interaction may provide mechanisms whereby the gut microbiota may induce metabolic, behavioral, mood and cognitive changes [65]. This field is still in its infancy but is being implicated as an etiologic factor in dictating eating habits, BDNF levels, HPA axis activity, inflammation and oxidative stress, all of which are important factors in the mechanisms of affective and cognitive dysfunction, as previously discussed [64, 65]. In brief, the gut may have bidirectional communication with the brain to induce behaviors that increase the risk of diabetes as well as may be the nidus of a chronic inflammatory state which may induce sickness behavior, hypercholesterolemia, hyperglycemia, hypercortisolemia and ultimately neural damage, affecting cognitive and emotional function [64, 65].

Microangiopathy
Microvascular (nephropathy, neuropathy, retinopathy) and macrovascular (stroke, myocardial infarction) complications of diabetes are well established in the literature [21]. Moreover, it has now been well-established that the brain has increased susceptibility to microvascular disease, independent of the presence of large vessel disease, in people with diabetes [66]. Postmortem and imaging analyses has revealed these microangiopathic changes to be associated with the development of depression, cognitive impairment and dementia, particularly vascular dementia and Al-

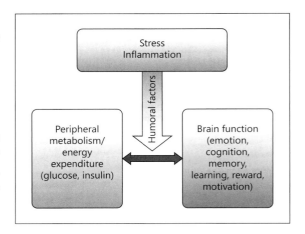

Fig. 2. Role of humoral factors in normal and pathological nexus between peripheral metabolism and brain functions. Reprinted with permission from Kaidanovich-Beilin et al. [17].

zheimer's disease [67]. Microangiopathic changes may be linked with amyloid-β oligomer formation [68]. The proposed mechanism and evidence in support of the microangiopathy-cognitive-affective connection have been reviewed elsewhere [66, 67, 69].

Common Psychosocial Determinants
A separate but not mutually exclusive explanation of the connection between diabetes, depression and dementia may be due to the psychosocial risk factors that are shared by these disease processes [17]. Epidemiological studies provide evidence for low socioeconomic status, childhood adversity, medical comorbidities, addiction and psychiatric comorbidities as being common risk factors for type 2 diabetes and major depressive disorder [70–72]. Therefore, one potential explanation for the observed association may be common etiologic factors [17]. As shown in figure 2, both common biological and psychosocial factors may be creating a pathological nexus between peripheral metabolism and brain function. Taken together, certain life circumstances may predispose individuals to the development of both type

2 diabetes and major depressive disorder, which could synergistically damage the neural circuits of emotion and cognition, thereby increasing the risk of cognitive impairment and dementia [17].

Implications for Treatment and Prevention

As shown, numerous mechanisms may be involved in the interaction of diabetes, depression and dementia, and may present new therapeutic targets. Therefore, in this section, the focus will be placed on selected new and novel therapeutic and preventative options that target components of the mechanisms previously discussed. Emphasis will be placed on (1) the benefit of early detection and treatment of major depressive disorder and diabetes, (2) the importance of lifestyle modifications, namely exercise and dietary changes, and (3) novel metabolic therapeutic options which hold promise for improving mood and cognition in the context of major depressive disorder, type 2 diabetes and Alzheimer's disease.

As previously discussed, no disease-modifying agents are currently identified for Alzheimer's disease [10]. Therefore, prevention through risk factor modification has been a focus of Alzheimer's disease research and public health efforts [10, 73]. Understanding the pathophysiology of Alzheimer's disease as occurring over a lifetime, rather than only in old age when symptoms begin to manifest, is essential to this preventative approach. Epidemiologic and mechanistic data strongly suggest both depression and diabetes to be modifiable risk factors of Alzheimer's disease. Therefore, screening programs to allow for early detection and treatment of both major depressive disorder and type 2 diabetes may be extremely helpful in the prevention of Alzheimer's disease. Indeed, evidence suggests that an estimated 10–15% of Alzheimer's disease cases are attributable to depression and a 25% reduction in depression prevalence would result in approximately 830,000 fewer Alzheimer's disease

cases worldwide [74]. Similarly for type 2 diabetes, appropriate therapy achieving adequate glycemic, lipid and blood pressure control has been shown to decrease the risk of cognitive impairment, Alzheimer's disease and vascular dementia [75, 76]. Taken together, screening for major depressive disorder in people with type 2 diabetes and vice versa would thus have clear benefits for early detection and treatment for both conditions while reducing the risk of developing Alzheimer's disease [77].

From a public health perspective, exercise and a healthy diet have been promoted because of their positive impact on cardiovascular health [78]. Evidence consistently documents the importance of exercise and a healthy diet and their impact on diabetes, depression and dementia [14, 79–83]. For example, exercise has been shown repeatedly to have a positive effect on mood and cognition in individuals with depression [32, 83]. Likewise, among individuals with Alzheimer's disease, exercise has been shown to improve mood and cognition both in the short and long term [80, 81]. In type 2 diabetes, lifestyle management has long been a part of first-line therapy with clear effects on cognition, mood and Alzheimer's disease prevention [10, 84, 85]. Therefore, lifestyle management should also be emphasized from a mental health perspective, rather than only for its cardiovascular benefits.

From a pharmacologic perspective, increasing interest has been developing for the use of diabetic medications for improvement of mood and cognition. For example, recent studies have been conducted investigating the role of insulin in mood and cognition [22]. As previously discussed, CNS insulin plays a key role in brain function, and CNS insulin levels are reduced in people with Alzheimer's disease [27]. Intravenous administration of insulin has been investigated for its effects on cognition and emotion. Several investigators have shown that in both human and animal models, intravenous insulin administration can increase hippocampal neural activity and improve mood and cognition (most reproducibly declarative memory) in the short and long term [86, 87]. However, concerns of the systemic effects and risks, namely hypoglycemic events, were a limiting factor to their wider promotion [88, 89]. Therefore, interest has shifted to intranasal insulin administration, whereby insulin directly enters the CNS, bypassing the blood-brain barrier, presumably via the olfactory and trigeminal nerves [88, 89]. Intranasal administration has been shown to increase the level of insulin in the CNS while not affecting the systemic concentration of insulin or glucose [88–90]. Furthermore, in human and animal studies, intranasal insulin has been shown to improve mood and cognition reproducibly in healthy, obese and Alzheimer's disease subjects [91]. Moreover, intranasal insulin has benefited disparate measures of neurocognition in adults with bipolar disorder, a group highly susceptible to cognitive dysfunction [92].

Oral diabetic medication, particularly thiazolidinediones and incretins have also produced interesting results. Pioglitazone, a thiazolidinedione, is an insulin sensitizer that has been shown to also have effects on cognition [87, 93]. Indeed, cognitive improvements as well as a reduction in the development of Alzheimer's disease have been observed in people with type 2 diabetes treated with pioglitazone [87, 93]. Incretins, gastrointestinal hormones which delay gastric emptying and increase insulin release from the pancreas, have also shown great promise to treat metabolic, cognitive and affective symptoms simultaneously [22, 94]. In a recent review by McIntyre et al. [94], the positive effects of incretins, specifically glucagon-like peptide-1, were discussed. In brief, glucagon-like peptide-1 may improve glycemic control, improve cognition and mood, and decrease the risk of Alzheimer's disease through its neuroprotective effects, ability to reduce amyloid-β load and through promotion of long-term potentiation and neuroplasticity [22, 94].

Bariatric surgery produces vastly improved glycemic control and significant sustained reduction in weight far beyond the effects of medical therapy alone [95–97]. This significant improvement in diabetic control, in theory, may decrease the risk of depression and cognitive impairment later in life by preventing neural degeneration from the previously described mechanisms. However, to the authors' knowledge, there have been no studies to assess the effect of bariatric surgery on mood, cognition and risk of Alzheimer's disease development. Therefore, this effect may be an interesting topic for future research.

Conclusion

Several mechanisms have been proposed to account for the well-documented association between diabetes, depression and dementia. The metabolic-brain axis appears to be a key mediator connecting these conditions. Brain regions important for cognition and emotional regulation may be damaged by the effects of hyperglycemia and insulin resistance. Indeed, a decreased insulin effect and thus decreased intracellular glucose levels in frontal and subcortical regions results in neurotoxicity, decreased neuroplasticity, decreased signaling and decreased synaptic connectivity resulting in an overall effect of dysfunctional neural circuits. Major depressive disorder may further facilitate neural circuit damage through the inflammatory pathway, HPA axis deregulation, monoamine changes and lowering of central BDNF levels. Stress and psychosocial determinants of health may also be key mediators and etiologic factors in these interactions. Taken together, several mechanistic pathways may be involved, presenting new potential drug targets for the treatment and prevention of dementia using a lifetime approach. Systemic and intranasal insulin, insulin sensitizers, incretins, exercise, dietary changes, bariatric surgery, improved screening and early treatment practices of type 2 diabetes and major depressive disorder have all been implicated for potential use in the treatment and prevention of dementia. Further research is most definitely indicated as the literature reviewed here shows great promise for further studies of the metabolic-brain axis which could revolutionize the understanding, treatment and prevention of cognitive and affective disorders.

References

1 WHO: Depression fact sheet. 2012. http://www.who.int/mediacentre/factsheets/fs369/en/.
2 Ramasubbu R, Taylor VH, Samaan Z, Sockalingham S, Li M, Patten S, et al: The Canadian Network for Mood and Anxiety Treatments (CANMAT) Task Force recommendations for the management of patients with mood disorders and select comorbid medical conditions. Ann Clin Psychiatry 2012;24:91–109.
3 WHO: Diabetes fact sheet. 2013. http://www.who.int/mediacentre/factsheets/fs312/en/.
4 Kan C, Silva N, Golden SH, Rajala U, Timonen M, Stahl D, et al: A systematic review and meta-analysis of the association between depression and insulin resistance. Diabetes Care 2013;36:480–489.
5 Profenno LA, Porsteinsson AP, Faraone SV: Meta-analysis of Alzheimer's disease risk with obesity, diabetes, and related disorders. Biol Psychiatry 2010;67:505–512.
6 Byers AL, Yaffe K: Depression and risk of developing dementia. Nat Rev Neurol 2011;7:323–331.
7 Katon W, Lyles CR, Parker MM, Karter AJ, Huang ES, Whitmer RA: Association of depression with increased risk of dementia in patients with type 2 diabetes: the Diabetes and Aging Study. Arch Gen Psychiatry 2012;69:410–417.
8 WHO: Dementia fact sheet. 2012. http://www.who.int/mediacentre/factsheets/fs362/en/.
9 Hebert LE, Scherr PA, Bienias JL, Bennett DA, Evans DA: Alzheimer disease in the US population: prevalence estimates using the 2000 census. Arch Neurol 2003;60:1119–1122.
10 Mayeux R, Stern Y: Epidemiology of Alzheimer disease. Cold Spring Harb Perspect Med 2012;2:pii:a006239.

11 Cummings JL, Banks SJ, Gary RK, Kinney JW, Lombardo JM, Walsh RR, et al: Alzheimer's disease drug development: translational neuroscience strategies. CNS Spectr 2013;18:128–138.
12 Diniz BS, Butters MA, Albert SM, Dew MA, Reynolds CF 3rd: Late-life depression and risk of vascular dementia and Alzheimer's disease: systematic review and meta-analysis of community-based cohort studies. Br J Psychiatry 2013;202:329–335.
13 Rapp MA, Schnaider-Beeri M, Wysocki M, Guerrero-Berroa E, Grossman HT, Heinz A, et al: Cognitive decline in patients with dementia as a function of depression. Am J Geriatr Psychiatry 2011;19:357–363.
14 Umegaki H, Hayashi T, Nomura H, Yanagawa M, Nonogaki Z, Nakshima H, et al: Cognitive dysfunction: an emerging concept of a new diabetic complication in the elderly. Geriatr Gerontol Int 2013;13:28–34.
15 Wood JN, Grafman J: Human prefrontal cortex: processing and representational perspectives. Nat Rev Neurosci 2003;4:139–147.
16 Caraci F, Copani A, Nicoletti F, Drago F: Depression and Alzheimer's disease: neurobiological links and common pharmacological targets. Eur J Pharmacol 2010;626:64–71.
17 Kaidanovich-Beilin O, Cha DS, McIntyre RS: Crosstalk between metabolic and neuropsychiatric disorders. F1000 Biol Rep 2012;4:14.
18 Zhou H, Lu W, Shi Y, Bai F, Chang J, Yuan Y, et al: Impairments in cognition and resting-state connectivity of the hippocampus in elderly subjects with type 2 diabetes. Neurosci Lett 2010;473:5–10.
19 Musen G, Jacobson AM, Bolo NR, Simonson DC, Shenton ME, McCartney RL, et al: Resting-state brain functional connectivity is altered in type 2 diabetes. Diabetes 2012;61:2375–2379.

20 Reijmer YD, Brundel M, de Bresser J, Kappelle LJ, Leemans A, Biessels GJ, et al: Microstructural white matter abnormalities and cognitive functioning in type 2 diabetes: a diffusion tensor imaging study. Diabetes Care 2013;36:137–144.
21 Kahn CR, Joslin EP: Joslin's Diabetes Mellitus, ed 14. Philadelphia, Lippincott Williams & Willkins, 2005.
22 McIntyre RS, Vagic D, Swartz SA, Soczynska JK, Woldeyohannes HO, Voruganti LP, et al: Insulin, insulin-like growth factors and incretins: neural homeostatic regulators and treatment opportunities. CNS Drugs 2008;22:443–453.
23 Banks WA, Owen JB, Erickson MA: Insulin in the brain: there and back again. Pharmacol Ther 2012;136:82–93.
24 Peters A, Schweiger U, Pellerin L, Hubold C, Oltmanns KM, Conrad M, et al: The selfish brain: competition for energy resources. Neurosci Biobehav Rev 2004;28:143–180.
25 Unger JW, Betz M: Insulin receptors and signal transduction proteins in the hypothalamo-hypophyseal system: a review on morphological findings and functional implications. Histol Histopathol 1998;13:1215–1224.
26 McNay EC, Recknagel AK: Brain insulin signaling: a key component of cognitive processes and a potential basis for cognitive impairment in type 2 diabetes. Neurobiol Learn Mem 2011;96:432–442.
27 Craft S, Peskind E, Schwartz MW, Schellenberg GD, Raskind M, Porte D Jr: Cerebrospinal fluid and plasma insulin levels in Alzheimer's disease: relationship to severity of dementia and apolipoprotein E genotype. Neurology 1998;50:164–168.
28 Craft S, Watson GS: Insulin and neurodegenerative disease: shared and specific mechanisms. Lancet Neurol 2004;3:169–178.

29 Reagan LP: Neuronal insulin signal transduction mechanisms in diabetes phenotypes. Neurobiol Aging 2005; 26(suppl 1):56–59.

30 Rodgers EE, Theibert AB: Functions of PI 3-kinase in development of the nervous system. Int J Dev Neurosci 2002; 20:187–197.

31 McNay EC, Ong CT, McCrimmon RJ, Cresswell J, Bogan JS, Sherwin RS: Hippocampal memory processes are modulated by insulin and high-fat-induced insulin resistance. Neurobiol Learn Mem 2010;93:546–553.

32 Fotuhi M, Do D, Jack C: Modifiable factors that alter the size of the hippocampus with ageing. Nat Rev Neurol 2012;8: 189–202.

33 S Roriz-Filho J, Sa-Roriz TM, Rosset I, Camozzato AL, Santos AC, Chaves ML, et al: (Pre)diabetes, brain aging, and cognition. Biochim Biophys Acta 2009; 1792:432–443.

34 Attwell D, Laughlin SB: An energy budget for signaling in the grey matter of the brain. J Cereb Blood Flow Metab 2001;21:1133–1145.

35 Li Y, Liu Y, Li J, Qin W, Li K, Yu C, et al: Brain anatomical network and intelligence. PLoS Comput Biol 2009; 5:e1000395.

36 Madsen PL, Hasselbalch SG, Hagemann LP, Olsen KS, Bulow J, Holm S, et al: Persistent resetting of the cerebral oxygen/glucose uptake ratio by brain activation: evidence obtained with the Kety-Schmidt technique. J Cereb Blood Flow Metab 1995;15:485–491.

37 Hitze B, Hubold C, van Dyken R, Schlichting K, Lehnert H, Entringer S, et al: How the selfish brain organizes its supply and demand. Front Neuroenergetics 2010;2:7.

38 Mansur RB, Cha DS, Asevedo E, McIntyre RS, Brietzke E: Selfish brain and neuroprogression in bipolar disorder. Prog Neuropsychopharmacol Biol Psychiatry 2013;43:66–71.

39 Bullmore E, Sporns O: The economy of brain network organization. Nat Rev Neurosci 2012;13:336–349.

40 Artola A, Kamal A, Ramakers GM, Biessels GJ, Gispen WH: Diabetes mellitus concomitantly facilitates the induction of long-term depression and inhibits that of long-term potentiation in hippocampus. Eur J Neurosci 2005;22:169–178.

41 Ferreira ST, Klein WL: The Aβ oligomer hypothesis for synapse failure and memory loss in Alzheimer's disease. Neurobiol Learn Mem 2011;96:529–543.

42 Janson J, Laedtke T, Parisi JE, O'Brien P, Petersen RC, Butler PC: Increased risk of type 2 diabetes in Alzheimer disease. Diabetes 2004;53:474–481.

43 Gasparini L, Netzer WJ, Greengard P, Xu H: Does insulin dysfunction play a role in Alzheimer's disease? Trends Pharmacol Sci 2002;23:288–293.

44 Farris W, Mansourian S, Chang Y, Lindsley L, Eckman EA, Frosch MP, et al: Insulin-degrading enzyme regulates the levels of insulin, amyloid beta-protein, and the beta-amyloid precursor protein intracellular domain in vivo. Proc Natl Acad Sci USA 2003;100:4162–4167.

45 Zhao WQ, De Felice FG, Fernandez S, Chen H, Lambert MP, Quon MJ, et al: Amyloid beta oligomers induce impairment of neuronal insulin receptors. FASEB J 2008;22:246–260.

46 Chen H, Epstein J, Stern E: Neural plasticity after acquired brain injury: evidence from functional neuroimaging. PM R 2010;2(12 suppl 2):S306–S312.

47 Maritim AC, Sanders RA, Watkins JB 3rd: Diabetes, oxidative stress, and antioxidants: a review. J Biochem Mol Toxicol 2003;17:24–38.

48 Reichenberg A, Yirmiya R, Schuld A, Kraus T, Haack M, Morag A, et al: Cytokine-associated emotional and cognitive disturbances in humans. Arch Gen Psychiatry 2001;58:445–452.

49 McNamara RK, Lotrich FE: Elevated immune-inflammatory signaling in mood disorders: a new therapeutic target? Expert Rev Neurother 2012;12: 1143–1161.

50 Moylan S, Maes M, Wray NR, Berk M: The neuroprogressive nature of major depressive disorder: pathways to disease evolution and resistance, and therapeutic implications. Mol Psychiatry 2013; 18:595–606.

51 Miller AH, Haroon E, Raison CL, Felger JC: Cytokine targets in the brain: impact on neurotransmitters and neurocircuits. Depress Anxiety 2013;30:297–306.

52 Kraft AD, Harry GJ: Features of microglia and neuroinflammation relevant to environmental exposure and neurotoxicity. Int J Environ Res Public Health 2011;8:2980–3018.

53 Weitz TM, Town T: Microglia in Alzheimer's disease: it's all about context. Int J Alzheimers Dis 2012;2012:314185.

54 Turnbull AV, Rivier CL: Regulation of the hypothalamic-pituitary-adrenal axis by cytokines: Actions and mechanisms of action. Physiol Rev 1999;79:1–71.

55 Gillespie CF, Phifer J, Bradley B, Ressler KJ: Risk and resilience: genetic and environmental influences on development of the stress response. Depress Anxiety 2009;26:984–992.

56 Roozendaal B: Stress and memory: opposing effects of glucocorticoids on memory consolidation and memory retrieval. Neurobiol Learn Mem 2002;78: 578–595.

57 Sorrells SF, Sapolsky RM: An inflammatory review of glucocorticoid actions in the CNS. Brain Behav Immun 2007;21: 259–272.

58 Krabbe KS, Nielsen AR, Krogh-Madsen R, Plomgaard P, Rasmussen P, Erikstrup C, et al: Brain-derived neurotrophic factor (BDNF) and type 2 diabetes. Diabetologia 2007;50:431–438.

59 Sheline YI, Mintun MA, Barch DM, Wilkins C, Snyder AZ, Moerlein SM: Decreased hippocampal 5-HT(2A) receptor binding in older depressed patients using [18F]altanserin positron emission tomography. Neuropsychopharmacology 2004;29:2235–2241.

60 Alagiakrishnan K, Sclater A: Psychiatric disorders presenting in the elderly with type 2 diabetes mellitus. Am J Geriatr Psychiatry 2012;20:645–652.

61 Chamberlain SR, Robbins TW: Noradrenergic modulation of cognition: therapeutic implications. J Psychopharmacol 2013;27:694–718.

62 Cowen P, Sherwood AC: The role of serotonin in cognitive function: evidence from recent studies and implications for understanding depression. J Psychopharmacol 2013;27:575–583.

63 Cole DM, Beckmann CF, Oei NY, Both S, van Gerven JM, Rombouts SA: Differential and distributed effects of dopamine neuromodulations on resting-state network connectivity. Neuroimage 2013; 78:59–67.

64 Bested AC, Logan AC, Selhub EM: Intestinal microbiota, probiotics and mental health: From metchnikoff to modern advances: part I – autointoxication revisited. Gut Pathog 2013;5:5.

65 Cryan JF, Dinan TG: Mind-altering microorganisms: the impact of the gut microbiota on brain and behaviour. Nat Rev Neurosci 2012;13:701–712.

66 Bourdel-Marchasson I, Mouries A, Helmer C: Hyperglycaemia, microangiopathy, diabetes and dementia risk. Diabetes Metab 2010;36(suppl 3):S112–S118.

67 Schneider R, Kiesewetter H: The significance of microcirculatory disturbances in the pathogenesis of vascular dementia. Pharmacopsychiatry 1988; 21(suppl 1):11–16.

68 Kalaria RN: Neurodegenerative disease: diabetes, microvascular pathology and Alzheimer disease. Nat Rev Neurol 2009; 5:305–306.

69 Perlmutter LS, Chui HC: Microangiopathy, the vascular basement membrane and Alzheimer's disease: a review. Brain Res Bull 1990;24:677–686.

70 Dallman MF, Pecoraro N, Akana SF, La Fleur SE, Gomez F, Houshyar H, et al: Chronic stress and obesity: a new view of 'comfort food'. Proc Natl Acad Sci USA 2003;100:11696–11701.

71 Everson SA, Maty SC, Lynch JW, Kaplan GA: Epidemiologic evidence for the relation between socioeconomic status and depression, obesity, and diabetes. J Psychosom Res 2002;53:891–895.

72 Talbot F, Nouwen A: A review of the relationship between depression and diabetes in adults: is there a link? Diabetes Care 2000;23:1556–1562.

73 Carrillo MC, Brashear HR, Logovinsky V, Ryan JM, Feldman HH, Siemers ER, et al: Can we prevent Alzheimer's disease? Secondary 'prevention' trials in Alzheimer's disease. Alzheimers Dement 2013;9:123–131.e1.

74 Enache D, Winblad B, Aarsland D: Depression in dementia: epidemiology, mechanisms, and treatment. Curr Opin Psychiatry 2011;24:461–472.

75 Awad N, Gagnon M, Messier C: The relationship between impaired glucose tolerance, type 2 diabetes, and cognitive function. J Clin Exp Neuropsychol 2004; 26:1044–1080.

76 Messier C: Impact of impaired glucose tolerance and type 2 diabetes on cognitive aging. Neurobiol Aging 2005; 26(suppl 1):26–30.

77 Hermanns N, Caputo S, Dzida G, Khunti K, Meneghini LF, Snoek F: Screening, evaluation and management of depression in people with diabetes in primary care. Prim Care Diabetes 2013;7:1–10.

78 Topp R, Fahlman M, Boardley D: Healthy aging: health promotion and disease prevention. Nurs Clin North Am 2004;39:411–422.

79 Conn VS: Anxiety outcomes after physical activity interventions: meta-analysis findings. Nurs Res 2010;59:224–231.

80 Rolland Y, Abellan van Kan G, Vellas B: Physical activity and Alzheimer's disease: from prevention to therapeutic perspectives. J Am Med Dir Assoc 2008;9:390–405.

81 Rolland Y, Abellan van Kan G, Vellas B: Healthy brain aging: role of exercise and physical activity. Clin Geriatr Med 2010; 26:75–87.

82 Conn VS: Depressive symptom outcomes of physical activity interventions: meta-analysis findings. Ann Behav Med 2010;39:128–138.

83 Cooney GM, Dwan K, Greig CA, Lawlor DA, Rimer J, Waugh FR, et al: Exercise for depression. Cochrane Database Syst Rev 2013;9:CD004366.

84 Nolan CJ, Damm P, Prentki M: Type 2 diabetes across generations: from pathophysiology to prevention and management. Lancet 2011;378:169–181.

85 Fiocco AJ, Scarcello S, Marzolini S, Chan A, Oh P, Proulx G, et al: The effects of an exercise and lifestyle intervention program on cardiovascular, metabolic factors and cognitive performance in middle-aged adults with type II diabetes: a pilot study. Can J Diabetes 2013;37:214–219.

86 Rotte M, Baerecke C, Pottag G, Klose S, Kanneberg E, Heinze HJ, et al: Insulin affects the neuronal response in the medial temporal lobe in humans. Neuroendocrinology 2005;81:49–55.

87 Strachan MW: Insulin and cognitive function in humans: experimental data and therapeutic considerations. Biochem Soc Trans 2005;33:1037–1040.

88 Benedict L, Nelson CA, Schunk E, Sullwold K, Seaquist ER: Effect of insulin on the brain activity obtained during visual and memory tasks in healthy human subjects. Neuroendocrinology 2006;83: 20–26.

89 Benedict C, Hallschmid M, Schultes B, Born J, Kern W: Intranasal insulin to improve memory function in humans. Neuroendocrinology 2007;86:136–142.

90 Born J, Lange T, Kern W, McGregor GP, Bickel U, Fehm HL: Sniffing neuropeptides: a transnasal approach to the human brain. Nat Neurosci 2002;5:514–516.

91 Shemesh E, Rudich A, Harman-Boehm I, Cukierman-Yaffe T: Effect of intranasal insulin on cognitive function: a systematic review. J Clin Endocrinol Metab 2012;97:366–376.

92 McIntyre RS, Soczynska JK, Woldeyohannes HO, Miranda A, Vaccarino A, Macqueen G, et al: A randomized, double-blind, controlled trial evaluating the effect of intranasal insulin on neurocognitive function in euthymic patients with bipolar disorder. Bipolar Disord 2012;14:697–706.

93 Seaquist ER, Miller ME, Fonseca V, Ismail-Beigi F, Launer LJ, Punthakee Z, et al: Effect of thiazolidinediones and insulin on cognitive outcomes in ACCORD-MIND. J Diabetes Complications 2013; 27:485–491.

94 McIntyre RS, Powell AM, Kaidanovich-Beilin O, Soczynska JK, Alsuwaidan M, Woldeyohannes HO, et al: The neuroprotective effects of GLP-1: possible treatments for cognitive deficits in individuals with mood disorders. Behav Brain Res 2013;237:164–171.

95 Schauer PR, Burguera B, Ikramuddin S, Cottam D, Gourash W, Hamad G, et al: Effect of laparoscopic Roux-en Y gastric bypass on type 2 diabetes mellitus. Ann Surg 2003;238:467–484, discussion 484–485.

96 Buchwald H, Avidor Y, Braunwald E, Jensen MD, Pories W, Fahrbach K, et al: Bariatric surgery: a systematic review and meta-analysis. JAMA 2004;292: 1724–1737.

97 Maggard-Gibbons M, Maglione M, Livhits M, Ewing B, Maher AR, Hu J, et al: Bariatric surgery for weight loss and glycemic control in nonmorbidly obese adults with diabetes: a systematic review. JAMA 2013;309:2250–2261.

Roger S. McIntyre, MD, FRCPC
Mood Disorders Psychopharmacology Unit (MDPU), University Health Network, University of Toronto
399 Bathurst Street, MP 9-325
Toronto, ON M5T 2S8 (Canada)
E-Mail roger.mcintyre@uhn.ca

Sartorius N, Holt RIG, Maj M (eds): Comorbidity of Mental and Physical Disorders.
Key Issues Ment Health. Basel, Karger, 2015, vol 179, pp 54–65 (DOI: 10.1159/000365531)

Cardiovascular Disease and Severe Mental Illness

Richard I.G. Holt

Human Development and Health Academic Unit, Faculty of Medicine, University of Southampton,
University Hospital Southampton NHS Foundation Trust, Southampton, UK

Abstract

People with schizophrenia or bipolar disorder have increased morbidity and shortened life expectancy compared with the general population. The prevalence of many physical illnesses is increased in people with severe mental illness and accounts for around three quarters of all deaths; cardiovascular disease is the most common cause of death. The increased prevalence of cardiovascular disease is explained, at least in part, by increased rates of traditional cardiovascular risk factors including diabetes, dyslipidaemia, obesity and smoking, but mental illness is an independent risk factor for cardiovascular disease and mortality. Despite national and international guidance and an increasing awareness of physical health issues in people with severe mental illness, the level of screening for and management of cardiovascular risk factors remains poor. While there are additional challenges in managing cardiovascular risk in people with severe mental illness, the principles are similar to those in the general population. A multidisciplinary approach involving healthcare professionals within psychiatry, general practice and medical specialties as well as and clear patient pathways are needed to reduce the health inequalities experienced by people with severe mental illness.

© 2015 S. Karger AG, Basel

Cardiovascular disease is the leading cause of mortality worldwide, accounting for approximately 30% of all deaths. Similarly, mental illness is also common, affecting 1 in 10 people at any one time. A degree of comorbidity is therefore to be expected but it is clear that mental illness occurs more commonly among people with cardiovascular disease than expected and vice versa [1].

The relationship between cardiovascular disease and mental illness is complex and bi-directional, with mental illness being both a cause and consequence of cardiovascular disease. For example, cross-sectional studies have shown that the prevalence of depression is increased in people with cardiovascular disease with up to 40% of people having either major or minor depression following a myocardial infarction [2]. Furthermore, longitudinal studies indicate that depression increases the risk of myocardial infarction, coronary heart disease, cerebrovascular disease and other cardiovascular diseases by up to 2-fold in both men and women, independent of other risk factors [3, 4], and increases mortality following a myocardial infarction [5, 6]. Similarly, anxiety is an independent risk factor for incident coronary heart disease and cardiac mortality [7].

Table 1. Estimated prevalence of modifiable cardiovascular risk factors in people with schizophrenia and bipolar disorder, and relative risk compared with the general population (adapted from De Hert et al. [10])

Modifiable risk factor	Schizophrenia		Bipolar disorder	
	prevalence	relative risk	prevalence	relative risk
Smoking	50–80%	2–3	54–68%	2–3
Dyslipidaemia	25–69%	≤5	23–38%	≤3
Diabetes	10–15%	2–3	8–17%	1.5–3
Hypertension	19–58%	2–3	35–61%	2–3
Obesity	45–55%	1.5–2	21–49%	1–2
Metabolic syndrome	37–63%	2–3	30–49%	2–3

This chapter, however, will review the association between severe mental illness (schizophrenia and bipolar disorder) and cardiovascular disease as an example of this complex relationship. It will explore the reasons for the comorbidity and the steps needed to reduce cardiovascular disease in people with severe mental illness. Severe mental illness is associated with a 3-fold increased risk of premature death and shortened life expectancy by approximately 10–20 years [8]. Although suicide accounts for the highest *relative* risk of mortality, being up to 20-fold more common than the general population, a range of physical illnesses occurs more frequently in people with severe mental illness and which are the cause of approximately three quarters of all deaths, with cardiovascular disease being the most common cause of death [8].

Epidemiology of Cardiovascular Disease in Severe Mental Illness

Cardiovascular morbidity and mortality are increased approximately 2- to 3-fold in people with severe mental illness [8]. The *relative* risk is more markedly increased in younger individuals with severe mental illness, in whom the prevalence of cardiovascular disease is 3.6-fold higher compared with a 2.1-fold increase in people who are older than 50 years [9]. While the morbidity and mortality associated with cardiovascular disease have fallen in the general population over the last 20 years, these benefits have not been shared by people with severe mental illness, which has led to a widening health inequality gap.

Aetiology of Cardiovascular Disease in Severe Mental Illness

There are numerous reasons for the increased rate of cardiovascular disease in people with severe mental illness, including an increased prevalence of modifiable cardiovascular risk factors, such as obesity, smoking, diabetes and dyslipidaemia (table 1), as well as intrinsic biological changes that occur during psychosis [10]. Not only do modifiable cardiovascular risk factors occur more commonly, but they appear at a younger age; in the US Clinical Antipsychotic Trials of Intervention Effectiveness (CATIE), over a quarter of men with schizophrenia, aged 20–29 years, at baseline had metabolic syndrome, a proxy for cardiovascular risk, compared with fewer than 10% in the general US population [11]. The implication of this finding is that healthcare professionals need to pay attention to cardiovascular risk factor management in people with severe mental illness from diagnosis.

Obesity

The global prevalence of obesity has increased dramatically over the last three decades, driven by changes in diet and physical activity. These demographic changes appear to have affected people with severe mental illness to a greater extent than the general population as studies that predate the 1980s did not consistently report higher rates of obesity in those with severe mental illness [12]. By contrast, more recent studies have shown that obesity is approximately 2-fold more common in people with schizophrenia or bipolar disorder. The mean baseline BMI in the CATIE study was 29.7 kg/m^2, with 37% of men and 73% of women having central obesity as defined by a waist circumference in excess of 102 and 88 cm, respectively.

Obesity occurs early in the natural history of schizophrenia with a significant proportion of people with first-episode psychosis being overweight prior to any treatment. Weight gain frequently occurs rapidly following treatment initiation. Seventeen per cent of people with schizophrenia in the European First Episode Schizophrenia Trial were overweight at baseline prior to treatment and 37–86% had gained more than 7% of their initial body weight during the first year of treatment, depending on medication choice [13].

Body composition is also altered in people with severe mental illness; higher waist-to-hip ratios and increased visceral fat have been found even in people with first episode psychosis; other studies have not replicated these findings, but note marked weight gain and increasing girth during treatment with antipsychotic medication [12].

The cause of obesity in people with schizophrenia includes genetic and lifestyle factors as well as illness and treatment effects. Individuals with schizophrenia are more likely to consume a diet that is rich in fat and refined carbohydrates while containing less fibre, fruit and vegetables than the general population [14]. The lower levels of physical activity and social and urban deprivation experienced by those with schizophrenia may contribute further to the increased obesity rates.

Diabetes

It is estimated that between 10 and 15% of people with severe mental illness have diabetes [10]. The onset occurs on average 10 years earlier, with women appearing to have a greater risk of diabetes than men [15]. Type 1 diabetes is not increased and so the 2- to 3-fold excess is explained by an increase in type 2 diabetes. The prevalence of undiagnosed diabetes is also considerably higher in people with schizophrenia than the general population with as many as 70% of cases being undiagnosed. This may reflect a reluctance of people with severe mental illness to volunteer symptoms and the overlap between some symptoms of diabetes and mental illness, leading to less screening in people with severe mental illness.

Like obesity, the rates of diabetes may be increased because of lifestyle factors, but there is also evidence of a genetic link between the two conditions. There is a high prevalence of metabolic abnormalities in the first degree relatives of people with severe mental illness, and between 17 and 50% of people with schizophrenia have a family history of type 2 diabetes [15]. Although these findings may result from shared familial environment, genome-wide association studies have suggested a shared genetic linkage between severe mental illness and diabetes [16].

Dyslipidaemia and Hypertension

A meta-analysis including 11 papers on dyslipidaemia showed that the major lipid abnormalities seen in people with severe mental illness are lower levels of HDL cholesterol and hypertriglyceridaemia, although not all studies have shown this [17]. By contrast, total cholesterol was not higher in people with severe mental illness. Overall, dyslipidaemia is reported in 25–69% of people with severe mental illness. The same meta-analysis included 12 papers on hypertension and found a non-significant 11% increase in the prevalence of hypertension (1.11, 95% CI: 0.91–1.35) [17].

Smoking

Smoking rates are high in people with severe mental illness (50–80%). In the USA, 68% of 689 schizophrenia patients who took part in the CATIE study were smokers compared to 35% of age-matched controls. In the UK general population, 20% of men and 19% of women are current smokers, but the odds of people with schizophrenia being current smokers are 5.3 times higher and the odds are greater for men than women at 7.2 and 3.3, respectively [18]. People with severe mental illness are also heavier smokers both in terms of total number of cigarettes smoked and amount of smoke inhaled.

Intrinsic Biological Changes in Severe Mental Illness

Severe mental illnesses are associated with a number of biological changes that affect intermediate metabolism and consequently cardiovascular risk [15]. These include hypothalamic-pituitary-adrenal axis dysfunction, manifesting as subclinical hypercortisolism and blunted diurnal cortisol rhythm, altered immune function (e.g. altered cytokine expression) and altered platelet function.

Antipsychotic Medication and Cardiovascular Disease

There are concerns that antipsychotics may contribute to cardiovascular risk by inducing weight gain and worsening lipid profile and blood glucose. Weight gain is the most common side effect seen with second-generation antipsychotics, affecting between 15 and 72% of patients [12]. Most weight gain occurs early in treatment, but patients may continue to gain weight for at least 4 years after the initiation of treatment, albeit at a slower rate. There is a hierarchy of weight gain between second-generation antipsychotics, with clozapine and olanzapine being associated with the greatest weight gain, but no agent should be considered as weight neutral. There is an intermediate risk of weight gain with quetiapine and risperidone, while aripiprazole, amisulpride and ziprasidone have little effect on weight. Some first-generation antipsychotics, for example chlorpromazine, and other psychotropic medications, such as certain antidepressants, are also associated with a high risk of weight gain.

Predicting weight gain with treatment is difficult because there is marked inter-individual variation in treatment-induced weight change. Other factors associated with weight gain are younger age, lower initial BMI, family history of obesity, concomitant cannabis use and a tendency to overeat at the time of stress [12]. The best predictor of long-term weight gain is the change in the first 4–6 weeks of treatment, emphasising the need for regular weight measurement during the early phase of treatment.

The relationship between antipsychotics and diabetes is complex because of the long natural history of diabetes and the potential confounding effects of other diabetes risk factors in people with severe mental illness [19]. The earliest case report linking antipsychotics with diabetes was in 1956 when a man developed haemolytic anaemia and diabetes 2 weeks after stopping chlorpromazine [20]. Since then, cases of diabetes and diabetic ketoacidosis have been seen in people receiving various first- and second-generation antipsychotics [19]. Although these studies provide evidence of causality, particularly when the glucose was measured before treatment initiation and where the diabetes entered remission after treatment discontinuation, the small numbers make it difficult to determine whether these are isolated cases or whether they can be extrapolated to the wider body of people receiving antipsychotic medication.

A large number of pharmaco-epidemiological studies have indicated that people receiving antipsychotics have a higher prevalence of diabetes than the general population and that people receiving second-generation drugs have a slightly increased risk of diabetes compared with those receiving first-generation drugs. One meta-analysis found that the relative risk of diabetes in those prescribed a second-generation antipsychotic was 32% (15–51%) higher than those receiving a first-generation antipsychotic. There was, however, considerable variation between studies [21], and a further systematic review of cohort studies found no consistent difference in diabetes risk between second-generation antipsychotics either as a group when compared with first-generation antipsychotics or between individual drugs [22].

Over the last decade, randomised controlled trials reporting treatment-emergent diabetes have begun to appear in the literature. A systematic review of 22 of these trials found no consistent significant difference in treatment-emergent glucose abnormalities between antipsychotics, either when compared with other antipsychotics or with placebo [23]. However, caution is needed when interpreting this analysis as the primary aim of many of these studies was to assess antipsychotic efficacy rather than metabolic side effects, and as such are underpowered to address this issue. The reporting of metabolic data was inconsistent and duration of many studies was too short to assess diabetes risk. Furthermore, several studies have shown small increases in glucose concentration in people receiving second-generation antipsychotics during the studies, which may translate into meaningful differences in the rate of diabetes over the many years that people with severe mental illness take antipsychotics [24]. A more recent meta-analysis comparing the metabolic side effects of different second-generation antipsychotics found that olanzapine produced a greater increase in glucose than amisulpride, aripiprazole, quetiapine, risperidone and ziprasidone, but a similar increase as clozapine [24].

Overall it appears that there is a causative link between antipsychotics and diabetes, but the risk is probably low and the majority of people receiving antipsychotics will not develop diabetes as a result of their medication [19].

Antipsychotic treatment is also associated with increases in LDL cholesterol and triglycerides and decreased HDL cholesterol. In a meta-analysis of 48 studies comparing different second-generation antipsychotics, olanzapine produced a greater increase in total cholesterol than aripiprazole, risperidone and ziprasidone, but no differences with amisulpride, clozapine and quetiapine were seen [24]. These differences may reflect the propensity to weight gain, but there may be other direct mechanisms as hypertriglyceridaemia may occur following treatment despite only modest weight gain.

The effect of antipsychotics on blood pressure is variable; although weight gain may lead to increased blood pressure, this may be offset by adrenergic blockade by the antipsychotics [17].

Overall it appears that many antipsychotics have an adverse effect on cardiovascular risk factors. However, it is important to understand that these are surrogate markers and may not translate into increased cardiovascular events and mortality. Indeed, the opposite is suggested by several large epidemiological studies. A UK study of over 46,000 people found that while exposure to first-generation antipsychotics, particularly high doses, was associated with excess cardiovascular mortality, this increase was not seen in people receiving second-generation antipsychotics [9]. Similarly in a large Finnish study of 66,881 people with schizophrenia, total mortality was lowest in individuals receiving clozapine and olanzapine, with no difference in cardiovascular mortality between drugs [25]. A more recent Finnish study examining the impact of the first- and second-generation antipsychotics on mortality in people with first-onset schizophrenia found that the use

Table 2. Recommended screening based on currently available guidelines

	Baseline	2–3 months	Annual	Target
Medical history to include family history, ethnicity, smoking, alcohol, diet, exercise	✓	✓	✓	
Height	✓			
Weight[1]	✓	Every week during first 6–8 weeks of treatment and at every clinic visit thereafter, but at least quarterly	✓	BMI <25 kg/m²
Blood pressure	✓	✓	✓	<140/90 mm Hg
Glucose[2]	✓	✓	✓	Fasting glucose <6.0 mmol/l Non-fasting glucose <7.8 mmol/l
Glycated haemoglobin[3]	✓	✓	✓	<6.0% (42 mmol/mol) if no history of diabetes; target should be individualised for people with diabetes but likely 6.5–7.5% (47–58 mmol/mol)
Lipid profile[4]	✓	✓	✓	Total cholesterol <5.0 mmol/l, <4.0 mmol/l if established CVD or diabetes LDL-cholesterol <3.0 mmol/l, <2.0 mmol/l if established CVD or diabetes 30% reduction in patient starting statins
Electrocardiogram	✓	✓	✓	To assess QTc interval

[1] Additional information can be obtained by measuring waist circumference; target men <94 cm, women <80 cm. Lower values should be sought in people from non-white European populations. [2] Either a fasting or non-fasting sample can be used. Fasting samples are more reproducible, but may be logistically more difficult to obtain. A formal 75-gram oral glucose tolerance test is only needed rarely. [3] Note glycated haemoglobin may be normal in situations where there is a rapid onset of diabetes and so is less suited to the 2- to 3-month sample. [4] Either a fasting or non-fasting sample can be used. Fasting samples are needed to assess LDL cholesterol and triglycerides, but cardiovascular risk can be calculated using the total:HDL cholesterol ratio which is largely unaffected by eating.

of second-generation antipsychotics, especially clozapine, olanzapine and quetiapine, was associated with reduced risk of all-cause mortality in people with schizophrenia [26]. By contrast, first-generation antipsychotics, specifically levomepromazine, thioridazine and clorprothixene, were associated with increased risk of all-cause mortality and levomepromazine with an increased likelihood for cardiovascular death. As these studies are both observational, there may be other explanations or confounders underlying the results [25, 26].

Screening for Cardiovascular Risk Factors

The increased prevalence of cardiovascular disease and its modifiable risk factors in people with severe mental illness provides a strong rationale to screen for cardiovascular risk factors. Screening should begin prior to the onset of treatment or as soon as is reasonably possible, 2–3 months later to assess the acute metabolic effects of the antipsychotics, and thereafter on an annual basis unless significant treatment changes are contemplated (table 2).

Cardiovascular risk assessment should include a detailed medical history to assess risk factors, physical examination to include weight and blood pressure, a blood test to assess lipids and glycaemia, and an electrocardiogram [10]. It is known that waist circumference is more closely associated with cardiovascular disease than BMI, but in some settings, such as within the UK primary care, there has been reluctance to undertake this measurement. The close correlation between weight and waist circumference for most of the population would suggest that while additional information may be obtained from a waist measurement, weight is a pragmatic and practical alternative.

A fasting blood sample is required to interpret a full lipid profile, but a non-fasting sample is acceptable where logistical difficulties prevent the patient from attending in a fasting state. The sensitivity and specificity for diabetes, particularly if the glucose measurement is combined with glycated haemoglobin, does not differ greatly and most 10-year cardiovascular risk engines use the total and HDL cholesterol, which are largely unaffected by eating. Although it may be easier to obtain a non-fasting sample, clinicians should not assume that patients with severe mental illness are unable to attend fasted as several studies have shown that this is feasible [27].

Current Screening Practises
Despite clear guidance from both national and international bodies [10, 28–30], it is clear that many people with severe mental illness are not being screened for cardiovascular risk factors. In an audit of 50 in-patients and 50 out-patients with severe mental illness in Hampshire, UK, documented evidence that blood pressure had been measured was found in only 32% of case notes, and glucose (16%), lipids (9%) and weight (2%) were assessed even less frequently [31]. This was despite a high prevalence of metabolic syndrome in these patients and a significant number at high risk of cardiovascular disease.

The effectiveness of national guidelines and campaigns has been questioned by a study of US psychiatrists which showed that US Food and Drug Administration guidelines and a joint position statement of the American Psychiatric Association, American Diabetes Association and North American Association for the Study of Obesity had no effect on screening rates for diabetes [32]. There is a lack of clarity among mental healthcare professionals about whose responsibility physical health screening is [33]. In some countries, such as the UK, the responsibility for screening is placed within primary care [28]. This may be appropriate because many people with mental illness have frequent contact with their primary care doctor and primary care doctors have all the skills and training to address this issue. However, some people with severe mental illness only see their mental health team and under this circumstance it is important the screening occurs in this setting. It is clear that good communication is needed between primary care and mental health teams to ensure that the patient does not fall between the two settings. Mental healthcare professionals have also expressed concern about their lack of understanding about what should be measured and when and how to interpret the results [33]. Lack of access to necessary equipment may be a further barrier.

It is well recognised that people with severe mental illness are less likely to take advantage of health screening [34] and health services. Since to a large extent care is not offered unless requested, people with severe mental illness may be disadvantaged. The Disability Rights Commission has highlighted that instead of receiving holistic care, many people with mental illness describe how their physical illnesses are overshadowed by the mental illness, with healthcare professionals concentrating on the latter to the detriment of the former [35].

Assessment of Cardiovascular Risk
Cardiovascular risk is usually assessed by the use of locally relevant risk engines. These have not been validated in people with severe mental illness who are typically younger, have higher blood pressure and are more likely to smoke than the

populations used to derive cardiovascular disease risk scoring systems, such as Framingham and QRISK. As traditional risk factors only partially explain the excess cardiovascular disease seen in people with severe mental illness, it is possible that these traditional risk engines may underestimate cardiovascular risk in people with severe mental illness. However, pending further research, they provide a guide for the initiation of primary preventative measures.

Managing Cardiovascular Risk Factors

While there are additional challenges in ensuring that the person with severe mental illness understands the aims and rationale for treatment, cardiovascular risk factor management is essentially along similar lines to the general population.

Smoking
Healthcare professionals should provide smokers with information about the risks of smoking and encourage them to quit. Interventions for smoking cessation range from basic advice to pharmacotherapy coupled with either individual or group psychological support. Smokers with schizophrenia are less likely to quit than the general population, with one meta-analysis reporting the smoking cessation rate for people with schizophrenia to be 9% compared with 14–49% in the general population (OR 0.19, 95% CI: 0.14–0.24) [18]. This lower rate is partly attributable to an increased severity of nicotine dependence, fewer attempts to stop smoking, lower motivation to quit and less access to interventions [36, 37]. However, the rates of smoking cessation in people with schizophrenia can be increased with appropriate support [38].

The three main pharmacotherapies are nicotine replacement therapy, the antidepressant bupropion and the nicotinic receptor partial agonist varenicline. Of these, bupropion is both safe and effective in increasing the rates of abstinence in people with schizophrenia. A meta-analysis showed that those taking bupropion with co-interventions (group therapy alone or in combination with nicotine replacement therapy) for up to 12 weeks were 3 times more likely to be abstinent 6 months after starting treatment, compared with those taking a placebo [39]. Bupropion, however, is contraindicated in people with bipolar disorder. Varenicline may also improve smoking cessation rates in people with schizophrenia, but there have been reports of suicidal ideation and behaviours from people on varenicline.

Obesity
The pessimism surrounding treatment of obesity in people with severe mental illness has been challenged by a number of recent observational studies and randomised controlled trials of lifestyle and pharmacological interventions. A recently published meta-analysis of non-pharmacological interventions in people with schizophrenia has shown that these led to a mean reduction in weight of 3.12 kg over a period of 8–24 weeks [40]. In addition, there were commensurate reductions in waist circumference and improvements in other cardiovascular risk factors. The benefits of these programmes were seen irrespective of the duration of mental illness treatment, whether the intervention was delivered to an individual or in a group setting, whether the intervention was based on cognitive behavioural therapy or a nutritional intervention, or whether it was designed to promote weight loss or prevent weight gain. Out-patient interventions appeared more effective than in-patient settings. The meta-analysis acknowledges a number of limitations of the trials, including the small numbers of participants and the lack of long-term follow-up. Most studies do not extend beyond 12 weeks and hence their applicability to the long-term nature of schizophrenia remains uncertain. The few studies reporting long-term effects suggest that these may be persistent after the end of the programme for up to 1 year, but others suggest that long-term behaviour change is difficult to achieve [41].

There are several longer-term observational studies of the effects of weight management programmes. Menza et al. [42] showed that a 52-week multimodal weight control programme led to significant improvements in weight, BMI, glycated haemoglobin, blood pressure, levels of exercise and nutritional knowledge in 20 of the 31 participants who completed the programme. Another study of 33 people with schizophrenia in Taiwan demonstrated a mean 3.7 and 2.7 kg reduction in body weight after 6 months and 1 year, respectively, following a 10-week multimodal weight control program [43]. A long-term (8 years) observational study of a group intervention demonstrated that further weight loss is achievable with ongoing support [44]. In this study of well-motivated patients, there was a progressive statistically significant reduction in mean weight and BMI throughout the follow-up with no suggestion of a plateau. The mean weight loss was approximately 10% at 1 year (approx. 10 kg), with 61% achieving a 7% weight loss. By the end of the programme, 92% (n = 130) had lost some weight. The only predictor of weight loss was the number of sessions attended; gender, age, diagnosis and treatment were not related to weight loss. This suggests that an intervention of greater intensity or stronger focus may be needed in people with severe mental illness compared with the general population. Although previous studies have suggested that lifestyle interventions are hard to maintain in people with schizophrenia without support [41], there may be other factors that contributed to the achieved weight loss in this clinic. The model of care offered a multimodal programme that incorporated nutrition, exercise and some degree of behavioural interventions on the premise that weight management should not be viewed in isolation and is best combined with a holistic approach to lifestyle management. The clinic first utilised a group approach as a pragmatic low cost way forward, but the group setting and peer support was also appreciated by many participants. Lifestyle changes were not imposed on patients by healthcare professionals, but were chosen by the participants themselves. Furthermore, many of the initial health behaviours, such as high intake of sugary carbonated beverages, were readily amenable to change. The stepwise change made the process simple, achievable and sustainable.

Several pharmacological agents have been tried to reverse or prevent antipsychotic-induced weight gain [45]. No drug has been found to be particularly effective, but a recent systematic review showed that there was preliminary evidence that metformin may attenuate weight gain in both adult and adolescent patients taking second generation antipsychotics [46]. The review included 14 articles, 8 of which were double-blind, placebo-controlled studies. The studies lasted 8–16 weeks and used doses ranging from 500 to 2,550 mg daily. Most of these studies showed a modest reduction in weight with metformin (approx. 1 kg), while those treated with placebo gained weight. Where it was measured, insulin resistance appeared to improve in those treated with metformin. The review concluded that although there was no clear substantial evidence that metformin, as an adjuvant to second generation antipsychotic use, will decrease weight gain and improve metabolic effects, the results are encouraging and additional studies of longer duration were recommended.

Dyslipidaemia
Although target levels of total cholesterol and LDL cholesterol are the same as the general population (<5.0 and <3.0 mmol/l, respectively), tighter goals of <4.0 and <2.0 mmol/l may be appropriate for individuals with established cardiovascular disease or diabetes. No cardiovascular disease outcome trials with statins have been performed specifically in people with severe mental illness, but these drugs are as effective in lowering total and LDL cholesterol as the general population [47]. Furthermore, there is no evidence that lipid-lowering medication is associated with suicide or traumatic deaths in people with severe mental illness.

Diabetes

The treatment of diabetes in people with severe mental illness should follow currently available treatment algorithms, although oral antidiabetes agents that induce less weight gain may have advantages given the high prevalence of obesity in people with severe mental illness [48]. The additional challenges of managing comorbid diabetes and mental illness, however, require close collaboration between mental and diabetes services. As hyperglycaemia is associated with an increased risk of diabetes complications, neuropathy, retinopathy and nephropathy, glycaemic targets should be determined for each individual with diabetes. The precise target is dependent on a number of factors including disease duration, risk of hypoglycaemia, life expectancy and comorbidities including macrovascular disease as well as patient attitude and resources; however, glycated haemoglobin targets between 6.5 and 7.5% (48–58 mmol/mol) would be usual [48].

Prevention of diabetes is also an important consideration as lifestyle intervention programmes involving dietary modification, weight loss and increased physical activity have been shown to reduce the incidence of type 2 diabetes [49]. As these programmes share many features with lifestyle weight loss programmes used in people with severe mental illness, it is hoped that the programmes may also lead to diabetes prevention, although this has not been formally assessed. Metformin may also be considered [10].

Hypertension

The management of hypertension in severe mental illness should follow the same treatment algo-rithms as the general population, with recommended target blood pressure levels of <140/90 mm Hg. Patients should be advised to reduce smoking and salt intake. European and UK guidelines emphasise the need to choose antihypertensive agents best suited to the individual patient's needs as the achieved blood pressure is more important than the agent used to achieve this.

Conclusion

The increased rates of cardiovascular disease in people with severe mental illness provide a clinical imperative to screen and manage cardiovascular risk factors with a systematic approach. In the past, the physical health needs of people with severe mental illness have largely been ignored, creating significant heath inequalities. Contrary to expectation, individuals with severe mental illness are as motivated about their physical health as the rest of the population, but often lack awareness and fail to prioritise physical well-being [50]. Providing a supportive environment in which cardiovascular risk factors can be managed systematically is likely to have a significant impact on cardiovascular morbidity and mortality in people with severe mental illness.

Disclosure Statement

Professor Holt has lectured on cardiovascular risk in people with severe mental illness for Sanofi-Aventis, Eli Lilly, Otsuka, Lundbeck and Bristol-Myers Squibb.

References

1 Katon WJ: Epidemiology and treatment of depression in patients with chronic medical illness. Dialogues Clin Neurosci 2011;13:7–23.

2 Carney RM, Freedland KE: Depression, mortality, and medical morbidity in patients with coronary heart disease. Biol Psychiatry 2003;54:241–247.

3 Nicholson A, Kuper H, Hemingway H: Depression as an aetiologic and prognostic factor in coronary heart disease: a meta-analysis of 6362 events among 146 538 participants in 54 observational studies. Eur Heart J 2006;27:2763–2774.

4 Van der Kooy K, van Hout H, Marwijk H, Marten H, Stehouwer C, Beekman A: Depression and the risk for cardiovascular diseases: systematic review and meta analysis. Int J Geriatr Psychiatry 2007; 22:613–626.

5 Sorensen C, Brandes A, Hendricks O, Thrane J, Friis-Hasche E, Haghfelt T, et al: Psychosocial predictors of depression in patients with acute coronary syndrome. Acta Psychiatr Scand 2005;111: 116–124.

6 van Melle JP, de Jonge P, Spijkerman TA, Tijssen JG, Ormel J, van Veldhuisen DJ, et al: Prognostic association of depression following myocardial infarction with mortality and cardiovascular events: a meta-analysis. Psychosom Med 2004;66:814–822.

7 Roest AM, Martens EJ, de Jonge P, Denollet J: Anxiety and risk of incident coronary heart disease: a meta-analysis. J Am Coll Cardiol 2010;56:38–46.

8 Brown S, Kim M, Mitchell C, Inskip H: Twenty-five year mortality of a community cohort with schizophrenia. Br J Psychiatry 2010;196:116–121.

9 Osborn DP, Levy G, Nazareth I, Petersen I, Islam A, King MB: Relative risk of cardiovascular and cancer mortality in people with severe mental illness from the United Kingdom's General Practice Research Database. Arch Gen Psychiatry 2007;64:242–249.

10 De Hert M, Dekker JM, Wood D, Kahl KG, Holt RI, Moller HJ: Cardiovascular disease and diabetes in people with severe mental illness position statement from the European Psychiatric Association (EPA), supported by the European Association for the Study of Diabetes (EASD) and the European Society of Cardiology (ESC). Eur Psychiatry 2009; 24:412–424.

11 McEvoy JP, Meyer JM, Goff DC, Nasrallah HA, Davis SM, Sullivan L, et al: Prevalence of the metabolic syndrome in patients with schizophrenia: baseline results from the Clinical Antipsychotic Trials of Intervention Effectiveness (CATIE) schizophrenia trial and comparison with national estimates from NHANES III. Schizophr Res 2005;80: 19–32.

12 Holt RI, Peveler RC: Obesity, serious mental illness and antipsychotic drugs. Diabetes Obes Metab 2009;11:665–679.

13 Kahn RS, Fleischhacker WW, Boter H, Davidson M, Vergouwe Y, Keet IP, et al: Effectiveness of antipsychotic drugs in first-episode schizophrenia and schizophreniform disorder: an open randomised clinical trial. Lancet 2008;371: 1085–1097.

14 McCreadie RG: Diet, smoking and cardiovascular risk in people with schizophrenia: descriptive study. Br J Psychiatry 2003;183:534–539.

15 Holt RI, Peveler RC, Byrne CD: Schizophrenia, the metabolic syndrome and diabetes. Diabet Med 2004;21:515–523.

16 Gough SC, O'Donovan MC: Clustering of metabolic comorbidity in schizophrenia: a genetic contribution? J Psychopharmacol 2005;19(6 suppl):47–55.

17 Osborn DP, Wright CA, Levy G, King MB, Deo R, Nazareth I: Relative risk of diabetes, dyslipidaemia, hypertension and the metabolic syndrome in people with severe mental illnesses: systematic review and metaanalysis. BMC Psychiatry 2008;8:84.

18 de Leon J, Diaz FJ: A meta-analysis of worldwide studies demonstrates an association between schizophrenia and tobacco smoking behaviors. Schizophr Res 2005;76:135–157.

19 Holt RI, Peveler RC: Antipsychotic drugs and diabetes – an application of the Austin Bradford Hill criteria. Diabetologia 2006;49:1467–1476.

20 Cooperberg AA, Eidlow S: Haemolytic anemia, jaundice and diabetes mellitus following chlorpromazine therapy. Can Med Assoc J 1956;75:746–749.

21 Smith M, Hopkins D, Peveler RC, Holt RI, Woodward M, Ismail K: First- v. second-generation antipsychotics and risk for diabetes in schizophrenia: systematic review and meta-analysis. Br J Psychiatry 2008;192:406–411.

22 Citrome LL, Holt RI, Zachry WM, Clewell JD, Orth PA, Karagianis JL, et al: Risk of treatment-emergent diabetes mellitus in patients receiving antipsychotics. Ann Pharmacother 2007;41: 1593–1603.

23 Bushe CJ, Leonard BE: Blood glucose and schizophrenia: a systematic review of prospective randomized clinical trials. J Clin Psychiatry 2007;68:1682–1690.

24 Rummel-Kluge C, Komossa K, Schwarz S, Hunger H, Schmid F, Lobos CA, et al: Head-to-head comparisons of metabolic side effects of second generation antipsychotics in the treatment of schizophrenia: a systematic review and metaanalysis. Schizophr Res 2010;123: 225–233.

25 Tiihonen J, Lonnqvist J, Wahlbeck K, Klaukka T, Niskanen L, Tanskanen A, et al: 11-year follow-up of mortality in patients with schizophrenia: a population-based cohort study (FIN11 study). Lancet 2009;374:620–627.

26 Kiviniemi M, Suvisaari J, Koivumaa-Honkanen H, Hakkinen U, Isohanni M, Hakko H: Antipsychotics and mortality in first-onset schizophrenia: prospective Finnish register study with 5-year follow-up. Schizophr Res 2013;150:274–280.

27 van Winkel R, De Hert M, Wampers M, Van Eyck D, Hanssens L, Scheen A, et al: Major changes in glucose metabolism, including new-onset diabetes, within 3 months after initiation of or switch to atypical antipsychotic medication in patients with schizophrenia and schizoaffective disorder. J Clin Psychiatry 2008;69:472–479.

28 National Collaborating Centre for Mental Health: The NICE Guideline on Core Interventions in the Treatment and Management of Schizophrenia in Adults in Primary and Secondary Care CG82. London, British Psychological Society and Royal College of Psychiatrists, 2010.

29 Consensus development conference on antipsychotic drugs and obesity and diabetes. J Clin Psychiatry 2004;65:267–272.

30 Citrome L, Yeomans D: Do guidelines for severe mental illness promote physical health and well-being? J Psychopharmacol 2005;19(6 suppl):102–109.

31 Holt RI, Abdelrahman T, Hirsch M, Dhesi Z, George T, Blincoe T, et al: The prevalence of undiagnosed metabolic abnormalities in people with serious mental illness. J Psychopharmacol 2010; 24:867–873.

32 Morrato EH, Newcomer JW, Kamat S, Baser O, Harnett J, Cuffel B: Metabolic screening after the American Diabetes Association's consensus statement on antipsychotic drugs and diabetes. Diabetes Care 2009;32:1037–1042.

33 Barnes TR, Paton C, Cavanagh MR, Hancock E, Taylor DM: A UK audit of screening for the metabolic side effects of antipsychotics in community patients. Schizophr Bull 2007;33:1397–1403.

34 Lindamer LA, Wear E, Sadler GR: Mammography stages of change in middle-aged women with schizophrenia: an exploratory analysis. BMC Psychiatry 2006;6:49.

35 Disability Rights Commission: Equal Treatment: Closing the Gap. A Formal Investigation into Physical Health Inequalities Experienced by People with Learning Difficulties and Mental Health Problems. London, Disability Rights Commission, 2006.

36 Foulds J, Gandhi KK, Steinberg MB, Richardson DL, Williams JM, Burke MV, et al: Factors associated with quitting smoking at a tobacco dependence treatment clinic. Am J Health Behav 2006;30:400–412.

37 Siru R, Hulse GK, Tait RJ: Assessing motivation to quit smoking in people with mental illness: a review. Addiction 2009;104:719–733.

38 El-Guebaly N, Cathcart J, Currie S, Brown D, Gloster S: Public health and therapeutic aspects of smoking bans in mental health and addiction settings. Psychiatr Serv 2002;53:1617–1622.

39 Tsoi DT, Porwal M, Webster AC: Interventions for smoking cessation and reduction in individuals with schizophrenia. Cochrane Database Syst Rev 2013; 2:CD007253.

40 Caemmerer J, Correll CU, Maayan L: Acute and maintenance effects of non-pharmacologic interventions for antipsychotic associated weight gain and metabolic abnormalities: a meta-analytic comparison of randomized controlled trials. Schizophr Res 2012;140:159–168.

41 McCreadie RG, Kelly C, Connolly M, Williams S, Baxter G, Lean M, et al: Dietary improvement in people with schizophrenia: randomised controlled trial. Br J Psychiatry 2005;187:346–351.

42 Menza M, Vreeland B, Minsky S, Gara M, Radler DR, Sakowitz M: Managing atypical antipsychotic-associated weight gain: 12-month data on a multimodal weight control program. J Clin Psychiatry 2004;65:471–477.

43 Chen CK, Chen YC, Huang YS: Effects of a 10-week weight control program on obese patients with schizophrenia or schizoaffective disorder: a 12-month follow up. Psychiatry Clin Neurosci 2009;63:17–22.

44 Holt RI, Pendlebury J, Wildgust HJ, Bushe CJ: Intentional weight loss in overweight and obese patients with severe mental illness: 8-year experience of a behavioral treatment program. J Clin Psychiatry 2010;71:800–805.

45 Baptista T, ElFakih Y, Uzcategui E, Sandia I, Talamo E, Araujo de Baptista E, et al: Pharmacological management of atypical antipsychotic-induced weight gain. CNS Drugs 2008;22:477–495.

46 Miller LJ: Management of atypical antipsychotic drug-induced weight gain: focus on metformin. Pharmacotherapy 2009;29:725–735.

47 Hanssens L, De Hert M, Kalnicka D, van Winkel R, Wampers M, Van Eyck D, et al: Pharmacological treatment of severe dyslipidaemia in patients with schizophrenia. Int Clin Psychopharmacol 2007;22:43–49.

48 Inzucchi SE, Bergenstal RM, Buse JB, Diamant M, Ferrannini E, Nauck M, et al: Management of hyperglycaemia in type 2 diabetes: a patient-centered approach. Position statement of the American Diabetes Association (ADA) and the European Association for the Study of Diabetes (EASD). Diabetologia 2012;55:1577–1596.

49 Norris SL, Kansagara D, Bougatsos C, Fu R: Screening adults for type 2 diabetes: a review of the evidence for the U.S. Preventive Services Task Force. Ann Intern Med 2008;148:855–868.

50 Buhagiar K, Parsonage L, Osborn DP: Physical health behaviours and health locus of control in people with schizophrenia-spectrum disorder and bipolar disorder: a cross-sectional comparative study with people with non-psychotic mental illness. BMC Psychiatry 2011;11: 104.

Prof. Richard I.G. Holt, MA, MB, BChir, PhD, FRCP, FHEA
Human Development and Health Academic Unit, Faculty of Medicine
University of Southampton, University Hospital Southampton NHS Foundation Trust
IDS Building (MP887), Tremona Road, Southampton SO16 6YD (UK)
E-Mail R.I.G.Holt@southampton.ac.uk

Sartorius N, Holt RIG, Maj M (eds): Comorbidity of Mental and Physical Disorders.
Key Issues Ment Health. Basel, Karger, 2015, vol 179, pp 66–80 (DOI: 10.1159/000365532)

Multiple Comorbidities in People with Eating Disorders

Palmiero Monteleone[a, b] · Francesca Brambilla[c]

[a]Department of Medicine and Surgery, University of Salerno, Salerno, [b]Department of Psychiatry, University of Naples SUN, Naples, and [c]Department of Psychiatry, San Paolo Hospital, Milan, Italy

Abstract

Eating disorders, including anorexia nervosa and bulimia nervosa, are complex psychiatric diseases characterized by severe disturbances in eating behavior, often resulting in dramatic consequences for the physical health of patients. Even though appearing after the beginning of an eating disorder and therefore not representing their primary cause, physical impairments play an important role in the development of psychopathology, its course and prognosis, and in the most severe cases may also represent a significant threat to the patient's life. They contribute, together with suicide, to the high mortality of patients with eating disorders. Indeed, anorexia nervosa has the highest mortality of any psychiatric diagnosis, estimated at 10% within 10 years of diagnosis, while mortality for bulimia nervosa is lower, occurring at approximately 1% within 10 years of diagnosis. With a few exceptions, the physical complications resolve with the recovery of body weight and the discontinuation of aberrant eating and purging behaviors. The burden of physical complications demands prompt clinical consideration and appropriate treatment.   © 2015 S. Karger AG, Basel

Eating disorders, including anorexia nervosa and bulimia nervosa, are complex psychiatric diseases characterized by severe disturbances in eating behavior often resulting in dramatic consequences for the physical health of patients. Anorexia nervosa is characterized by restricted eating, obsessive fears of being fat and the voluntary pursuit of thinness with an inability to maintain a normal healthy body weight. Despite increasing emaciation and a body weight below 85% of the ideal, individuals with anorexia are dissatisfied with the perceived size and shape of their body, and engage in unhealthy behaviors to perpetuate weight loss or prevent weight gain. There are two subtypes of anorexia nervosa: anorexia nervosa binge-eating/purging subtype, where patients engage in binge-eating/purging behaviors, and anorexia nervosa restricting subtype, where patients exclusively restrict their food intake.

Bulimia nervosa is characterized by recurrent episodes of uncontrolled binge eating coupled with inappropriate compensatory behaviors, such as vomiting, laxative abuse, food restriction and/or excessive exercising, in order to prevent weight gain due to the patient's pathological fear of becoming fat. Generally, because of the ingestion of some food in the course of bingeing, people with bulimia nervosa have a normal body weight.

Anorexia and bulimia are perhaps the most intriguing combinations of psychological and physical pathology. Even though appearing after the beginning of an eating disorder and therefore not representing their primary cause, physical comorbidity plays an important role in the development of psychopathology, its course and prognosis, possibly through the essential contribution that nutritional alterations typical of these diseases exert on the brain biochemical function. The physical complications observed in eating disorders have been considered a consequence of nutritional derangements because of the similarities with the alterations observed in simple starvation. People with bulimia are not starving, but the loss of food from vomiting or use of laxatives, the biased selection of macro-/micronutrients typical of the bingeing episodes, and the alternation of gorging and severe dieting might lead to malnutrition, resulting in some of the adverse effects of simple starvation. What remain uncertain are the mechanisms by which starvation during anorexia and malnutrition with bulimia induces and maintains the physical complications of the syndromes. In particular, it is unclear why some patients show the full spectrum of physical complications while others with a very similar psychopathological picture do not. Moreover, it is not clear what influence is exerted by peripheral physical complications on the course, response to treatments and prognosis of eating disorders. These problems must be addressed in the future.

This chapter provides a brief review of the most common physical complications occurring in patients with eating disorders [1–5] (table 1).

Alterations of Skin and Related Organs

In both subtypes of anorexia nervosa, cutaneous alterations occur as a consequence of starvation, self-induced vomiting and abuse of purging drugs [6, 7].

Brittle hair and eyelashes and loss of hair and eyebrows are present in people with both subtypes of anorexia nervosa, while the skin is often covered by a fine, down-like hair known as 'lanugo', growing especially on the face, superior lip, back, arms and legs. Fragile nails and a dystrophic aspect of the skin, which is dry and scaling, pale or yellowish like old paper or brownish like dirt because of cornification, occur because of nutritional deficiencies and starvation-linked hypothyroidism that develops early in the disease. The yellowish color of the skin is partly due to the hypercarotenemia, which is typically observed in people with anorexia in contrast to involuntary starvation when hypocarotenemia is characteristic. In people with anorexia, the phenomenon is linked to the excessive consumption of carrots, pumpkins and similar yellowish vegetables, but possibly also to an acquired defect in the absorption, use or metabolism of carotene. Skin thickness and median collagen content are significantly reduced. Spontaneous cuts are frequently observed at the corners of the lips and near the nails.

The presence of skin trauma and calluses on the dorsal surface of hands, secondary to using the hands as an instrument to induce vomiting, is characteristic and was first described in 1979 by Russell (Russell sign) [7]. The lesions appear in people with anorexia nervosa binge-eating/purging subtype, and can be anywhere on the dorsum of the hand, but more frequently at the metacarpophalangeal joint of each finger. They rapidly progress to hyperpigmentation of the calluses and scarring. It has been reported that these lesions may disappear in the later course of the disease, as many patients train themselves to vomit reflexively. Poor wound healing is frequent. Facial dermatitis, seborrheic dermatitis and acne are occasionally observed.

Peripheral edema, especially pretibial, may occur in 20% of people with anorexia mostly of the restrictive subtype, often during the refeeding phase. A mild form may occur in people with the restrictive subtype of anorexia without a clear etio-

Table 1. The most common physical complications of eating disorders

Anorexia nervosa

Skin and related organs: yellow-orange dry and dystrophic skin (especially on the palmar surfaces of hands and on the plantar surfaces of feet), lanugo hair, especially on the face and on the back, brittle falling out hair, Russell's sign

Oral cavity: tooth enamel erosion, caries, gingivitis, salivary gland hypertrophy

Gastrointestinal system: gastroesophageal reflux disease, esophagitis, delayed gastric emptying, esophageal erosions and ulcers, hepatomegaly, fatty liver disease, constipation, hemorrhoids, rectal prolapse

Cardiovascular system: bradycardia, hypotension, tricuspid and mitral valve prolapse, arrhythmias caused by electrolyte abnormalities, electrocardiographic alterations (low voltage, prolonged QRS and QT interval, T wave and ST segment depression, T wave inversion), reduced cardiac output

Skeletal system: osteopenia, osteoporosis, muscle wasting, bone fractures

Metabolic changes: hypoglycemia, hypothermia, dehydration, hypercholesterolemia, ketosis, ketonuria, hyperuricemia, hypoproteinemia, metabolic alkalosis

Electrolyte alterations: hypochloremia, hypokalemia, hyponatremia, hypomagnesemia, hypophosphatemia

Hematologic changes: vitamin B_{12} and/or iron deficiency anemia, neutropenia

Endocrine system: amenorrhea, lower T_3, hypercortisolism, high GH and reduced IGF-I

Bulimia nervosa

Skin and related organs: dry and dystrophic skin, Russell's sign, peripalpebral petechiae, conjunctival hemorrhages, perioral ulcerations

Oral cavity: tooth enamel erosion, caries, gingivitis, salivary gland hypertrophy

Gastrointestinal system: gastritis, esophagitis, esophageal erosions and ulcers, gastroesophageal reflux, dysphagia and odynophagia, inflammations of the colon, hepatomegaly, fatty liver disease

Electrolyte alterations: hypokalemia

Cardiovascular system: bradycardia, hypotension, cardiac arrhythmias

logical cause in those with normal plasma proteins, and in particular albumin levels. A more severe form is associated with purging and chronic laxative abuse, which leads to marked hypoproteinemia and subsequent lowering of plasma osmotic pressure and passage of fluids from the vascular tree into tissues. This severe form of edema is rapid in onset and may lead to life-threatening shock, renal infarction and cardiovascular collapse due to an inability to maintain fluid volume [1].

In people with the binging subtype of anorexia, vomiting strain may lead to the appearance of cutaneous petechiae, especially on the face, and hemorrhage of the conjunctiva, possibly linked to fragility of venous and capillary walls, reduced platelet number and increased capillary vessel permeability. With repeated vomiting, subcutaneous emphysema of the neck has been described, in some cases associated with spontaneous pneumomediastinum.

Stable erythema, linked to the abuse of phenolphthalein-containing laxatives or ipecac, has been reported in people with anorexia. Cutaneous alterations linked to vitamin deficiency, including scurvy or pellagra, have been infrequently reported. More frequent are signs of self-injury, such as excoriated acne and erythema ab igne.

In bulimia, lesions of the skin, hair and other annexes are similar to those observed in anorexia, only occurring less frequently [8]. The most frequent alteration is the Russell sign, which is due to self-induced vomiting. Peripheral edema may be seen although less frequently than in anorexia, possibly due to the loss of electrolytes through vomiting and the relative poor consumption of proteins in these patients. Subcutaneous emphysema may be present secondary to recurrent severe vomiting strain. Signs of self-injury are frequent.

Oral Pathology

Dental caries is frequent in anorexia, being related to starvation in the restricting type and to both vomiting and excessive carbohydrate intake in the bingeing-purging type [9]. There is delayed formation and missing tooth enamel, as well as erosion (perimolysis) of the maxillary lingual surfaces, especially of the anterior teeth. A frequent oral pathology is angular cheilosis, a stomatitis characterized by pallor and maceration of the mucosa at the corners of the mouth, which may result in painful linear fissures and consequent scars. It is mostly observed in the binging subtype of anorexia, and is caused by the caustic effect of regurgitated gastric acid content, but may also be an expression of an underlying vitamin deficiency, especially of riboflavin (B_2) and pyridoxine (B_6) – in this case being seen also in the restrictive subtype of anorexia.

Gingival health is impaired in anorexia, possibly due to the chronic irritation produced by the regurgitated gastric acid content, often associated with painful pharyngeal erythema. Hypertrophy of the salivary glands (sialadenosis) is common in the binging subtype of anorexia, again linked to repeated vomiting, with occlusion of the salivary ducts by fragments of nondigested food. Generally the hypertrophy is painless, mostly bilateral, and more frequent in the parotids, which may enlarge up to five times their normal size. The hypertrophy of the glands may be more evident in the case of concomitant masseteric hypertrophy, especially present in people with the binging subtype of anorexia affected by bruxism [10].

The oral alterations reported for the binging subtype of anorexia are also present in bulimia nervosa [10]. Most of the dental problems are related to the frequent vomiting resulting in enamel injury and dental caries, which may also be induced by the ingestion of large amounts of carbohydrates. Enamel biopsies (postmortem) reveal a preserved thickness of the surface, with normal hardness measurements suggesting that oral hygiene and use of fluoride may minimize the erosive effect of vomiting on tooth enamel. Sialadenitis is extremely frequent in bulimia, and is often related to hyperamylasemia. The phenomenon has been attributed to excessive food intake and a reflex stimulation of the glands during vomiting.

Gastrointestinal Complications

The esophagus is frequently affected in both types of anorexia nervosa. Pathologies include stenosis, esophagitis (which causes epigastric or substernal burning pain radiating to the jaw or down both arms), erosions and ulcers of the gastroesophageal junction and esophageal rupture. These lesions are due mostly to vomiting, the frequently spastic motility of the esophagus and a neuropathy linked to vitamin deficiencies. Superior mesenteric artery syndrome occurs frequently in anorexia [11].

In the restrictive type of anorexia, gastric volume is normal or reduced, the wall's smooth muscle is atrophic and atonic, and antral mobility is abnormally low; gastric emptying is always slow and delayed for solid food and hypertonic liquids [11]. These abnormalities are partly responsible for the postprandial early feeling of gastric fullness and the very frequent belching observed in people with anorexia. Complications secondary to binging in the bulimic type of anorexia include gastric dilatation, which is rarely associated with rupture.

During refeeding, gastric bloating and other nonspecific abdominal discomforts usually persist. Complaints of esophageal reflux may occur even without self-induced vomiting, and is generally secondary to diminished competence of the gastroesophageal sphincter.

Gastritis and pyloric erosions are not frequent, but dilatation of the proximal duodenum and jejunum are frequently reported. Gastric perforation is a rare complication of the restrictive type of anorexia.

Constipation, mostly due to the drastically reduced caloric intake, constantly follows weight loss in anorexia, and is generally worsened by the abuse of laxatives. Abdominal pain is generally diffuse but without tenderness. Decreased colonic transit and pelvic floor dysfunction occur in undernourished people with anorexia, and normalize after refeeding. Colonic lesions are mostly secondary to chronic constipation and laxative abuse. Inflammation, atony and dilatation and the so-called cathartic colon characterized by thinness, atrophy and superficial ulcers of the mucosa, retention cysts and mononuclear infiltration of the submucosa are very frequent observations. Occasionally, ischemic necrosis of the segmental ileum and cecum has been reported, possibly resulting from poor blood supply linked to severe malnutrition and dehydration. Rectal prolapse occurs, possibly due to constipation or increased intra-abdominal pressure from forced vomiting [12].

Esophagitis, disordered esophageal motility including lower than normal esophageal sphincter pressure, relaxed sphincter pressure, reduced mean esophageal body contraction and amplitude, altered waveform morphology, and reduced progression occur infrequently in bulimia nervosa, while gastroesophageal reflux, dysphagia and odynophagia are often observed [13].

Gastric capacity is generally increased in relation to the frequency and severity of the binging and the amount of daily food intake [14]. The sensation of maximal fullness occurs sooner than the maximally tolerated gastric pain, which is mostly reduced. Intragastric pressure reached at maximum tolerance is normal. Gastric emptying is slower in bulimia nervosa than in normal subjects,

probably due to reduced intragastric pressure for a given volume and a lower gradient between the stomach and duodenum. Rectal prolapse has been reported to occur secondary to constipation, laxative abuse, overzealous exercise and increased intra-abdominal pressure from forced vomiting.

Hepatic and Pancreatic Pathology

In both types of anorexia nervosa, deficiencies of many specific food components may lead to hepatic abnormalities, including hepatomegaly, increases in serum concentrations of lactate dehydrogenase, aspartate and alanine transaminase, and reduction of cholinesterase and plasma proteins. Diffuse liver steatosis may be observed in the most severe forms of the disorder, occasionally evolving in cirrhosis and disappearing with refeeding. Lower than normal plasma concentrations of glutathione are observed, with higher than normal levels of homocysteine, glycine and glutamine, which points to a decreased utilization of these amino acids for glutathione synthesis and an impairment of transsulfuration [15].

Morphological and functional pancreatic abnormalities are frequent in both types of anorexia, sometimes persisting long after recovery [16]. Morphological changes include atrophy with reduced acinar cells and zymogen granules, increases of fibrous interstitial tissue, cystic dilatation of pancreatic ducts and diffuse calcification. The most specific functional abnormality is a reduction of pancreatic enzyme secretion. Amylase and elastase-1 serum concentrations, specific indices of pancreatic dysfunction, are increased. Pancreatitis may be present, but occurs more frequently during refeeding. Amylase levels are generally elevated, correlating with vomiting frequency. The occurrence of pancreatitis may be facilitated by the duodenal stasis followed by duodenal-pancreatic reflux.

Similar alterations may be present in bulimia nervosa [16].

Cardiovascular Complications

Cardiovascular abnormalities occur in up to 87% of people with anorexia [17]. They include sinus bradycardia and much less frequently tachycardia, ventricular arrhythmia resulting from electrolyte disturbances, lower than normal heart rate variation between supine and standing posture, lower than normal ratios of low- and mid-frequency to high-frequency power (which may represent a balance between the activities of the cardiac sympathetic symptoms), cardiac failure, reduced atrial and left ventricular volume, reduced mean cardiac output, and reduced mean ascending aortic velocity. Bradycardia of less than 60 beats/min during the day and around 30 beats/min at night, related to an energy-conserving slowing of the metabolic rate, is possibly linked to vagal hypertonus. Heart rate variability correlates inversely with BMI [18].

As reported in simple starvation, electrocardiographic alterations occur frequently in people with both types of anorexia [19]. They are represented by low voltage, prolonged Q time, increased QT dispersion, longer QRS intervals, a shift to the right of the QRS axis, diminished amplitude of the QRS complex and T wave, depression of the ST tract, inversion of the T wave, occasional U waves linked to hypokalemia and hypomagnesemia, and premature atrial and ventricular heart beats. Ventricular tachyarrhythmias, however, are less frequent. The inversion of the T wave and the prolonged Q time, which increases the risk of tachyarrhythmias, prevail in people with the bingeing subtype of anorexia, with more severe hypokalemia and hypomagnesemia. Sometimes, however, electrocardiographic impairments occur also in people without evident electrolytic alterations, possibly linked to hypertonus of the central autonomic system. Most of the electrocardiographic changes are reversible, often improving rapidly with correction of electrolytic disturbances and a return to normal nutrition and hydration. During the refeeding period, a too rapid weight gain may lead to congestive heart failure and arrhythmias, possibly related to hypophosphatemia occurring during the first weeks of nutritional rehabilitation.

Hypotension, both systolic and diastolic, of less than 90/60 mm Hg occurs in up to 85% of people with anorexia [20], usually as a result of chronic volume depletion and orthostatic changes resulting in frequent bouts of dizziness and occasionally frank syncope. Decreased thickness of ventricular walls, with consequent decreased myocardial contractility and subsequent hypovolemia and reduction of cardiac cavities concur to decrease blood pressure.

People with bulimia may show some of the cardiovascular changes seen in anorexia nervosa, but these are much less frequent and less severe [21]. A slightly longer mean QT has been reported. Hypotension is very uncommon in this disorder. Arrhythmias due to electrolytic disturbances may occur in people with severe purging behaviors.

Pulmonary Disease

Pulmonary alterations do not occur frequently in anorexia nervosa [22], but can occur as a consequence of vomiting or refeeding phenomena. Pneumomediastinum has been observed in the bulimic subtype of anorexia with and without vomiting. The pathology is due to alveolar rupture and subsequent tracking of air along perivascular planes to the mediastinum and subcutaneous area. Subcutaneous emphysema is diagnosed by palpation of the skin overlying the thorax, which reveals a 'crunchy' sensation, and is also heard over the pericardium being synchronous to systole. During rapid refeeding, pulmonary edema may result from congestive heart failure with dyspnea, orthopnea and paroxysmal nocturnal dyspnea. On examination, dullness to percussion of the lung fields and crackles or wheeze on auscultation may be found.

Pulmonary alterations are infrequent in bulimia nervosa [22], and are linked mainly to vomiting and ingestion of the material in the lungs or to a rapid increase in intra-alveolar pressure with alveolar rupture and pneumomediastinum. Pulmonary edema due to congestive heart failure is generally observed only in long-lasting and extremely severe cases.

Renal Disease

Impaired renal function occurs in 70% of starving people with anorexia, with alterations of glomerular filtration rate and concentration capacity, acute or chronic renal failure, increased blood urea, pitting edema, hypokalemic nephropathy, pyuria, hematuria, and proteinuria. An increased risk of urolithiasis has been noted, possibly linked to a combination of high dietary oxalate intake (from tea, spinach, rhubarb, almonds and cashew nuts), chronic dehydration, low urinary excretion and purging. Hypokalemic nephropathy due to the chronic abuse of diuretics or laxatives may occur. This pathology can lead to chronic renal failure with polyuria, polydipsia and increased serum creatinine concentration. High serum levels of uric acid have been seen and along with increased creatinine are considered a poor prognostic feature of the disease [22].

Renal impairment is not frequent in bulimia nervosa [22], unless the pathology is extremely severe; in such cases, abnormalities similar to anorexia are seen.

Musculoskeletal Abnormalities

The most common alterations of the muscular system observed in people with anorexia are muscular weakness, hypotonia and atrophy, which become evident when starvation is markedly severe [23]. A primary myopathy with prominent atrophy of type II fibers is the major abnormality and differs from that observed in simple starvation, which is represented by a mix of type I and II fiber atrophy. Electromyographic studies have revealed increased polyphasic potentials parallel to increases in plasma creatinine-phosphokinase concentrations. Possible causes of this myopathy are the reduced total body potassium levels and caloric and protein deficiency, together with increased physical activity. No muscular alterations have been reported in people with bulimia.

When anorexia has its onset in childhood, patients have reduced skeletal growth, resulting in short stature. Bone accretion and maturation, characteristic of adolescence, are generally retarded, and bone maturation may even totally cease during active phases of the disease [24]. Treatment and weight restoration induce a growth catch-up, which, however, does not reach the expected growth rate. Around a quarter to a third of people with anorexia suffer from osteoporosis, represented by reduced peak bone mass, decreased mineral density, decreased total body mineral content, pathological fractures and vertebral collapse. These alterations correlate with illness duration and BMI. It is not clear whether strenuous weight-bearing exercise can improve bone density in people with anorexia. Osteoporosis and osteopenia also occur in men with anorexia, but with greater severity than in women. Bilateral osteonecrosis of the talus has been reported in anorexia [25].

Increased bone fractures are also observed in bulimia, although less frequently than in anorexia. It is unknown whether the phenomenon is related to osteoporosis (which generally has not been demonstrated in bulimia) or to increased behavioral impulsivity [26].

Hematological Changes

In two thirds of patients with anorexia, neutropenia and reduced monocytes occur, with white blood cell numbers lower than 5,000/mm^3. Relative lymphocytosis and multilobular polymorphonuclear leukocytes are very frequently seen. This alteration could result from bone marrow hypoplasia and its gelatinous transformation with markedly reduced cell production. Gelatinous transformation and cellular necrosis derive from insufficient medullar nutrition, the former occurring when the caloric deficiency develops gradually and the latter when the starvation is acute and extremely rapid, or when other threatening events (e.g. a severe infection) occur concomitantly. People with anorexia may have bone marrow suppression secondary to excessive consumption of phenolphthalein-containing laxatives. The alteration disappears with normal nutrition and weight recovery [23, 27].

Anemia, usually of the normochromic and normocytic type with preserved hemoglobin, is observed in at least one third of people with anorexia [27]. Occasionally, macrocytic anemia may be observed, with elevated mean cell volume due to vitamin B_{12} deficiency. Acanthocytosis, a disorder of the red blood cell membrane, is also observed and is likely linked to abnormalities of cholesterol metabolism. Iron deficiency anemia occurring in anorexia may be normochromic when hemoglobin is above 11 g/dl, or microcytic, hypochromic and with anisocytosis when hemoglobin is below 11 g/dl. Thrombocytopenia has been described in nearly one third of people with anorexia. Purpura and petechiae are infrequent in anorexia.

People with bulimia do not seem to have significant hematological abnormalities.

Metabolic Changes

In anorexia, glucose metabolism is impaired and, even though glucose concentration may be low-normal, the glucose response to a glucose tolerance test is diabetic-like or flat. Insulin and glucagon concentrations are normal or reduced, and inversely correlated with the degree of weight loss. Glucose ingestion results in prolonged insulin peaks [28].

Lipid alterations occur in 50% of people with anorexia, with hypercholesterolemia linked to an increase in LDL cholesterol and elevated fasting free fatty acid concentration [29]. The cholesterol alteration does not correlate with thyroid dysfunction, severity of weight loss, type of food consumption, vomiting or laxative abuse. It may be related to diminished activity of the 5-α-reductase enzyme system. Decreased concentrations of n–6 polyunsaturated fatty acids have been found. Plasma levels of HDL cholesterol, VLDL cholesterol and triglycerides are normal or increased.

Hypercholesterolemia has been observed in bulimia [1].

People with anorexia generally have a reduced concentration of total blood proteins [15]. In particular, globulin levels, more than albumin, are lower than normal. Muscular mass destruction, typical of the disease, is responsible for protein catabolism. Dehydration, hypovolemia, diminished plasma renal flow and diminished glomerular filtration induce an increase of serum urea. Reduced urinary excretion of methylhistidine, a specific index of muscular catabolism, has been observed. Very low albumin levels seem to be highly predictive of death. Reduced blood levels of the essential amino acids, threonine, valine, isoleucine, leucine, and normal or reduced tryptophan levels (including normal or reduced tryptophan to neutral amino acid ratio) have been reported. The tryptophan/neutral amino acid ratio seems to be higher in people with anorexia who are actively exercising. Uric acid is often elevated as an expression of strenuous physical activity combined with starvation resulting in muscle destruction.

No significant protein alterations have been observed in bulimia nervosa.

Electrolyte and Vitamin Alterations

In anorexia, electrolytic alterations occur frequently as a consequence of starvation and malnutrition, vomiting, and laxative and diuretic abuse, with ensuing fluid depletion and hypovolemia [30, 31]. Hypokalemia, hypochloremia and hypochloremic metabolic alkalosis with increased pCO_2 are the most frequently observed alterations. Phosphate and calcium concentrations are generally normal, but vomiting, diarrhea and abuse of diuretics may result in severe hypophosphatemia, which may also be seen during refeeding as a result of transfer of phosphate into cells for phosphorylation of glucose and for protein synthesis. A quarter of people with anorexia [32] develop hypomagnesemia, refractory hypocalcemia caused by increased urinary calcium excretion with renal calculi production, and hypokalemia, which return to normal after magnesium replacement. Iron deficiency and decreased total iron-binding capacity may occur, generally as a consequence of a lack of iron-rich foods. Zinc is low in plasma, urine and tissues linked to the duration and severity of the disease, and zinc deficiency is due to starvation, reduced intestinal absorption of the metal or increased excretion through sweating. Zinc deficiency per se induces anorexia with related weight loss, delayed growth and sexual development, depressed mood, loss of taste, hair loss, and skin alterations resembling those of anorexia. All metal alterations normalize after nutritional rehabilitation.

Hypercarotenemia, normal plasma levels of vitamin A binding protein and retinol-binding protein are observed especially in the restrictive subtype of anorexia following severe starvation and weight loss [33]. Riboflavin and pyridoxine deficiencies have been reported. Vitamin B_{12} and folate concentrations in blood are generally low. Vitamin B_{12} and vitamin C-related pellagra and scurvy have been infrequently reported. Blood 25-hydroxyvitamin D, 1,25-dihydroxyvitamin and 24,25-dihydroxyvitamin concentrations are reduced while vitamin D-binding protein values are normal.

Endocrine Consequences

Hypothalamic-Pituitary-Gonad Axis

Amenorrhea is the most frequent clinical endocrine alteration occurring in underweight women with anorexia, and has long been considered a key criterion for the diagnosis of anorexia [34, 35]. Only recently has it been excluded from the definition of the disorder in the fifth edition of the Diagnostic and Statistical Manual of Mental Disorders, since it has been recognized that menstruation may still occur even in severely malnourished patients or, on the contrary, it may be absent even when body weight is normal. Hypogonadotropic hypogonadism with reduced secretion of luteinizing hormone (LH), follicle-stimulating hormone (FSH), estrogens and progesterone are at the basis of amenorrhea. In the acute phase of anorexia, circadian gonadotropin secretion is similar to that of the prepubertal stage, with secretory pulses almost completely absent during the day and occasionally present at night. The hypothalamic-pituitary-gonad (HPG) axis response to the administration of the gonadotropin-releasing hormone (GnRH) results in low or absent secretion of LH and FSH (with a preponderance of the FSH response over the LH), as occurs before pubertal maturation. Since estrogens are synthesized from androgens in the fat tissue and exert a positive feedback on hypothalamic GnRH secretion, a critical minimum amount of fat tissue seems to be necessary for normal HPG axis functioning [36]. Therefore, in low-fat tissue patients with anorexia, a lack of aromatization of androgens to estrogens, with a consequent hypoestrogenemia is probably responsible for HPG axis dysfunction. However, since in some women amenorrhea precedes weight loss or persists after the recovery of body weight [37], factors other than weight changes may be involved in the HPG axis dysfunction, including the exaggerated physical activity of some women with anorexia. Indeed, in female athletes, menstrual dysfunction has been found to correlate with the intensity of physical exercise rather than with fat mass.

Men with anorexia nervosa are characterized by low levels of testosterone and LH, but normal response of the HPG axis to the administration of GnRH [38, 39]. Moreover, the exocrine testis function seems to be preserved as suggested by the occurrence of normal blood concentrations of inhibin B, which is a marker of gonadal exocrine activity [39]. Therefore, in men with anorexia nervosa, malnutrition seems to have less impact on the gonadal axis.

Oligomenorrhea or amenorrhea occur in almost half of women with bulimia [35], especially when there is a chronic course of bulimic attacks. Normal or decreased levels of plasma gonadotropins, with reduced circadian pulsatility, and diminished concentrations of estrogens and progesterone may be observed. LH secretion is more deranged in its amplitude than in the frequency of secretory pulses, and the LH response to GnRH is normal or even enhanced. These irregularities have been ascribed to food deficiency and especially to protein malnutrition. In addition, since binging episodes increase plasma prolactin levels, it is possible that repeated hyperprolactinemia could impair HPG axis activity due to the inhibitory action of this hormone on GnRH release.

Hypothalamic-Prolactin Axis
Normal baseline concentrations of prolactin are generally observed in people with anorexia, even though slightly reduced or increased plasma levels may be found [40]. Normal diurnal and increased nocturnal concentrations of prolactin have been observed in acutely ill patients. The prolactin response to thyrotropin-releasing hor-

mone (TRH) is normal. Paradoxical responses to both GnRH and GHRH have been detected in the acute phase of the disease [41].

Normal, decreased or increased baseline prolactin levels can be observed in people with bulimia, with a prolactin response to TRH that is generally normal [41].

Hypothalamic-Pituitary-Thyroid Axis
In acutely ill patients with anorexia, triiodothyronine (T_3) levels are lower than normal, reversed T_3 (rT_3) levels (which are biologically inactive) are increased, and thyroxine and thyroid-stimulating hormone (TSH) levels are normal [42]. The lower T_3 levels have been attributed to a reduced peripheral deionization of thyroxine with a simultaneous increased formation of rT_3, which delineates a 'low T_3 syndrome'. This represents a metabolic adaptation to the chronic reduction in caloric intake since it decreases resting energy expenditure [43]. In spite of the reduced secretion of T_3, TSH is not increased in acutely ill patients with anorexia. This could be due to the fact that during low-energy expenditure, a reduction in endogenous metabolic processes occurs in all cells of the organism, including pituitary thyrotropes, which respond as if the low T_3 levels are sufficient for metabolic needs; in such a condition, TSH secretion does not increase. Even if TSH secretion is unaltered in anorexia, its central regulation is deranged. The TSH response to exogenous TRH is delayed and sometimes lower than normal. Finally, atrophy of the thyroid gland may occur in underweight people with anorexia. This alteration has been related to the low insulin-like growth factor-I (IGF-I) levels since thyroid size is clearly influenced by this peptide.

Basal thyroxine and T_3 concentrations are preserved in people with bulimia, even though low circulating T_3 levels have been observed. Baseline concentrations of TSH are mostly normal in bulimia, whereas the TSH response to TRH can be found to be either normal, blunted or delayed [1].

Hypothalamic Growth Hormone-IGF-I Axis

In emaciated people with anorexia, plasma levels of growth hormone (GH) are increased and the plasma concentration of IGF-I and GH-binding protein is reduced [44]. The concentration of the IGF-binding proteins, especially that of the IGF-binding protein-3, is reduced during starvation, although increased levels of circulating IGF-binding proteins resulting in a decrease of free IGF-I have also been reported [45]. In underweight people with anorexia, the decreased IGF-I production increases GH secretion because of diminished negative feedback. Concomitantly, primary or secondary hypothalamic or suprahypothalamic changes may further affect GH production. Increased GH levels correlate negatively with the amount of calories ingested and decrease with improved nutritional intake even before significant weight recovery has taken place. Since GH-binding protein represents the GH receptor extracellular domain, its reduced blood levels mirror a reduced sensitivity to GH. The decrements of IGF-I and GH-binding protein in severely undernourished people with anorexia, an expression of a resistance to GH, are probably the reason why GH hypersecretion in these individuals does not result in acromegalic symptomatology.

The hypothalamic GH-IGF-I axis dysregulation may contribute to the development of osteopenia since IGF-I has a trophic effect on the bone. In prepubertal subjects, the 'resistance' to GH may be one of the causes for the growth delay or cessation persisting following treatment, resulting in a final height lower than that genetically determined [46]. Recombinant human IGF-I or GH have been used in people with anorexia to prevent bone loss or bone fractures, and to facilitate a more rapid metabolic recovery. Recombinant human IGF-I in severely osteopenic women with anorexia increases bone turnover markers in the short term, leading to amelioration of bone density after 9 months, with the latter effect being potentiated by concomitant oral contraceptive administration. Moreover, it has been shown that the recombinant human GH in people with anorexia achieves medical and cardiovascular stability more rapidly [47].

Normal or increased GH levels with a normal circadian rhythm are reported in people with bulimia, while circulating IGF-I is reduced [1].

Hypothalamic-Pituitary-Adrenal Axis

Abnormalities of the hypothalamic-pituitary-adrenal (HPA) axis are frequently present in people with anorexia, including increased plasma levels of cortisol with normal blood concentrations of adrenocorticotropic hormone (ACTH), and increased urinary cortisol levels in the acute phase of the disease [48]. The circadian rhythm of ACTH is well preserved, but plasma cortisol concentrations are higher than normal throughout the day and have an increased number and amplitude of cortisol secretory bursts, especially during the middle afternoon when values of the hormone should be at their lowest point. These data suggest that the HPA axis in the acute phase of anorexia is hyperactive. Dynamic studies of HPA axis function tend to demonstrate that hypothalamic and/or suprahypothalamic alterations may cause the higher than normal activity of the axis [49]. Indeed, most people with anorexia cannot suppress cortisol production during the dexamethasone suppression test; the cortisol responses to ACTH stimulation are enhanced while the ACTH response to corticotropin-releasing factor (CRF) is reduced/normal in underweight individuals with anorexia [50]. Since these alterations revert with the recovery of body weight, they are considered a consequence of malnutrition, although this is controversial [51]. In experimental animals, CRF provokes anorexia, increased physical activity and reduced sexual behavior, which would support a role for this peptide in the development and/or maintenance of some anorexic symptoms. Clinically, it is intriguing that the hypercortisolemia of people with anorexia never leads to the development of Cushingoid features.

The adrenal glands also secrete androgen dehydroepiandrosterone (DHEA) and DHEA sulfate (DHEAS) under the regulation of the CRF-ACTH system. Evidence for a decreased production of both DHEA and DHEAS in underweight people with anorexia has been widely reported, with a dissociation in the adrenal secretion between cortisol and androgen similar to that observed in the pubertal stage of sexual maturation [52]. This suggests that people with postpubertal acute anorexia may regress to a prepubertal secretory aspect of the reproductive axis (see below), also affecting the HPA androgen system. This reduction, together with the increase in cortisol levels, leads to decreased DHEA to cortisol and DHEAS to cortisol ratios similar to that occurring in the pubertal stage of sexual maturation [53].

In people with bulimia, HPA axis activity is only slightly altered, with morning plasma cortisol concentrations either normal or increased, while urinary excretion of free cortisol and 17-hydroxycorticosteroids as well as cortisol responses to CRF or ACTH are normal. The most widely reported alteration of the HPA axis in bulimia is the nonsuppression of cortisol to a dexamethasone challenge in 20–60% of patients, without significant correlations with severity and chronicity of the illness, concomitant depressive symptoms, or previous history of anorexia. This alteration disappears after successful treatment of bulimia, and is not predictive of treatment outcome [54].

Conclusions

In people with eating disorders, physical complications are very common and usually occur as consequences of nutritional derangements secondary to aberrant eating and abnormal compensatory behaviors. In the most severe cases, these complications represent a significant threat to the patient's life. In emaciated people with anorexia, especially in those who vomit and/or abuse diuretics and laxatives, immediate

Table 2. Main signs and symptoms of the physical complications of anorexia and bulimia nervosa

Anorexia nervosa
Signs
    Hypothermia
    Bradycardia (<60 beats/min)
    Hypotension (<90 mm Hg systolic pressure)
    Dry skin
    Brittle hair
    Brittle nails
    Hair loss
    Yellow-orange dry and dystrophic skin (especially on the palmar surfaces of hands and on the plantar surfaces of feet)
    Lanugo hair
    Edema (ankles, around eyes)
    Cardiac murmur (caused by mitral prolapse)
Symptoms
    Amenorrhea
    Fatigue
    Faintness
    Dizziness
    Abdominal pain
    Sensation of fullness
    Polyuria
    Cold intolerance
    Constipation
    Polydipsia

Bulimia nervosa
Signs
    Russell's sign (calluses on knuckles)
    Salivary gland hypertrophy
    Tooth enamel erosion
    Perioral ulcerations
    Petechiae
    Lanugo hair
    Hematemesis (vomiting of blood)
    Edema (ankles, around eyes)
    Abdominal bloating
    Dysregulated heart beat
Symptoms
    Dysregulated menses
    Heart palpitations
    Esophagus burning pain
    Abdominal pain
    Abdominal bloating
    Faintness
    Constipation or diarrhea
    Hands and feet swelling
    Sensitive teeth

risks come from electrolytic perturbations and starvation-induced cardiovascular and renal complications. These complications may lead to the development of severe arrhythmias and sudden death. Individuals with a chronic course of anorexia are exposed to consequences of the progressive impairment in bone density, which increases the likelihood of pathological fractures. On the other hand, some of the somatic alterations occurring in the acute phase of anorexia seem to have a protective effect. Indeed, in emaciated people with anorexia, the impaired function of the reproductive axis and the reduced activity of thyroid gland aim to preserve residual energy stores for vital functions and reduce basal metabolic needs.

In bulimia, physical complications are less severe and occur less frequently than in anorexia. Therefore, they rarely represent a serious threat to the patient's life. The most harmful complications are represented by esophageal and/or gastric ruptures, secondary to the massive ingestion of food in the course of binge episodes, and cardiac arrhythmias induced by severe electrolytic imbalance following vomiting and diuretic or laxative abuse.

Although, with a few exceptions, physical complications resolve with the recovery of body weight and the discontinuation of aberrant behaviors, they contribute, together with suicide, to the high mortality of patients with eating disorders. Indeed, anorexia has the highest mortality of any psychiatric diagnosis, estimated at 10% within 10 years of diagnosis, and is the leading cause of death in young females 15–24 years of age. Mortality for bulimia is approximately 1% within 10 years of diagnosis. It is important to remember that even if most of the physical complications of eating disorders do not represent life-threatening conditions, they increase the patients' burden of suffering, impair their quality of life and, therefore, need clinical consideration and appropriate treatment. Therefore, psychiatrists who have patients with anorexia nervosa and bulimia nervosa should be alerted to identify those signs and symptoms that express malnutrition-related physical complications (table 2) and collaborate with medical experts who specialize in the treatment of physical alterations. This will ensure the simultaneous correction of psychopathological and physical aberrations in order to obtain a full and fast recovery from the diseases.

References

1 Brambilla F, Monteleone P: Physical complication and physiological aberrations in eating disorders: a review; in Maj M, Halmi K, Lopez-Ibor J, Sartorius N (eds): Eating Disorders. Chichester, Wiley & Sons, 2003, pp 139–222.
2 Carney CP, Andersen AE: Eating disorders: guideline to medical evaluation and complications. Psychiatr Clin North Am 1996;19:657–679.
3 Crow S: Physical complications of eating disorders; in Wonderlich S, Mitchell J, de Zwaan M, Steiger H (eds): Eating Disorders Review, Part 1. Oxford, Radcliffe Publishing, 2005, pp 127–137.
4 Patrik L: Eating disorders: a review of the literature with emphasis on physical complications and clinical nutrition. Altern Med Rev 2002;7:184–202.
5 Schwabe AD, Lippe BM, Chang RJ, Pops MA, Yager J: Anorexia nervosa. Ann Intern Med 1981;94:371–381.
6 Strumia R, Varotti E, Manzato E, Gualandi M: Skin signs in anorexia nervosa. Dermatology 2001;203:314–317.
7 Russell G: Bulimia nervosa: an ominous variant of anorexia nervosa. Psychol Med 1979;9:429–448.
8 Gupta MA, Gupta AK, Haberman HF: Dermatologic signs in anorexia nervosa and bulimia nervosa. Arch Dermatol 1987;123:1386–1390.
9 Clark DC: Oral complications of anorexia nervosa and/or bulimia: with a review of the literature. J Oral Med 1985;40: 134–138.
10 Sharp CW, Freeman CP: The physical complications of anorexia nervosa. Br J Psychiatry 1993;162:452–462.
11 Waldholtz B, Andersen AE: Gastrointestinal symptoms in anorexia nervosa: a prospective study. Gastroenterology 1990;98:1415–1419.
12 Chiarioni G, Bassotti G, Monsignori A, Menegotti M, Saladini C, Di Matteo G, Vantini I, Whitehead WE: Anorectal dysfunction in constipated women with anorexia nervosa. Mayo Clin Proc 2000; 75:1015–1019.

13 Anderson L, Shaw JM, McCargar L: Physiological effects of bulimia nervosa on the gastrointestinal tract. Can J Gastroenterol 1997;11:451–459.

14 Geliebter A, Hashim SA: Gastric capacity in normal, obese, and bulimic women. Physiol Behav 2001;74:743–746.

15 Umeki S: Biochemical abnormalities of the serum in anorexia nervosa. J Nerv Ment Dis 1988;176:503–506.

16 Kobayashi N, Tamai H, Uehata S, Komaki G, Mori K, Matsubayashi S, Nakagawa T: Pancreatic abnormalities in patients with eating disorders. Psychosom Med 1988;50:607–614.

17 Fohlin L: Body composition, cardiovascular and renal function in adolescent patients with anorexia nervosa. Acta Paediat Scand 1977;268(suppl):1–20.

18 Arik TH, Dresser KB, Benchimol A: Cardiac complications of intensive dieting and eating disorders. Ariz Med 1985;42:72–74.

19 Webb JG, Birmingham CL, MacDonald IL: Electrocardiographic abnormalities in anorexia nervosa. Int J Eat Disord 1988;7:785–790.

20 Warren MP, Vande Wiele RL: Clinical and metabolic features of anorexia nervosa. Am J Obstet Gynecol 1973;117:435–449.

21 Panagiotopoulos C, McCrindle BW, Hick K, Katzman DK: Electrocardiographic findings in adolescents with eating disorders. Pediatrics 2000;105:1100–1105.

22 Palla B, Litt IF: Physical complications of eating disorders in adolescents. Pediatrics 1988;81:613–623.

23 Alloway R, Shur E, Obrecht R, Russell GF: Physical complications in anorexia nervosa. Haematological and neuromuscular changes in 12 patients. Br J Psychiatry 1988;153:72–75.

24 Crisp AH: Some skeletal measurements in patients with primary anorexia nervosa. J Psychosom Res 1969;13:125–142.

25 Rigotti NA, Nussbaum SR, Herzog DB, Neer RM: Osteoporosis in women with anorexia nervosa. N Engl J Med 1984;311:1601–1606.

26 Carmichael KA, Carmichael DH: Bone metabolism and osteopenia in eating disorders. Medicine (Baltimore) 1995;74:254–267.

27 Lambert M, Hubert C, Depresseux G, Vande Berg B, Thissen JP, Nagant de Deuxchaisnes C, Devogelaer JP: Hematological changes in anorexia nervosa are correlated with total body fat mass depletion. Int J Eat Disord 1997;21:329–334.

28 Silverman JA: Clinical and metabolic aspects of anorexia nervosa. Int J Eat Disord 1983;2:159–166.

29 Crisp AH, Blendis LM, Pawan GL: Aspects of fat metabolism in anorexia nervosa. Metabolism 1968;17:1109–1118.

30 Fonseca V, Havard CW: Electrolyte disturbances and cardiac failure with hypomagnesaemia in anorexia nervosa. Br Med J 1985;291:1680–1682.

31 Mars DR, Anderson NH, Riggall FC: Anorexia nervosa: a disorder with severe acid-base derangement. South Med J 1982;75:1038–1042.

32 Mitchell JE, Bantle JP: Metabolic and endocrine investigations in women of normal weight with the bulimia syndrome. Biol Psychiatry 1983;18:355–365.

33 Casper RC, Kirschner B, Sandstead HH, Jacob RA, Davis JM: A evaluation of trace metals, vitamins, and taste function in anorexia nervosa. Am J Clin Nutr 1980;33:1801–1808.

34 Brown GM, Garfinkel PE, Jeuniewic N, Moldofsky H, Stancer HC: Endocrine profiles in anorexia nervosa; in Vigersky RA (ed): Anorexia Nervosa. New York, Raven Press, 1977, pp 123–136.

35 Frisch RE, McArthur JW: Menstrual cycles: fatness as a determinant of minimum weight for height necessary for their maintenance or onset. Science 1974;185:949–951.

36 Jeuniewic N, Brown GM, Garfinkel PE, Moldofsky H: Hypothalamic function as related to body weight and body fat in anorexia nervosa. Psychosom Med 1978;40:187–198.

37 Copeland PM, Natalie R, Sacks MS, Herzog DB: Longitudinal follow-up of amenorrhea in eating disorders. Psychosom Med 1995;57:121–126.

38 Tomova A, Kumanov P: Sex differences and similarities of hormonal alterations in patients with anorexia nervosa. Andrologia 1999;31:143–147.

39 Galusca B, Leca V, Garmain N, Frere D, Khalfallah Y, Lang F, Estour B: Normal inhibin B levels suggest partial preservation of gonadal function in adult male patients with anorexia nervosa. J Sex Med 2012;9:1442–1447.

40 Monteleone P, Brambilla F, Bortolotti F, Maj M: Serotoninergic dysfunction across the eating disorders: relationship to eating behaviour, purging behaviour, nutritional status and general psychopathology. Psychol Med 2000;30:1099–1110.

41 Kiriike N, Nishiwaki S, Izuniya Y, Maeda Y, Kawakitia Y: Thyrotropin, prolactin and growth hormone responses to thyrotropin-releasing hormone in anorexia nervosa and bulimia. Biol Psychiatry 1987;22:167–176.

42 Burman KD, Virgesky RA, Loriaux DL, Strum D, Djuh YY, Wright FD, Wartofsky L: Investigations concerning deiodinative pathways in patients with anorexia nervosa; in Vigersky RA (ed): Anorexia Nervosa. New York, Raven Press, 1977, pp 255–262.

43 Moore R, Mills IH: Serum T3 and T4 levels in patients with anorexia nervosa showing transient hyperthyroidism during weight gain. Clin Endocrinol 1979;10:443–448.

44 Counts DR, Gwirtsman H, Carlsson LM, Lesem M, Cuttler GB Jr: The effect of anorexia nervosa and refeeding on growth hormone-binding protein, the insulin-like growth factors (IGFs) and IGF-binding proteins. J Clin Endocrinol Metab 1992;75:762–767.

45 Argente J, Caballo N, Barrios V, Munoz MT, Pozo J, Chowen JA, Morande G, Hernandez M: Multiple endocrine abnormalities of the growth hormone and insulin-like growth factor axis in patients with anorexia nervosa: effects of short- and long-term weight recuperation. J Clin Endocrinol Metab 1997;82:2084–2092.

46 Nussbaum M, Baird D, Sonnenblick M, Cowan K, Shenker IR: Short stature in anorexia nervosa patients. J Adolesc Health Care 1985;6:453–455.

47 Grinspoon S, Thomas L, Miller K, Herzog D, Klibanski A: Effects of recombinant human IGF-I and oral contraceptive administration on bone density in anorexia nervosa. J Clin Endocrinol Metab 2002;87:2883–2891.

48 Bliss E, Migeon CJ: Endocrinology of anorexia nervosa. J Clin Endocrinol Metab 1957;17:766–776.

49 Walsh BT, Katz JL, Levin J, Kream J, Fukushima DK, Hellman LD, Weiner H, Zumoff B: Adrenal activity in anorexia nervosa. Psychosom Med 1978;40:499–506.

50 Müller E, Cavagnini F, Panerai AE, Massironi R, Ferrari E, Brambilla F: Neuroendocrine measures in anorexia nervosa: comparisons with primary affective disorders. Adv Biochem Psychopharmacol 1987;43:261–271.

51 Herpetz Dahlmann B, Remschmidt H: The prognostic value of the dexamethasone suppression test for the course of anorexia nervosa in comparison with depressive diseases (in German). Z Kinder Jugenpsychiatr 1990;18:5–11.

52 Zumoff B, Walsh BT, Katz JL, Levin J, Rosenfeld RJ, Kream J, Weiner H: Subnormal plasma dehydroisoandrosterone to cortisol ratio in anorexia nervosa: a second hormonal parameter of ontogenic regression. J Clin Endocrinol Metab 1983;56:668–672.

53 Winterer J, Gwirtsman HE, George DT, Kaye WH, Loriaux DL, Cutler GB: Adrenocorticotropin stimulated adrenal androgen secretion in anorexia nervosa: impaired secretion at low weight with normalization after long term weight recovery. J Clin Endocrinol Metab 1985; 61:693–697.

54 Walsh BT, Roose SR, Lindy DC, Gladis M, Glassman AH: Hypothalamic-pituitary-adrenal axis in bulimia; in Hudson JI, Pope HG (eds): The Psychobiology of Bulimia. Washington, American Psychiatric Press, 1987, pp 3–11.

Palmiero Monteleone, MD
Department of Medicine and Surgery
University of Salerno
Via S. Allende, IT–84081 Baronissi, Salerno (Italy)
E-Mail monteri@tin.it

Sartorius N, Holt RIG, Maj M (eds): Comorbidity of Mental and Physical Disorders.
Key Issues Ment Health. Basel, Karger, 2015, vol 179, pp 81–87 (DOI: 10.1159/000365538)

Anxiety and Related Disorders and Physical Illness

Catherine Kariuki-Nyuthe[a] · Dan J. Stein[b]

[a] Eastern Health Outer East Mobile Support and Treatment Service, Ringwood East, Vic., Australia;
[b] Department of Psychiatry and Mental Health, University of Cape Town, Cape Town, South Africa

Abstract

Anxiety and related disorders are the most prevalent mental disorders in the general population. There is a strong bidirectional association between anxiety and related disorders and co-occurring general medical conditions. The co-occurrence of anxiety and related disorders and general medical conditions is associated with significant impairment, morbidity and economic costs. At the same time, recognition of anxiety and related disorders in people with medical illness may be challenging when comorbid with physical illness due in part to overlap in symptomatology. Furthermore, there is a relatively limited evidence base of randomized controlled trials in this population. Additional work is needed to improve screening for anxiety and related disorders in medical illness, to enhance diagnosis and assessment, and to optimize treatment.   © 2015 S. Karger AG, Basel

Anxiety disorders, obsessive-compulsive and related disorders, and trauma- and stressor-related disorders are the most prevalent psychiatric disorders in the general population [1, 2], with generalized anxiety disorder the most common anxiety disorder in primary care populations [3]. Indeed, these anxiety and related disorders occur frequently with a range of general medical disorders [4, 5], including gastrointestinal disease [6], pulmonary disease [7, 8], cardiovascular disease [9], endocrine disorders [10], dermatological disorders [11] and cancer [12], as well as neuropsychiatric disorders such as chronic pain [13, 14], migraines [15], dementia [16] and Parkinson's disease [17]. In this chapter we review the epidemiology of comorbid anxiety and related disorders and physical illness, the growing evidence of a bidirectional relationship between these sets of conditions [18] and relevant randomized controlled trials in this area.

Epidemiology

Anxiety and related disorders are the most common psychiatric disorders worldwide, with a 12-month prevalence worldwide of between 4 and 20% [2]. The onset of anxiety and related disorders usually happens in childhood or adolescence, with many individuals first presenting with physical symptoms in primary care settings

Table 1. Common medical conditions associated with anxiety

Endocrine disorders	diabetes mellitus [32], thyroid disease [10], catecholamine-secreting pheochromocytoma
Gastrointestinal disorders	peptic ulcers [27], celiac disease [33], irritable bowel syndrome [26]
Musculoskeletal disorders	fibromyalgia/chronic fatigue syndrome [34], arthritis [35]
Neurological disorders	migraines [15], epilepsy, neurodegenerative illness [17]
Cardiorespiratory disease	asthma [30], angina [25], chronic obstructive pulmonary disease [7], mitral valve prolapse [36], cystic fibrosis [8], obesity [24, 37, 38]
Chronic pain	burns [14], cancer [12]
Infectious disease	HIV [39], tuberculosis [39]

[4]. Anxiety and related disorders are prevalent throughout life [19–22]. Furthermore, while the prevalence of comorbid anxiety and related disorders in those with chronic medical illness is not as well studied as depression in medical conditions, studies which have been done indicate it is as common [22–25]. A large cross-sectional study demonstrated that generalized anxiety disorder was the most prevalent anxiety disorder in primary care settings [3].

Systematic reviews have established that anxiety disorders are particularly prevalent in gastrointestinal disorders, pulmonary disease, cardiovascular disease, endocrine disease and cancer, as well as neuropsychiatric disorders such as chronic pain and migraines. In irritable bowel syndrome, up to 95% of patients have generalized anxiety disorder or panic disorder [26]. Similarly, panic disorder and generalized anxiety disorder were more prevalent in those with peptic ulcer disease [27]. In asthma, anxiety disorders occur in at least 25% of patients [28, 29]. In multiple studies of adolescents and adults with asthma, the prevalence of panic disorder and agoraphobia is almost three times that of the general population [30, 31]. Another anxiety disorder that co-occurs with respiratory illness is generalized anxiety disorder [31]. Table 1 outlines medical conditions associated with anxiety symptoms and disorders.

The co-occurrence of anxiety and general medical conditions is associated with significant impairment, morbidity and economic costs [36, 40–42]. For example, in a study of almost 500 medically ill persons diagnosed with anxiety disorders, those with posttraumatic stress disorder, panic disorder and social anxiety disorder were found more likely to be frequent consumers of healthcare, and to remain unable to maintain their roles and responsibilities, including work [43]. Medical comorbidities with anxiety disorders have also been shown to elevate suicide risk [44]. Adequate management of anxiety symptoms can improve outcomes of physical ill-health, and reduce the use of healthcare resources [4, 45]. In addition, some work suggests that quality of life and functional ability may be improved with optimal treatment of comorbid general medical and anxiety disorders [46–48].

Etiology

There is a growing body of evidence for a strong bidirectional association between anxiety and related disorders and co-occurring general medical conditions [14, 29, 49]. On the one hand, medical disorders may lead to fears about diagnosis, hospitalization, painful procedures and a foreshortened lifespan, while certain medical disorders may be linked physiologically to the development of anxiety and related disorders [50]. On the other hand, anxiety and related disorders may lead to vulnerability for various medical conditions. There may also be underlying factors that contribute to susceptibility for both anxiety disorders and physical conditions [51].

There is ongoing work to determine the precise nature of the relationships between anxiety disorders and physical illness in a number of areas. Thus, in irritable bowel syndrome, it has been suggested that infection or inflammation of the gastrointestinal tract lead to anxiety [29], while in asthma it has been postulated that increased partial pressure of carbon dioxide is responsible for panic attacks [52]. On the other hand, neurotransmitter disturbances and hypothalamic-pituitary-adrenal axis dysfunction have been postulated to play a key role in explaining how anxiety symptoms and disorders lead to medical illnesses [53].

The common underlying factors that may contribute to both anxiety disorders and comorbid physical illness have also received ongoing study. Genetic factors may, for example, predispose to both general medical conditions and anxiety disorders [54, 55]. In the World Mental Health Surveys, there were strong relationships between early adversity and subsequent onset of both anxiety disorders and various physical disorders, including chronic spinal pain, chronic headache, heart disease, asthma, diabetes and hypertension [56, 57].

Clinical Features

Recognition of anxiety disorders in people with medical illness can be challenging for several reasons. Firstly, anxiety symptoms are an understandable response to the diagnosis of medical conditions. A medical condition can be sufficient enough to be a stressor for an individual to develop an adjustment disorder, and in some cases even posttraumatic stress disorder. Secondly, anxiety symptoms may overlap with symptoms of an underlying medical disorder; thus, since patients with cancer may have insomnia and fatigue, conditions such as generalized anxiety disorder are overlooked. Similarly, medications used in the treatment of physical disorders may lead to anxiety symptoms [20, 49, 58].

In a patient with anxiety symptoms, a range of different diagnoses can be considered. Table 2 tabulates the main features of key anxiety and related disorders. Posttraumatic stress disorder is the anxiety and related disorder that is most commonly associated with gastrointestinal, cardiac, endocrine, chronic pain, migraines and Parkinson's disease [14, 22]. Symptoms of generalized anxiety disorder arguably most closely resemble those of many general medical conditions, particularly in the older population [20]. Panic disorder may, however, mimic a number of physical illnesses. Indeed, a broad range of different anxiety and related disorders have been associated with various physical illnesses.

Management

Early identification of anxiety symptoms and disorders in individuals with chronic illness is important in determining better outcomes for individuals with both sets of disorders [60–62]. The therapeutic alliance and collaboration between medical professionals may contribute to successful management of symptoms [50]. There is, however, a paucity of robust evidence in the treatment of chronically ill patients with comorbid anxiety and related disorders [51].

Cognitive behavioral therapy has been undertaken in a number of studies of individuals with medical illness and anxiety and related disorders. A systematic review of 32 psychotherapy

Table 2. Anxiety and related disorders commonly seen in medically ill adult patients [14, 59]

Generalized anxiety disorder	characterized by a pervasive and excessive worry about everyday life events; this worry is difficult to control and is accompanied by somatic symptoms which impair the individual's functioning
Specific phobia	characterized by excessive, irrational and persistent fear of specific objects, situations or activities such as heights, flying and spiders
Social anxiety disorder	characterized by an intense and excessive fear of scrutiny and humiliation in social situations which then leads to avoidance of these situations, or development of panic attacks when the situations are endured
Panic disorder	characterized by recurrent unexpected panic attacks described as discrete events in which the individual experiences symptoms that peak within a few minutes and resolve spontaneously, coupled with anticipatory anxiety about future panic attacks
Posttraumatic disorder	a disorder in which the individual experiences a traumatic event; the disorder is then characterized by recurrent distressing re-experiencing phenomena, increased arousal, persistent avoidance of reminders and stimuli associated with the event, and negative cognitions and mood
Hypochondriasis	characterized by preoccupation with having a severe disease; the individual cannot be reassured despite medical investigations
Obsessive-compulsive disorder	characterized by recurrent intrusive distressing thoughts or images (obsessions) which are neutralized by some other thought or repetitive mental act/behavior (compulsions)
Substance/medication-induced anxiety disorder	characterized by anxiety symptoms which are directly related to the physiological effects of a substance or medication
Adjustment disorder with anxiety	characterized by a time-limited, maladaptive anxiety response to an identifiable stressor
Separation anxiety disorder	characterized by excessive, developmentally inappropriate anxiety upon separation of the child from the home or from significant attachment figures
Anxiety disorder not otherwise specified	diagnosed when the individual's symptoms are severe and distressing but do not meet diagnostic criteria for any other anxiety disorder

trials in patients with irritable bowel syndrome and anxiety disorders indicates the efficacy of cognitive behavioral therapy in reducing somatic distress [63–65]. A systematic review of 20 studies of cognitive-behavioral interventions in nearly 3,000 participants found that they may be effective in the management of HIV-/AIDS-associated anxiety [66]. Cognitive behavioral therapy has also been shown to reduce anxiety symptoms and distress in patients with cardiac disease and anxiety in one randomized controlled trial [67].

Behavioral strategies in anxiety disorders and comorbid medical illnesses include biofeedback, relaxation training and meditation [68, 69]. Two randomized controlled trials examining the effects of biofeedback in the management of asthma [69], and another two randomized controlled trials looking at relaxation therapy showed a reduction in the use of bronchodilator agents and improved quality of life [70].

Hypnotherapy and interpersonal therapy are other treatment modalities showing promise in the management of pain related to procedures for

Kariuki-Nyuthe · Stein

cancer therapies [71, 72], but rigorous studies are lacking in this area [14, 64].

In patients with physical illness and anxiety and related disorders, there are relatively few randomized controlled trials to guide treatment choices. Thus, medications should be selected based on studies of efficacy in anxiety disorders, and on minimizing adverse events and drug-drug interactions. The selective serotonin reuptake inhibitors sertraline, citalopram and escitalopram have relatively few adverse events and are safe in interaction with other agents [73]. The serotonin-noradrenaline reuptake inhibitors venlafaxine and duloxetine have the potential advantage of being beneficial for pain symptoms, but venlafaxine has the disadvantage of requiring blood pressure monitoring [74]. Drugs such as mirtazapine and the tricyclic antidepressants may be efficacious in the treatment of some anxiety disorders, but carry a significant side-effect profile and may have worrisome drug-drug interactions [74]. Benzodiazepines and sedative-hypnotic agents may be helpful for anxiety symptoms, but should be used cautiously due to concerns of dependence [6]. The second-generation antipsychotic quetiapine is anxiolytic at low doses, and is efficacious in the treatment of some anxiety and related disorders [50], but its metabolic, cardiac and autonomic side-effect burden should be taken into consideration.

Conclusion

Anxiety and related disorders are frequently comorbid with chronic medical conditions. There is growing understanding of the bidirectional relationships between these sets of disorders. Recognition can be delayed due to the similarity of primary anxiety symptoms and anxiety secondary to general medical conditions. Pharmacotherapy management can be effective, but clinicians need to be aware of the side-effect burden of psychotropics in medical conditions as well as potential drug-drug interactions. There is a growing database of studies of cognitive-behavioral therapy showing efficacy in individuals with anxiety disorders and comorbid medical illness. Further work is needed to improve screening for anxiety and related disorders in medical illness, to enhance diagnosis and assessment, and to optimize treatment.

References

1 Kessler RC, Aguilar-Gaxiola S, Alonso J, et al: The global burden of mental disorders: an update from the WHO World Mental Health (WMH) Surveys. Epidemiol Psichiatr Soc 2009;18:23–33.

2 Kessler RC, Berglund P, Demler O, et al: Lifetime prevalence and age-of-onset distributions of DSM-IV disorders in the National Comorbidity Survey Replication. Arch Gen Psychiatry 2005;62:593–602.

3 Fava GA, Porcelli P, Rafanelli C, et al: The spectrum of anxiety disorder in the medically ill. J Clin Psychiatry 2010;71:910–914.

4 Mago R, Gomez JP, Gupta N, et al: Anxiety in medically ill patients. Curr Psychiatry Rep 2006;8:228–233.

5 Skodol AE: Anxiety in the medically ill: nosology and principles of differential diagnosis. Semin Clin Neuropsychiatry 1999;4:64–71.

6 Lydiard RB: Irritable bowel syndrome, anxiety and depression: what are the links? J Clin Psychiatry 2001;62:38–45.

7 Brenes GA: Anxiety and chronic obstructive pulmonary disease: prevalence, impact, and treatment. Psychosom Med 2003;65:963–970.

8 Cruz I, Marciel KK, Quittner AL, et al: Anxiety and depression in cystic fibrosis. Semin Respir Crit Care Med 2009;30:569–578.

9 Fan AZ, Strine TW, Jiles R, et al: Depression and anxiety associated with cardiovascular disease among persons aged 45 years and older in 38 states of the United States, 2006. Prev Med 2008;46:445–450.

10 Simon NM, Blacker D, Korbly NB, et al: Hypothyroidism and hyperthyroidism in anxiety disorders revisited: new data and literature review. J Affect Disord 2002;69:209–217.

11 Hayes J, Koo J: Psoriasis: depression, anxiety, smoking, and drinking habits. Dermatol Ther 2010;23:174–180.

12 Mitchell AJ, Chan M, Bhatti H, et al: Prevalence of depression, anxiety, and adjustment disorder in oncological, haematological, and palliative-care settings: a meta-analysis of 94 interview-based studies. Lancet Oncol 2011;12:160–174.

13 Williams LJ, Pasco JA, Jacka FN, et al: Pain and the relationship with mood and anxiety disorders and psychological symptoms. J Psychosom Res 2012;72: 452–456.

14 Jordan KD, Okifuji A: Anxiety disorders: differential diagnosis and their relationship to chronic pain. J Pain Palliat Care Psychother 2011;25:231–245.

15 Culpepper L: Generalized anxiety disorder and medical illness. J Clin Psychiatry 2009;70:20–24.

16 Wragg RE, Jeste DV: Overview of depression and psychosis in Alzheimer's disease. Am J Psychiatry 1989;146:577–587.

17 Stein MB, Heuser IJ, Juncos JL, et al: Anxiety disorders in patients with Parkinson's disease. Am J Psychiatry 1990; 147:217–220.

18 Sanna L, Stuart AL, Pasco JA, et al: Physical comorbidities in men with mood and anxiety disorders: a population-based study. BMC Med 2013;11: 110.

19 Hirsch JK, Walker KL, Chang EC, et al: Illness burden and symptoms of anxiety in older adults: optimism and pessimism as moderators. Int Psychogeriatr 2012;24:1614–1621.

20 Wetherell JL, Ayers CR, Nuovo R, et al: Medical conditions and depressive, anxiety, and somatic symptoms in older adults with and without generalized anxiety disorder. Aging Ment Health 2010;14:764–768.

21 Pao M, Bosk A: Anxiety in medically ill children/adolescents. Depress Anxiety 2011;28:40–49.

22 Scott KM, Bruffaerts R, Tsang A, et al: Depression-anxiety relationships with chronic physical conditions: results from the World Mental Health Surveys. J Affect Disord 2007;103:113–120.

23 Chou SP, Huang B, Goldstein R, et al: Temporal associations between physical illness and mental disorders – results from the Wave 2 National Epidemiologic Survey on Alcohol and Related Conditions (NESARC). Compr Psychiatry 2013;54:627–638.

24 Scott KM, McGee MA, Wells JE, et al: Obesity and mental disorders in the adult general population. J Psychosom Res 2008;64:97–105.

25 Beitman BD, Kushner MG, Basha I: Follow-up status of patients with angiographically normal coronary arteries and panic disorder. JAMA 1991;265: 1545–1549.

26 Whitehead WE, Palsson O, Jones KR: Systematic review of the comorbidity of irritable bowel syndrome with other disorders: what are the causes and implications? Gastroenterology 2002;122: 1140–1156.

27 Harter MC, Conway KP, Merikangas KR: Associations between anxiety disorders and physical illness. Eur Arch Psychiatry Clin Neurosci 2003;253:313–320.

28 Katon WJ: Panic Disorder in the Medical Setting. Publication No. 94-3482. Washington, National Institutes of Health, 1994.

29 Katon W, Lin EH, Kroenke K: The association of depression and anxiety with medical symptom burden in patients with chronic medical illness. Gen Hosp Psychiatry 2007;29:147–155.

30 Goodwin RD, Jacobi F, Thefeld W, et al: Mental disorders and asthma in the community. Arch Gen Psychiatry 2003; 60:1125–1130.

31 Smoller JW, Simon NM, Pollack MH, et al: Anxiety in patients with pulmonary disease: comorbidities and treatment. Semin Clin Neuropsychiatry 1999;4: 84–97.

32 Lin EH, Korff MV, Alonso J, et al: Mental disorders among persons with diabetes – results from the World Mental Health Surveys. J Psychosom Res 2008; 65:571–580.

33 Smith DF, Gerdes LU, et al: Meta-analysis on anxiety and depression in adult celiac disease. Acta Psychiatr Scand 2012;125:189–193.

34 Arnold LM: Antidepressants for fibromyalgia: latest word on the link to depression and anxiety. Curr Psychiatry 2002;1:49–54.

35 Smedstad LM, Vaglum P, Kvien TK, et al: The relationship between self-reported pain and sociodemographic variables, anxiety and depressive symptoms in rheumatoid arthritis. J Rheumatol 1995;22:514–520.

36 Zaubler T, Katon W: Panic disorder in the general medical setting. J Psychosom Res 1998;44:25–42.

37 Yanovski SZ, Nelson JE, Dubbert BK, et al: Association of binge eating disorder and psychiatric co-morbidity in obese subjects. Am J Psychiatry 1993;150: 1472–1479.

38 Vieweg WV, Julius DA, Benesek J, et al: Posttraumatic stress disorder and body mass index in military veterans. Preliminary findings. Prog Neuropsychopharmacol Biol Psychiatry 2006;30:1150–1154.

39 Van den Heuvel L, Chisinga N, Kinyanda E: Frequency and correlates of anxiety and mood disorders among TB- and HIV-infected Zambians. AIDS Care 2013;25:1527–1535.

40 Cully JA, Graham DP, Stanley MA, et al: Quality of life in patients with chronic obstructive pulmonary disease and comorbid anxiety and depression. Psychosomatics 2006;47:312–319.

41 Brenes GA: Anxiety, depression and quality of life in primary care patients. Prim Care Companion J Clin Psychiatry 2007;9:437–443.

42 Sareen J, Jacobi F, Cox BJ, et al: Disability and poor quality of life associated with comorbid anxiety disorder and physical conditions. Arch Intern Med 2006;166:2109–2116.

43 Stein MB, Roy-Byrne PP, Craske MG, et al: Functional impact and health utility of anxiety disorders in primary care outpatients. Med Care 2005;43:1164–1170.

44 Torres AR, Ramos-Cerqueira AT, Ferrao YA, et al: Suicidality in obsessive-compulsive disorder: prevalence and relation to symptom dimensions and comorbid conditions. J Clin Psychiatry 2011;72: 17–26.

45 Roy-Byrne PP, Davidson KW, Kessler RC, et al: Anxiety disorders and comorbid medical illness. Gen Hosp Psychiatry 2008;30:208–225.

46 Hofmeijer-Sevink MK, Batelaan NM, van Megen HJ, et al: Clinical relevance of comorbidity in anxiety disorders: a report from the Netherlands study of depression and anxiety (NESDA). J Affec Disord 2012;137:106–112.

47 Ginzburg K, Ein-Dor T, Solomon Z: Comorbidity of posttraumatic stress disorder, anxiety and depression: a 20-year longitudinal study of war veterans. J Affect Disord 2010;123:249–257.

48 O'Neil KA, Podell JL, Benjamin CL, et al: Comorbid depressive disorders in anxiety-disordered youth: demographic, clinical, and family characteristics. Child Psychiatry Hum Dev 2010;41:330–341.

49 Muller JE, Koen L, Stein DJ: Anxiety and medical disorders. Curr Psychiatry Rep 2005;7:245–251.

50 Hicks DW, Raza H: Facilitating treatment of anxiety disorders in patients with comorbid medical illness. Curr Psychiatry Rep 2005;7:228–235.

51 Clarke DM, Currie KC: Depression, anxiety and their relationship with chronic diseases: a review of the epidemiology, risk and treatment evidence. Med J Aust 2009;190:54–60.

52 Klein DF: False suffocation alarms, spontaneous panics, and related conditions. An integrative hypothesis. Arch Gen Psychiatry 1993;50:306–317.

53 Crowe RR, Noyes R, Pauls DL, et al: A family study of panic disorder. Arch Gen Psychiatry 1983;40:1065–1069.

54 Torgerson S: Genetic factors in anxiety disorders. Arch Gen Psychiatry 1983;40: 1085–1092.

55 Crowe RR, Goedken R, Samuelson S, et al: Genomewide survey of panic disorder. Am J Med Genet 2001;105:105–109.

56 Stein DJ, Scott K, Haro Abad JM, et al: Early childhood adversity and later hypertension: data from the World Mental Health Survey. Ann Clin Psychiatry 2010;22:19–28.

57 Scott KM, Von Korff M, Angermeyer MC: The association of childhood adversities and early onset mental disorders with adult onset chronic physical conditions. Arch Gen Psychiatry 2011;68: 838–844.

58 Kroenke K, Jackson JL, Chamberlain J: Depression and anxiety disorders in patients presenting with physical complaints: clinical predictors and outcome. Am J Med 1997;103:339–347.

59 Diagnostic and Statistical Manual of Mental Disorders, ed 5. Arlington, American Psychiatric Association, 2013.

60 Bruce S, Machan J, Dyck I, et al: Infrequency of 'pure' GAD: impact of psychiatric comorbidity on clinical course. Depress Anxiety 2001;14:219–225.

61 Andresscu C, Lenze EJ, Dew MA, et al: Effect of comorbid anxiety on treatment response and relapse risk in late-life depression: controlled study. Br J Psychiatry 2007;190:344–349.

62 Goes FS, McCusker MG, Bienvenu OJ, et al: Co-morbid anxiety disorders in bipolar disorder and major depression: familial aggregation and clinical characteristics of co-morbid panic disorder, social phobia, specific phobia and obsessive-compulsive disorder. Psychol Med 2012;42:1449–1459.

63 Levy RL, Olden KW, Naliboff BD, et al: Psychosocial aspects of the functional gastrointestinal disorders. Gastroenterology 2006;130:1447–1458.

64 Drossman DA, Toner BB, Whitehead WE, et al: Cognitive-behavioral therapy versus education versus desipiramine versus placebo for moderate to severe functional bowel disorders. Gastroenterology 2003;125:19–31.

65 Lachner JM, Morley S, Dowzer C, et al: Psychological treatments for irritable bowel syndrome: a systematic review and meta-analysis. J Consult Clin Psychology 2004;72:1100–1113.

66 Spies G, Asmal L, Seedat S: Cognitive-behavioural interventions for mood and anxiety disorders in HIV: a systematic review. J Affect Disord 2013;150:171–180.

67 Wulsin LR: Is depression a major risk factor for coronary disease? A systematic review of the epidemiologic evidence. Harv Rev Psychiatry 2004;12: 79–93.

68 McDonald-Haile J, Bradley LA, Bailey MA, et al: Relaxation training reduces symptom reports and acid exposure in patients with gastroesophageal reflux disease. Gastroenterology 1994;107: 619–620.

69 Acosta F: Biofeedback and progressive relaxation in weaning the anxious patient from the ventilator. Heart Lung 1988;17:299–301.

70 Yorke J, Fleming SL, Shuldham CM: Psychological interventions for adults with asthma. Cochrane Database Syst Rev 2006;1:CD002982.

71 Kellerman J, Zeltzer L, et al: Adolescents with cancer: hypnosis for the reduction of the acute pain and anxiety associated with medical procedures. J Adolesc Health Care 1983;4:85–90.

72 Richardson J, Smith JE, McCall G, et al: Hypnosis for procedure-related pain and distress in pediatric cancer patients: a systematic review of effectiveness and methodology related to hypnosis interventions. J Pain Symptom Manage 2006; 31:70–84.

73 Creed F, Fernandes L, Guthrie E, et al; North of England IBS Research Group: The cost-effectiveness of psychotherapy and paroxetine for severe irritable bowel syndrome. Gastroenterology 2003;124: 303–317.

74 Saarto T, Wiffen PJ: Antidepressants for neuropathic pain. Cochrane Database Syst Rev 2005;4:CD005454.

Dan J. Stein, BSc (Med), MBChB, FRCPC, FRSSAf, PhD, DPhil
Department of Psychiatry and Mental Health, University of Cape Town
Anzio Road, Rondebosch 7700
Cape Town (South Africa)
E-Mail dan.stein@uct.ac.za

Sartorius N, Holt RIG, Maj M (eds): Comorbidity of Mental and Physical Disorders.
Key Issues Ment Health. Basel, Karger, 2015, vol 179, pp 88–98 (DOI: 10.1159/000365541)

Cancer and Mental Illness

David Lawrence[a] · Kirsten J. Hancock[a] · Stephen Kisely[b]

[a]Telethon Kids Institute, Centre for Child Health Research, The University of Western Australia,
West Perth, W.A., [b]School of Medicine, The University of Queensland, Brisbane, Qld., Australia

Abstract

Over many years, it has been shown that cancer represents a significant proportion of excess mortality for people with mental illness. In this chapter, we probe this relationship in more detail, and examine the progression of factors that play a role in this finding. Against expectations, people with mental illness are no more likely to develop cancer, even though they have higher exposure to major risk factors including smoking, drug and alcohol use, and obesity. However, even though people with mental illness are just as likely to be diagnosed with cancer, they are more likely to die from it. The reasons for this are multifactorial, including lower rates of routine cancer screening (either because it is not recommended or people with mental illness do not follow through on the recommendation to do so), the increased length of time it takes to be diagnosed after presenting with symptoms, more advanced stage at diagnosis including metastatic cancer at diagnosis, and reduced likelihood of surgical intervention. We discuss the complexities associated with providing medical care for people with comorbid psychiatric disorders and the difficulties faced both by people with mental illness and the people who provide them with medical care.

© 2015 S. Karger AG, Basel

Overview of Excess Mortality and Mental Illness

It is well known that people with mental illness have higher mortality rates and reduced life expectancy compared to people without mental illness. Our own work using record linkage systems in Western Australia has shown that the gap in life expectancy for people with and without mental illness has increased since 1985, to 12 years for women and 16 years for men, principally because improvements in life expectancy for the general population have not extended to people with mental illness [1].

While mental illness is associated with an increased risk of suicide, much of the excess mortality associated with mental illness is actually due to common physical health conditions, in particular cardiovascular disease, respiratory diseases and cancer [1, 2]. With a particular focus on cancer – the topic of this chapter – we have previously reported that cancer diagnosis rates are comparable between people with and without mental illness; at the same time, however, not only is case fatality after a cancer is diagnosed substantially worse in

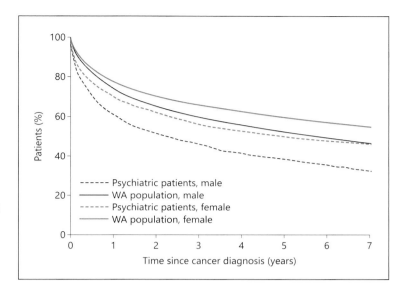

Fig. 1. Survival since diagnosis of all cancers by contact with mental health services. WA = Western Australia. Reproduced with permission from *JAMA Psychiatry* [3].

people with a history of mental illness, but survival times are also much shorter (fig. 1) [2–4]. In order to reduce the excess mortality attributable to cancer, it is important to understand the underlying factors as to why people with mental illness have worse case fatality associated with cancer. There are obvious and immediate avenues to examine, in particular whether lifestyle factors place people with mental illness at greater risk of developing cancer. For instance, are they less likely to participate in cancer screening activities, leading to differences in how soon diagnoses are made and therefore presenting with more advanced disease? Do people with mental illness receive differential treatment once they are diagnosed? Are they more likely to reject lifesaving treatments or not comply with aftercare requirements? All of these factors may go some way to developing a more rounded understanding of why people with mental illness experience greater cancer mortality. In this chapter we address each of these questions, reviewing the evidence as to where the greatest discrepancies lie and which aspects of cancer diagnosis and treatment deserve further attention.

The Evolution of Mental Illness and Cancer Research

Study of the relationship between poor physical health and high mortality in people with mental illness has a long history. In 1841, William Farr [5] reported to the Royal Statistical Society on mortality within the major asylums in England. At that time, high mortality was principally ascribed to infectious diseases and the generally poor conditions within asylums. Around the same time, the Commissioners in Lunacy were established to oversee the conditions and care provided in asylums and workhouses in England. The commissioners were among the first to note that in spite of the general poor health of people with mental illness, cancers were not often seen, and they suggested in their 1909 report that people with mental illness may have a certain immunity to cancer [6]. With the dawn of the computer age, new methods of research in mental illness became viable. The Oxford Record Linkage Study, established in the 1960s, was the first study to undertake a systematic analysis of the association between physical health problems and mental illness, using administrative data from mental health services in the Oxford region [7]. At that time, the main question of interest was whether an association between a physical illness and a mental illness could reveal something about the aetiology of both conditions. The relationships between cancer and schizophrenia and between rheumatoid arthritis and schizophrenia have received particular attention [8]. The strong negative correlation between these conditions led to hypotheses that there might be specific genes involved in the aetiology of these diseases.

As more data were accumulated over time and the pattern of association between schizophrenia and cancer was observed to be more complex, more nuanced hypotheses were advanced. These included the idea that certain neuroleptic drugs may have a tumour-suppressing effect, that this effect may vary depending on the stage of cancer during neuroleptic treatment, that the effect may vary depending on cancer morphology, or there may be an interaction between neuroleptics, levels of specific hormones and genetic susceptibility to certain types of tumours [9–12]. However, to date this line of investigation has not led to any significant advance in the understanding of the aetiology or treatment of either schizophrenia or cancer.

Cancer and Excess Mortality

While much of the early research focussed on the possibility of people with mental illness being at reduced risk for developing cancer, the possibility that cancer may be a cause of excess mortality was first reported by Katz et al. [13] in 1967, who found that cancer mortality amongst psychiatric patients in New York was higher than in the general population, though only for patients with shorter periods of hospitalisation. Patients with psychiatric hospital stays of more than 10 years had lower cancer mortality rates.

Since then, there have been numerous studies on cancer mortality and mental illness, and most studies published in the last decade have found higher standardised mortality ratios associated with cancer [3, 4, 14–17]. However, these findings have not always been consistent, and have varied according to the years of study, the mental illness and type of cancer examined, and the study populations and methodologies that each study used. For example, the results of earlier studies typically found no excess mortality attributable to cancer [18–21], and in some cases lower standardised mortality ratios were observed [22, 23].

Incidence and Case Fatality Rates

There is considerable research demonstrating that people with mental illness engage more frequently in behaviours that are associated with cancer risk. For example, people with mental illness have higher rates of smoking and smoke more cigarettes on average [24], and despite wanting to quit smoking find it much harder than people without mental illness to do so [25]. Drug and alcohol addiction is also more common in people with mental disorders [26], and many psychiatric disorders are treated with medications which, in addition to other lifestyle and diet factors, result in increased incidence of obesity [27]. Additionally, a common side effect of antipsychotic medications is hyperprolactinaemia, an excess of the hormone prolactin. Hyperprolactinaemia is also associated with an increased risk of breast cancer in women [28], and possibly prostate cancer in men [29], though others have noted that hyperprolactinaemia is also associated with hypogonadism, which may be protective against breast and prostate cancer [30].

Because of these lifestyle and medication side-effect risk factors, it may seem reasonable to hypothesise that increased exposure to these cancer risk factors would cause more cancers in people with mental illness. If this were the sole reason for worse cancer mortality, then we would expect that people with mental illness would be at greater *risk* of developing cancer, and as such we would see an increased *incidence* of cancer amongst people with mental illness. Despite the high rates of exposure to demonstrated carcinogens in people with mental illness, there is in fact no clear evidence that people with mental illness are more likely to develop cancer, or at least be any more likely to be diagnosed with cancer. Studies that have examined both cancer incidence and mortality in populations of people with mental illness indicate that cancer incidence rates for people with mental illness are generally comparable with the rest of the population, though this pattern appears to depend on the type of cancer and the severity of mental illness. Many studies have found that cancer rates are lower amongst people with schizophrenia in particular [31–34]. However, not all studies have found this pattern amongst people with schizophrenia [15], and as such, this pattern for people with schizophrenia may reflect methodological or cohort differences [35]. While some studies have found an increased incidence of smoking-related cancer, such as lung cancer, in people with mental illness [36, 37], the overwhelming majority of studies that examine psychiatric disorders, other than schizophrenia, have found no increased risk of cancer incidence in psychiatric populations [3, 4, 15, 36, 38–41]. In addition, people with severe mental illness do not have a greater incidence of melanoma, but have worse case fatality even though melanoma is a cancer that cannot be attributed to concurrent lifestyle factors such as diet, drugs, alcohol or tobacco, as it is mainly related to childhood sun exposure [3].

In the case of cancers that are associated with risk factors such as smoking, alcohol and other drugs, comparable rates of cancer incidence in people with and without mental illness may imply some other, as yet unknown, factor that reduces incidence of cancer in people with mental illness. Some exceptions are apparent, for example a systematic review of the incidence of breast cancer amongst women with schizophrenia found that while the incidence rates of breast cancer varied across the studies, those with larger samples and better quality indicators found higher rates of breast cancer in women with schizophrenia [42]. A possible explanation for this finding, if true, may relate to the increased likelihood of hyperprolactinaemia for people who are administered antipsychotic medication. However, we have not observed any increase in breast cancer in women with severe mental illness in our own work in Western Australia and Nova Scotia [2–4].

Brain tumours are a notable exception to the finding that the incidence of cancer is comparable in psychiatric and general populations. A number of studies have identified higher rates of brain cancer diagnosis following diagnosis of mental illness. A likely explanation for this finding is the general difficulty of diagnosing brain cancers, and the common early presentation of brain cancer sufferers with symptoms of mental distress including depression and memory impairment. This may lead to people with brain tumours being referred for mental health treatment prior to the diagnosis of their tumour [2, 43].

Factors Related to Higher Case Fatality

Less studied than cancer incidence, but more consistent in its findings, is the higher case fatality following cancer diagnosis in people with co-morbid mental illness. This has been consistently reported from a number of large record linkage and cohort studies including our own record linkage work using the populations of Western Australia and Nova Scotia [3, 4]. This worse case fatality from time of diagnosis deserves additional focus and attention. Here we examine the cancer screening rates for people with mental illness and further treatment discrepancies that occur following diagnosis.

Screening Rates

Another possible explanation for the comparable rate of cancer diagnosis in people with mental illness despite high exposure to known carcinogens is the hypothesis that cancers do occur more frequently in people with mental illness, but are less likely to be detected because of lower rates of screening and access to general healthcare. As life expectancy is substantially reduced in people with mental illness, and mortality from other causes of death is substantially higher, more people with mental illness who have cancer may die before that cancer is diagnosed. To date, the results about the extent to which people with mental illness receive routine cancer screening have been mixed. For example, in a study of privately insured women with, and without, claims for mental illness, women with a mental disorder were significantly less likely to receive mammography, particularly women with more severe disorders [44]. Similar patterns have been observed in other studies with different populations of patients [45–48], though others have found that women with mental illness were more likely [49], or at least equally likely, to receive mammography [50]. In a narrative review of 17 studies examining the uptake of screening services by people with mental illness, Happell et al. [51] showed a 20–30% reduced likelihood of breast, cervical and colorectal cancer screening for patients with severe mental illness in the majority of studies. The pattern was most commonly observed for people with more severe disorders, with up to a 60% reduced likelihood [52]. Taken together, the evidence suggests that people with mental illness are less likely to receive preventive cancer screening services than those without [53]. As a result, cancers may be more advanced by the time the diagnosis is made, with poorer outcomes associated with the delay in diagnosis.

The question of why people with mental illness may receive less cancer screening remains unresolved. For instance, some research points to the possibility that people with mental illness are less likely to be offered screening for cervical, breast, prostate or colorectal cancer by their primary physicians [54], or if screening is recommended, are less likely to adhere to recommended screening [55]. In their systematic review, Lord et al. [56] identified the relationship with the primary care physician as perhaps the most important factor to explain deficits in receipt of cancer screening and other preventive health measures. They note that proactive contact from the primary care physician, and the use of peer support workers, are two interventions where there is some evidence to support their effectiveness in boosting screening rates.

Delay to Diagnosis and Stage of Cancer at Diagnosis

Differences in screening rates aside, there is a growing body of literature documenting other disparities in cancer treatment for people with mental illness, including the length of time it takes to be diagnosed with cancer after presenting with symptoms. In a study of patients with oesophageal cancer, O'Rourke et al. [57] found that cancer patients who had a DSM-IV diagnosed psychiatric comorbidity waited a median of 90 days between reporting symptoms and receiving a diagnosis, compared to 35 days for patients without mental illness. They were also more likely to have advanced disease at the time of diagnosis (37 vs. 18%) and also had a decreased likelihood of receiving surgical therapy (38 vs. 59%). In other research, the proportion of people with cancer who had metastases at presentation was significantly higher in psychiatric patients (7.1 vs. 6.1%), though larger gaps were observed for specific types of cancer [3]. For example, for people with breast cancer the difference was 6.3 vs. 4.5%, and lung cancer 0.6 vs. 0.2%. No differences in rates of cancer with metastases were found for

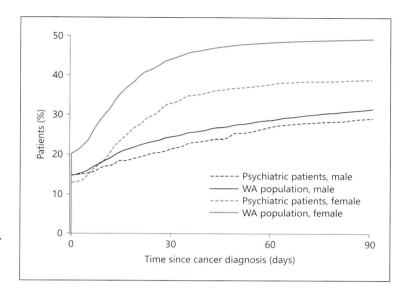

Fig. 2. Time from diagnosis to surgical removal of the tumour by contact with mental health services. WA = Western Australia. Reproduced with permission from *JAMA Psychiatry* [3].

other sites. Though statistically different, these difference rates are small in absolute terms, and cannot account for the significantly larger differences in case fatality for cancer patients. These patterns, reinforced by findings from another recent study [58], suggest that the elevated mortality associated with cancer is unlikely to be primarily the result of the cancer being more advanced by the time it is diagnosed.

Medical Care after Diagnosis: Surgical Intervention

There are apparent disparities in other ongoing treatment options, including rates of surgical intervention and the time it takes to get to surgery. In our recent work using the Western Australian Data Linkage System [3], psychiatric patients had a reduced likelihood of surgery after diagnosis for all types of cancer, and for those who did have surgery, the length of time between cancer diagnosis and surgery was longer (see fig. 2 for trends). Men were less likely to have a colorectal resection, and women were less likely to have surgery for colorectal, breast and cervical cancer. The psychiatric diagnosis also mattered –

colorectal resections occurred less frequently for patients who were diagnosed with dementia, affective psychoses, other psychoses and depression. Psychiatric patients also received 10.3 sessions of chemotherapy on average, compared to 12.1 for the general population, and were less likely to receive radiotherapy for breast cancer (2.6 vs. 4.1%), colorectal cancer (1.6 vs. 3.9%) and uterine cancer (13.0 vs. 21.1%). To summarise, although the cancer incidence in psychiatric patients is no higher than in the general population, psychiatric patients are more likely to have metastases at diagnosis and less likely to receive specialised interventions. Together, these may explain the greater case fatality found in people with a psychiatric disorder.

Though our focus here has been on cancer outcomes for people with a prior history of mental illness, for many people, the onset of mental illness can occur following cancer diagnosis and treatment [59], particularly post-traumatic stress disorder and depressive and anxiety disorders. Research indicates that people with comorbid diagnoses of cancer and mental illness have poorer outcomes and greater difficulty adhering to treatment regimens [60, 61]. In this respect, issues surrounding treatment disparities apply to all people with mental illness, irrespective of their psychiatric history prior to a cancer diagnosis. However, different types of mental illness offer different challenges to people with mental illness and to the practitioners who treat them, and the types of mental illness that arise following the development of cancer are somewhat narrower in scope than the range of illnesses that develop over a lifetime. Research that compares treatment outcomes for people whose onset of mental illness was before or after cancer may offer further insights as to why disparities occur.

Comorbidities and Challenges for Health and Mental Healthcare Providers

People with mental illness who also have physical health problems are often more likely to be among the more complex cases with multiple presenting symptoms and problems. For example, in a small-scale review of 29 people with schizophrenia and lung cancer [62], potentially curable cancers were identified in 17 individuals, with 5 of the 17 receiving less than best practice care. Issues that resulted in disparities in care included other physical comorbidities that complicated the treatment and ethical issues with patients not consenting to invasive treatments. Irrespective of the presence of mental illness, patients with complex needs who have multiple comorbidities have worse outcomes and are more poorly served by standard medical care [63]. With the high level of specialisation now required to deliver high-quality healthcare for any condition, it is clear that few healthcare providers are well equipped to deal effectively with diverse and challenging health problems simultaneously [64].

Equitable access to healthcare has become an important focus of research in the gaps in physical health outcomes associated with mental illness, and a number of contributing issues have

been noted in the literature [65, 66]. First, there is the long established separation of mental and physical healthcare, with many mental health service users not receiving ongoing physical healthcare, and many psychiatrists reluctant to diagnose and treat physical health conditions. Additionally, stigma is seen as a major issue in the equitable delivery and access to general healthcare. Unfortunately, mental illness can rob people of aspects of personality that others find most endearing, and even among health professionals there are many who find it difficult to provide the same level of concern and support to people with mental illness. Also, the way that healthcare is delivered in developed countries generally results in greater benefit to those who have the best understanding of health conditions and the healthcare system. People with mental illness may also have limited means to pay for healthcare or might not be covered by health insurance. Many mental illnesses are associated with cognitive impairments and disadvantages that can impact people's ability to maximise their use of healthcare options. These include smaller support networks and impacts on motivation, concentration, assertiveness and communications ability. In some cases these deficits have been used as justification not to provide health interventions. For instance, some cancer surgeries are highly invasive and debilitating, and pose substantial demands during recuperation. Similarly, chemotherapies and other more experimental drug treatments can have significant side effects and exact a toll on the patient.

The issue of obtaining informed ethical consent to risky treatments or treatments with substantial side effects also requires sensitive consideration. Some people with mental illness require a higher level of support to understand the implications of treatments, which may require more time commitment from the practitioner. Compliance with aftercare may also require a higher level of support. However, in the same way that physical disability is not a valid reason for not providing access to healthcare, any cognitive or behavioural impairment associated with mental illness should be recognised as a component of the illness that deserves support.

Finally, another aspect of medical care for people with both mental illness and cancer is end-of-life palliative care, which shares some similarities with the recovery model of mental healthcare that is based on respect, dignity, and valuing both life and the individual [67]. Results from limited research on this issue have been contradictory. Some work suggests that people with severe mental illness may be less likely to receive palliative care [67]. In contrast, our own preliminary work, using data from the Western Australian Data Linkage System for the period 1988–2007, indicates that people with a history of mental illness who were dying of cancer received the same level and duration of palliative care prior to death as the general population, with an average of 19 days of palliative care [unpubl. data]. In spite of the challenges that people with mental illness may pose to palliative care environments, they may especially benefit from such care when making difficult end-of-life decisions or deal with significant pain, as they are less likely to have strong personal support networks [67]. Again, the issue of stigma and the cognitive and behavioural consequences of mental illness can affect the way people are received and treated in the palliative care environment [68, 69].

Conclusions

With significant advances in the treatment and understanding of mental illness, and large-scale change in mental health service delivery to community-based care, there have been significant shifts in treatment goals and expectations. There are now effective treatments available for most mental health conditions [70], and a major focus of mental healthcare is on recovery from mental illness and valuing the contribution people with a history of mental illness make to their communities [71, 72]. This has led to a much greater focus on the human cost of the high physical comorbidity associated with mental illness, the wasted life seen in the substantial gaps in life expectancy [73].

Mental illnesses are common, and people with mental illness suffer a disproportionate burden associated with physical illness, including higher mortality from cancer. Bringmann et al. [74] estimate that up to one third of cancer patients have a psychiatric history. As such, dealing with comorbid mental illness is a significant component of cancer care. Though people with mental illness may not be at any higher risk than anyone else for developing cancers, the clearly worse outcomes once cancer is diagnosed highlight the role that preventive and treatment services are likely to play in reducing these disparities. There is insufficient research at present to definitively identify the contribution that individual issues make to the overall gaps in outcomes, but it is highly likely that a range of factors contribute. Further research into ways to improve health service delivery to people with comorbid mental health problems is required. It appears that reduced access to screening, delays in diagnosis, differential access to and uptake of treatment options, and impacts of other comorbidities may all play a role. Clearly, these issues are not straightforward to resolve as shown by the lack of major progress anywhere in the world. There is a small and developing evidence base supporting some directions for improving physical healthcare for people with mental illness, although none of this literature is specific to cancer. These include variations on the theme of more holistic care models including multidisciplinary teams and co-location, use of peer supporters and addressing stigma in the healthcare profession [66].

References

1 Lawrence D, Hancock KJ, Kisely S: The gap in life expectancy from preventable physical illness in psychiatric patients in Western Australia: retrospective analysis of population based registers. BMJ 2013;346:f2539.

2 Lawrence D, Holman CDJ, Jablensky AV: Preventable Physical Illness in People with Mental Illness. Perth, University of Western Australia, 2001.

3 Kisely S, Crowe E, Lawrence D: Cancer-related mortality in people with mental illness. JAMA Psychiatry 2013;70:209–217.

4 Kisely S, Sadek J, MacKenzie A, Lawrence D, Campbell LA: Excess cancer mortality in psychiatric patients. Can J Psychiatry 2008;53:753–761.

5 Farr W: Report upon the mortality of lunatics. J Stat Soc London 1841;4:17–33.

6 Commissioners in Lunacy for England and Wales: Annual Report. London, Her Majesty's Stationery Office, 1909.

7 Baldwin JA: Aspects of the epidemiology of mental illness: studies in record linkage. Boston, Little, Brown, 1971.

8 Torrey EF, Yolken RH: The schizophrenia-rheumatoid arthritis connection: infectious, immune, or both? Brain Behav Immun 2001;15:401–410.

9 Dalton SO, Mellemkjær L, Olsen JH, Mortensen PB, Johansen C: Depression and cancer risk: a register-based study of patients hospitalized with affective disorders, Denmark, 1969–1993. Am J Epidemiol 2002;155:1088–1095.

10 Dalton SO, Mellemkjær L, Thomassen L, Mortensen PB, Johansen C: Risk for cancer in a cohort of patients hospitalized for schizophrenia in Denmark, 1969–1993. Schizophr Res 2005;75:315–324.

11 Goldacre MJ, Kurina LM, Wotton CJ, Yeates D, Seagroat V: Schizophrenia and cancer: an epidemiological study. Br J Psychiatry 2005;187:334–338.

12 Hodgson R, Wildgust HJ, Bushe CJ: Cancer and schizophrenia: is there a paradox? J Psychopharmacol 2010;24:51–60.

13 Katz J, Kunofsky S, Patton RE, Allaway NC: Cancer mortality among patients in New York mental hospitals. Cancer 1967;20:2194–2199.

14 Capasso RM, Lineberry TW, Bostwick JM, Decker PA, St Sauver J: Mortality in schizophrenia and schizoaffective disorder: an Olmsted County, Minnesota cohort: 1950–2005. Schizophr Res 2008;98:287–294.

15 Lawrence D, Holman CDJ, Jablensky AV, Threfall TJ, Fuller SA: Excess cancer mortality in Western Australian psychiatric patients due to higher case fatality rates. Acta Psychiatr Scand 2000;101:382–388.

16 Musuuza JS, Sherman ME, Knudsen KJ, Sweeney HA, Tyler CV, Koroukian SM: Analyzing excess mortality from cancer among individuals with mental illness. Cancer 2013;119:2469–2476.

17 Piatt EE, Munetz MR, Ritter C: An examination of premature mortality among decedents with serious mental illness and those in the general population. Psychiatr Serv 2010;61:663–668.

18 Dutta R, Murray RM, Allardyce J, Jones PB, Boydell JE: Mortality in first-contact psychosis patients in the U.K.: a cohort study. Psychol Med 2012;42:1649–1661.

19 Haugland G, Craig TJ, Goodman AB, Siegel C: Mortality in the era of deinstitutionalization. Am J Psychiatry 1983;140:848–852.

20 Norton B, Whalley LJ: Mortality of a lithium-treated population. Br J Psychiatry 1984;145:277–282.

21 Osborn DP, Levy G, Nazareth I, Petersen I, Islam A, King MB: Relative risk of cardiovascular and cancer mortality in people with severe mental illness from the United Kingdom's General Practice Research Database. Arch Gen Psychiatry 2007;64:242–249.

22 Valenti M, Necozione S, Busellu G, Borrelli G, Lepore AR, Madonna R, et al: Mortality in psychiatric hospital patients: a cohort analysis of prognostic factors. Int J Epidemiol 1997;26:1227–1235.

23 Wood JB, Evenson RC, Cho DW, Hagan BJ: Mortality variations among public mental health patients. Acta Psychiatr Scand 1985;72:218–229.

24 Lasser K, Boyd JW, Woolhandler S, Himmelstein DU, McCormick D, Bor DH: Smoking and mental illness: a population-based prevalence study. JAMA 2000;284:2606–2610.

25 Lawrence D, Mitrou F, Zubrick SR: Non-specific psychological distress, smoking status and smoking cessation: United States National Health Interview Survey 2005. BMC Public Health 2011;11:256–268.

26 Regier DA, Farmer ME, Rae DS, Locke BZ, Keith SJ, Judd LL, Goodwin FK: Comorbidity of mental disorders with alcohol and other drug abuse. JAMA 1990;264:2511–2518.

27 Newcomer JW: Antipsychotic medications: metabolic and cardiovascular risk. J Clin Psychiatry 2007;68(suppl 4):8–13.

28 Tworoger SS, Eliassen AH, Sluss P, Hankinson SE: A prospective study of plasma prolactin concentrations and risk of premenopausal and postmenopausal breast cancer. J Clin Oncol 2007;25:1482–1488.

29 Harvey PW, Everett DJ, Springall CJ: Hyperprolactinaemia as an adverse effect in regulatory and clinical toxicology: role in breast and prostate cancer. Hum Exp Toxicol 2006;25:395–404.

30 Holt RI: Medical causes and consequences of hyperprolactinaemia. A context for psychiatrists. J Psychopharmacol 2008;22:28–37.

31 Barak Y, Levy T, Achiron A, Aizenberg D: Breast cancer in women suffering from serious mental illness. Schizophr Res 2008;102:249–253.

32 Catts VS, Catts SV, O'Toole BI, Frost AD: Cancer incidence in patients with schizophrenia and their first-degree relatives – a meta-analysis. Acta Psychiatr Scand 2008;117:323–336.

33 Chou FH, Tsai KY, Su CY, Lee CC: The incidence and relative risk factors for developing cancer among patients with schizophrenia: a nine-year follow-up study. Schizophr Res 2011;129:97–103.

34 Grinshpoon A, Barchana M, Ponizovsky A, Lipshitz I, Nahon D, Tal O, Weizman A, Levav I: Cancer in schizophrenia: is the risk higher or lower? Schizophr Res 2005;73:333–341.

35 Jablensky A, Lawrence D: Schizophrenia and cancer: is there a need to invoke a protective gene? Arch Gen Psychiatry 2001;58:579–580.

36 Goldacre MJ, Wotton CJ, Yeates D, Seagroatt V, Flint J: Cancer in people with depression or anxiety: record-linkage study. Soc Psychiatry Psychiatr Epidemiol 2007;42:683–689.

37 Whitley E, Batty GD, Mulheran PA, Gale CR, Osborn D, Tynelius P, Rasmussen F: Psychiatric disorder as a risk factor for cancer: different analytic strategies produce different findings. Epidemiology 2012;23:543–550.

38 Carney CP, Woolson RF, Jones L, Noyes RJ, Doebbeling BN: Occurrence of cancer among people with mental health claims in an insured population. Psychosom Med 2004;66:735–743.

39 Levav I, Kohn R, Barchana M, Lipshitz I, Pugachova I, Weizman A, Grinshpoon A: The risk for cancer among patients with schizoaffective disorders. J Affect Disord 2009;114:316–320.

40 Osborn DP, Limburg H, Walters K, Petersen I, King M, Green J, Watson J, Nazareth I: Relative incidence of common cancers in people with severe mental illness. Cohort study in the United Kingdom THIN primary care database. Schizophr Res 2013;143:44–49.

41 Truyers C, Buntinx F, De Lepeleire J, De Hert M, Van Winkel R, Aertgeerts B, Bartholomeeusen S, Lesaffre E: Incident somatic comorbidity after psychosis: results from a retrospective cohort study based on Flemish general practice data. BMC Fam Pract 2011;12:132.

42 Bushe CJ, Bradley AJ, Wildgust HJ, Hodgson RE: Schizophrenia and breast cancer incidence: a systematic review of clinical studies. Schizophr Res 2009;114:6–16.

43 Benros ME, Laursen TM, Dalton SO, Mortensen PB: Psychiatric disorder as a first manifestation of cancer: a 10-year population-based study. Int J Cancer 2009;124:2917–2922.

44 Carney CP, Jones LE: The influence of type and severity of mental illness on receipt of screening mammography. J Gen Intern Med 2006;21:1097–1104.

45 Druss BG, Rosenheck RA, Desai MM, Perlin JB: Quality of preventive medical care for patients with mental disorders. Med Care 2002;40:129–136.

46 Martens PJ, Chochinov HM, Prior HJ, Fransoo R, Burland E: Are cervical cancer screening rates different for women with schizophrenia? A Manitoba population-based study. Schizophr Res 2009; 113:101–106.

47 Owen C, Jessie D, De Vries Robbe M: Barriers to cancer screening amongst women with mental health problems. Health Care Women Int 2002;23:561–566.

48 Pirraglia PA, Sanyal P, Singer DE, Ferris TG: Depressive symptom burden as a barrier to screening for breast and cervical cancers. J Womens Health 2004;13:731–738.

49 Lasser KE, Zeytinoglu H, Miller E, Becker AE, Hermann RC, Bor DH: Do women who screen positive for mental disorders in primary care have lower mammography rates? Gen Hosp Psychiatry 2003;25:214–216.

50 Friedman LC, Puryear LJ, Moore A, Green CE: Breast and colorectal cancer screening among low-income women with psychiatric disorders. Psychooncology 2005;14:786–791.

51 Happell B, Scott D, Platania-Phung C: Provision of preventive services for cancer and infectious diseases among individuals with serious mental illness. Arch Psychiatr Nurs 2012;26:192–201.

52 Werneke U, Horn O, Maryon-Davis A, Wessely S, Donnan S, McPherson K: Uptake of screening for breast cancer in patients with mental health problems. J Epidemiol Community Health 2006;60:600–605.

53 Howard LM, Barley EA, Davies E, Rigg A, Lempp H, Rose D, Taylor D, Thornicroft G: Cancer diagnosis in people with severe mental illness: practical and ethical issues. Lancet Oncol 2010;11:797–804.

54 Xiong GL, Bermudes RA, Torres SN, Hales RE: Use of cancer-screening services among persons with serious mental illness in Sacramento County. Psychiatr Serv 2008;59:929–932.

55 Yee EF, White R, Lee S, Washington DL, Yano EM, Murata G, Handanos C, Hoffman RM: Mental illness: is there an association with cancer screening among women veterans? Womens Health Issues 2011;21:S195–S202.

56 Lord O, Malone D, Mitchell AJ: Receipt of preventive medical care and medical screening for patients with mental illness: a comparative analysis. Gen Hosp Psychiatry 2010;32:519–543.

57 O'Rourke RW, Diggs BS, Spight DH, Robinson J, Elder KA, Andrus J, Thomas CR, Hunter JG, Jobe BA: Psychiatric illness delays diagnosis of esophageal cancer. Dis Esophagus 2008;21:416–421.

58 Chang CK, Hayes RD, Broadbent MTM, Hotopf M, Davies E, Møller H, Stewart R: A cohort study on mental disorders, stage of cancer at diagnosis and subsequent survival. BMJ Open 2014; 4:e004295.

59 Gandubert C, Carrière I, Escot C, Soulier M, Hermès A, Boulet P, Ritchie K, Chaudieu I: Onset and relapse of psychiatric disorders following early breast cancer: a case-control study. Psychooncology 2009;18:1029–1037.

60 Colleoni M, Mandala M, Peruzzotti G, Robertson C, Bredart A, Goldhirsch A: Depression and degree of acceptance of adjuvant cytotoxic drugs. Lancet 2000; 356:1326–1327.

61 DiMatteo MR, Lepper HS, Croghan TW: Depression is a risk factor for noncompliance with medical treatment: metaanalysis of the effects of anxiety and depression on patient adherence. Arch Intern Med 2000;160:2101–2107.

62 Mateen FJ, Jatoi A, Lineberry TW, Aranguren D, Creagan ET, Croghan GA, Jett JR, Marks RS, Molina JR, Richardson RL: Do patients with schizophrenia receive state-of-the-art lung cancer therapy? A brief report. Psychooncology 2008;17:721–725.

63 Fortin M, Soubhi H, Hudon C, Bayliss EA, van den Akker M: Multimorbidity's many challenges. BMJ 2007;334:1016–1017.

64 Ogle KS, Swanson GM, Woods N, Azzouz F: Cancer and comorbidity. Cancer 2000;88:653–663.

65 Irwin KE, Henderson DC, Knight HP, Pirl WF: Cancer care for individuals with schizophrenia. Cancer 2014;120:323–334.

66 Lawrence D, Kisely S: Inequalities in healthcare provision for people with severe mental illness. J Psychopharmacol 2010;24:61–68.

67 Woods A, Willison K, Kington C, Gavin A: Palliative care for people with severe persistent mental illness: a review of the literature. Can J Psychiatry 2008;53:725–736.

68 Candilis PJ, Foti ME, Holzer JC: End-of-life care and mental illness: a model for community psychiatry and beyond. Community Ment Health J 2004;40:3–16.

69 Foti ME, Bartels SJ, Merriman MP, Fletcher KE, Van Citters AD: Medical advance care planning for persons with serious mental illness. Psychiatr Serv 2005;56:576–584.

70 Satcher D: Mental Health: A Report of the Surgeon General. Washington, Department of Health and Human Services, 1999.

71 Anthony WA: Recovery from mental illness: the guiding vision of the mental health service system in the 1990s. Psychosoc Rehabil J 1993;16:11.

72 Mental Health Council of Australia: Perspectives: Mental Health and Wellbeing in Australia. Canberra, MHCA, 2013.

73 Thornicroft G: Premature death among people with mental illness. BMJ 2013; 346:f2969.

74 Bringmann H, Singer S, Hockel M, Stolzenburg J, Kraub O, Schwarz R: Long-term course of psychiatric disorders in cancer patients: a pilot study. Psychosoc Med 2008;5:Doc03.

David Lawrence, PhD
Telethon Kids Institute
Centre for Child Health Research, The University of Western Australia
PO Box 855, West Perth, WA 6872 (Australia)
E-Mail david.lawrence@telethonkids.org.au

Sartorius N, Holt RIG, Maj M (eds): Comorbidity of Mental and Physical Disorders.
Key Issues Ment Health. Basel, Karger, 2015, vol 179, pp 99–113 (DOI: 10.1159/000365542)

Infectious Diseases and Mental Health

Norbert Müller

Department of Psychiatry and Psychotherapy, Ludwig-Maximilian University Munich, Munich, Germany

Abstract

Emil Kraepelin, the founder of modern psychiatric classification, and the Nobel laureate Julius Wagner von Jauregg highlighted the role of infections and the immune system in psychiatric disorders. It is well known that infections can trigger various psychiatric syndromes and influence the course of psychiatric disorders. Psychiatric symptoms during virulent infections, often presenting as encephalitis or meningitis, normally are diagnosed as mental disorders due to a general medical condition. On the other hand, an expanding research field underpins the view that infections and activation of the immune system may play a causative role in major psychiatric disorders such as schizophrenia or major depression. Also in other psychiatric syndromes, such as Tourette's syndrome, inflammation – partially based on infections – is involved. For this mild smoldering inflammatory process, the 'mild (chronic) encephalitis' concept was developed. In this chapter, findings related to immune activation and inflammation in schizophrenia, major depression and Tourette's syndromes as examples for this concept are described. Moreover, encouraging results from randomized clinical trials in schizophrenia and major depression showing a benefit of anti-inflammatory therapy in these psychiatric disorders are discussed as examples for immunomodulating treatment approaches in psychiatric disorders. Further immunotherapies used in Tourette's syndrome or pediatric autoimmune disorders associated with streptococci are highlighted as further examples for such a therapeutic approach.   © 2015 S. Karger AG, Basel

Humans are constantly being assaulted by infectious agents. Fortunately, we have evolved a complex process, the immune response, to help fight and clear infection [1]. The immune response evoked by an infectious agent may or may not generate clinical symptoms, depending on the exact type and degree of response. Infectious diseases are well known to provoke psychiatric symptoms. As early as 1890, Emil Kraepelin, one of the founders of modern psychiatry, described during an influenza epidemic 11 cases of psychiatric disorders that presented with different symptoms such as depressed mood, a paranoid and hallucinatory syndrome, involuntary movements, cognitive deterioration, and a delirious state [2]. Later, Kraepelin postulated in his pro-

Table 1. Diagnostic criteria DSM-IV: psychopathological states due to a general medical condition

293.0	Delirium due to a general medical condition
	Dementia due to a general medical condition
294.0	Amnestic disorder due to a general medical condition
293.8x	Psychotic disorder due to a general medical condition
293.83	Mood disorder due to a general medical condition
293.89	Anxiety disorder due to a general medical condition
	Sexual dysfunction due to a general medical condition
780.5x	Sleep disorder due to a general medical condition

grammatic essay 'Objectives and methods of psychiatric research' to make the immunological defense and adaption system a focus of psychiatric research [3, 4]. There are also numerous descriptions of an association between chronic inflammation of the central nervous system (CNS) and psychopathological states [5]. For example, symptoms of depression and schizophrenia have been described in a certain form of multiple sclerosis [6]. The same is true for viral CNS infection with herpes simplex virus types 1 [7] and 2 [8, 9] and measles [10]. Autoimmune processes, such as poststreptococcal disorders, lupus erythematodes and scleroderma, may present primarily as a psychopathological syndrome [11–18]. This line of evidence led to the concept of 'mild encephalitis' [19].

In modern diagnostics, psychiatric symptoms coexisting with severe infections are diagnosed as 'mental disorders due to a general medical condition'. Infections can cause a broad spectrum of psychiatric symptoms, e.g. delirium, psychotic disorder or mood disorder (table 1) [20].

Factors influencing the psychiatric presentation of infections are the subject of intense research and might include the pathogen, individual medical history and locus of infection. Infections of the CNS, such as meningitis and encephalitis, are believed to be more commonly associated with psychiatric symptoms than those of the peripheral organs, although peripheral infections are also well known to cause psychiatric

disturbances. An example is 'sickness behavior' as a model for depressive disorder, as described below.

The 'Sickness Behavior' Model in Major Depression

'Sickness behavior', the reaction of an organism to infection and inflammation, is well established as a model for depression in animals and humans [21, 22]. The model is based on the observation that increased levels of proinflammatory cytokines, such as tumor necrosis factor-α (TNF-α) and interleukin-6 (IL-6), are associated with depressive-like behavior in animals, including decreased drive and motivation, lack of energy and appetite, tiredness, and weight loss. The involvement of cytokines in the regulation of sickness behavior in humans has been studied by administering the bacterial endotoxin lipopolysaccharide to healthy volunteers [23]. Levels of anxiety, depression and cognitive impairment were found to be related to the levels of circulating cytokines [23, 24].

The findings of these studies, together with the sickness behavior model, have led to the hypothesis that 'cytokines sing the blues', i.e. cytokines and a proinflammatory immune state are involved in the pathogenesis of major depression [25, 26]. This view is supported by recent literature showing signs of a proinflammatory immune state in major depression.

Table 2. Components of the innate and adaptive immune system

Component	Innate	Adaptive
Cellular	Monocyte macrophages Granulocytes Natural killer cell γ-/δ-cells	T and B cells
Humoral	Complement, APP, mannose-binding lectin	Antibody

Components and Functions of the Immune System

The innate immune system, which includes natural killer cells and monocytes, for example, as the first barrier against infection, is phylogenetically the oldest part of the immune system. The adaptive immune response with the antibody-producing B lymphocytes and the T lymphocytes (helper T cells) is the pathogen- and antigen-specific component of the immune system. Cytokines regulate all cellular components of the immune system and are involved in both the innate and the adaptive immune response. Helper T cells are of two types: T helper 1 (Th-1) and 2 (Th-2). Th-1 cells produce the characteristic 'type 1' activating cytokines such as IL-2 and interferon-γ. However, since not only Th-1 cells, but also certain monocytes/macrophages (M1) and other cell types, produce these cytokines, this type of immune response is called the type 1 immune response. The humoral, antibody-producing arm of the adaptive immune system is mainly activated by the type 2 immune response. Th-2 and certain monocytes/macrophages (M2) produce mainly IL-4, IL-10 and IL-13 [27]. Another terminology system differentiates cytokines as being proinflammatory and anti-inflammatory. Proinflammatory cytokines such as TNF-α and IL-6 are primarily secreted from monocytes and macrophages, and activate other cellular components of the inflammatory response. While TNF-α mainly activates the type 1 response, IL-6 activates the type 2 response, including antibody production. Anti-inflammatory cytokines such as IL-4 and IL-10 help to downregulate the inflammatory immune response (table 2).

The Proinflammatory Immune State in Major Depression

Elevated plasma concentrations of C-reactive protein (CRP) are a common marker of an inflammatory process. CRP levels have been repeatedly observed to be higher in people with depression than in healthy controls, for example in severely depressed in-patients [28], and high CRP levels have been found to be associated with the severity of depression [29]. Higher CRP levels have also been found in both men [30, 31] and women [32, 33] in remission after a depressive state. In a sample of older healthy persons, CRP levels and IL-6 levels were predictive of cognitive symptoms of depression 12 years later [34]. In comparison to acute inflammatory diseases, such as pneumonia, however, the CRP increase is slight.

Characteristics of immune activation in major depression include increased numbers of circulating lymphocytes and phagocytic cells, upregulated serum levels of markers of immune activation, higher serum concentrations of positive

Table 3. Examples for immune markers reflecting immune activation in major depression

Disease-related markers	Markers for antidepressant response	Markers for response to immune related therapy
IL-6 [124]	IL-6 [28, 105]	IL-6 [105]
TNF-α [41]	Quinolinic acid	CRP [106]
CRP [28, 29]	[Müller et al., unpubl. data]	TNF-α [106]
Neopterin [47]	TNF-α [125]	TNFR1 [106, 126]
		TNFR2 [106]
		Kynurenine/tryptophan
		[Müller et al., unpubl. data]
		Kynurenine/quinolinic acid
		[Müller et al., unpubl. data]

acute phase proteins coupled with reduced levels of negative acute phase proteins, and increased release of proinflammatory cytokines such as IL-1β, IL-2, TNF-α and IL-6 (through activated macrophages) and interferon-γ (through activated T cells) [35–41]. Interferon-α is well documented to induce severe depressive symptoms, including suicidality, in about one third of patients [42]. Different research groups [43–45] have described increased numbers of peripheral mononuclear cells in major depression, and, in accordance with findings of increased monocytes and macrophages, an increased level of neopterin, a marker for activated macrophages, has also been described [46–49]. The role of cellular immunity, cytokines, and the innate and adaptive immune systems in depression has been recently reviewed [50, 51]. Table 3 summarizes several examples for immune markers in major depression.

Although immune activation is well established in major depression and infections are well known to trigger depressive symptoms, the association between infection and major depression has not been properly studied. In contrast, the etiology of immune activation in major depression is the subject of intense research.

Infections and Autoimmune Disorders as Risk Factors for Major Depression

The results of a prospective population-based Danish register study in 3.6 million people born between 1945 and 1996 support the view that an infection or autoimmune disease significantly increases the risk of a depressive disorder. Participants were followed up from 1977 to 2010, for a total of 78 million person-years. All people diagnosed with an affective disorder according to ICD-8, ICD-9 or ICD-10 and at least one in- or outpatient hospital contact due to an affective disorder (including bipolar disorder) were included. Every previous hospital contact due to an autoimmune disorder or infection (apart from HIV/AIDS) was then recorded. Over 91,000 cases of affective disorder were identified, of which approximately 30,000 had previously been diagnosed with infection and >4,000 with an autoimmune disease. The results show that hospitalization for infection significantly increased the risk for later mood disorder by 63% [incidence rate ratio (IRR) 1.63 (95% CI: 1.61–1.66)] and hospitalization for autoimmune disease significantly increased it by 45% [IRR 1.45 (95% CI: 1.39–1.52)]. Both risk factors interacted and increased the risk to an IRR of 2.35 (95% CI: 2.25–2.46). The findings do not support the hypothesis that primarily CNS infections result in later symptoms of mood disorders as, for example, the risks were higher for hepatitis infection [IRR 2.82 (95% CI: 2.58–3.08)] than for sepsis or CNS infections. Interestingly, the risk for mood disorder increased with the proximity of time to the infection, with the highest risk within the first year [IRR 2.70 (95% CI: 2.60–2.80)] [52]. Since only infections and autoimmune disorders resulting in a hospital contact were recorded, the risk for a mood disorder might be higher when all infections are considered.

Infection and Autoimmunity Presenting with Symptoms of Schizophrenia

There are numerous descriptions of an association between (chronic) inflammation of the CNS and schizophrenia [5]. For example, symptoms of schizophrenia have been described in the encephalitic form of multiple sclerosis [6], in viral CNS infection with herpes simplex virus types 1 [7] and 2 [8], and measles [10], and also in autoimmune processes such as poststreptococcal disorders [11–14], lupus erythematodes and scleroderma [15–18]. Schizophreniform symptoms in primary infectious diseases are diagnosed according to DSM-IV as a mental disorder due to a general medical condition (whereas in earlier times the diagnosis was 'organic brain disorder'). However, we do not know whether schizophreniform symptoms are 'secondary' to an infection or autoimmune process or the infection is a comorbid condition in a person with a 'primary' diagnosis of schizophrenia.

Inflammation and the Effect on Neurotransmission in Schizophrenia

Signs of inflammatory degradation products have been described in schizophrenic brain tissue [53] and in the cerebrospinal fluid of about 50% of people with schizophrenia [54]. Furthermore, a blunted type 1 and (compensatory) increased type 2 cytokine pattern have been repeatedly observed in people with unmedicated schizophrenia [55]. Recently published reviews on the imbalance of types 1 and 2 and pro- and anti-inflammatory immune systems as well as innate immunity, including the monocytic system, in schizophrenia have indicated that an inflammatory process plays an important role in the pathophysiology of (at least) a subgroup of people with schizophrenia [56, 57].

Over the last five decades, research on the neurobiology of schizophrenia has focused overwhelmingly on disturbances of dopaminergic neurotransmission [58]. A disturbance of the dopamine system is clearly involved in the pathogenesis of schizophrenia, although the mechanism is unclear and antipsychotic antidopaminergic drugs still show unsatisfactory therapeutic effects.

IL-1β, which can induce the conversion of rat mesencephalic progenitor cells into a dopaminergic phenotype [59–61], and IL-6, which is highly effective in decreasing the survival of fetal brain serotonergic neurons [62], seem to have an important effect on the development of the neurotransmitter systems specifically involved in schizophrenia, although the specificity of these cytokines is a matter of discussion. Maternal immune stimulation during pregnancy increased the number of mesencephalic dopaminergic neurons in the fetal brain, and the increase was probably associated with a dopaminergic excess in the midbrain [63]. Persistent pathogens might be key factors that drive imbalances of the immune reaction [18]. Nevertheless, many questions remain unanswered about how immunity and immune pathology in virus infections interact in order to show clinical symptoms [64].

Much evidence indicates that a lack of glutamatergic neurotransmission, mediated via NMDA antagonism, is a key mechanism in the pathophysiology of schizophrenia [65]. Kynurenic acid, the only NMDA receptor antagonist

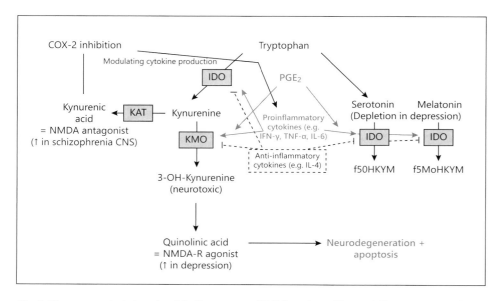

Fig. 1. The enzyme indoleamine 2,3-dioxygenase (IDO) is activated by proinflammatory cytokines [and prostaglandin E_2 (PGE_2)] and inhibited by anti-inflammatory cytokines. IDO degrades kynurenine, serotonin and melatonin, and influences the concentrations of these neuroactive metabolites and neurotransmitters. The enzyme KMO [kynurenine 3-monooxygenase (identical with kynurenine 3-hydroxylase)] drives the metabolism to the neurotoxic metabolite quinolinic acid. The enzyme KAT (kynurenine aminotransferase) drives the metabolism to kynurenic acid.

known to occur naturally in the human CNS [66], is one of at least three neuroactive intermediate products of the kynurenine pathway. In schizophrenia, a predominant type 2 immune response inhibits the enzyme indoleamine 2,3-dioxygenase, resulting in an increased production of kynurenic acid and consequently in NMDA receptor antagonism [65, 67]. The recent finding of NMDA receptor antibodies in about 10% of patients with acute and unmedicated schizophrenia is especially interesting in this regard (fig. 1).

Findings regarding kynurenic acid in schizophrenia vary. Elevated kynurenic acid has mainly been described in the cerebrospinal fluid [68–70] and in the brains of people with schizophrenia [71, 72], as well as in animal models of schizophrenia [73]. However, no increased kynurenic acid levels have been described in the peripheral blood of people with first-episode schizophrenia

[74] or in other groups of people with schizophrenia [75]. Increased neopterin values are to be mentioned here again [76]. Antipsychotic medication, however, affects kynurenine metabolites and has to be regarded as an interfering variable [74, 75, 77].

Infection as a Possible Pathogenetic Factor in Schizophrenia

The proposed involvement of immune activation and inflammation in the pathogenesis of schizophrenia has led to the hypothesis that infectious agents may be involved. Many recent studies have focused on members of the virus family of Herpesviridae [78], Borna virus [79], intracellular bacteria like *Chlamydia* [80] and the protozoan organism *Toxoplasma gondii* [81]. The roles of

Cytomegalovirus and *T. gondii* have been stressed for many years [82]. These agents are the focus of research because of their ability to establish persistent infections within the CNS and the occurrence of neurological and psychiatric symptoms in some individuals infected with these agents [83].

The group of Danish researchers mentioned above performed a study in schizophrenia similar to their study in affective disorders [127]. They found that severe infections and autoimmune disorders also additively increased the risk of schizophrenia and schizophrenia spectrum disorders. However, this large-scale study did not confirm infections in the parents, including intrauterine infections, as definite risk factors. Despite its large scale, the study's sensitivity was not very high because only infections associated with a contact to a Danish hospital were recorded, meaning that the risk factors which were identified may only have been the 'tip of the iceberg'.

Animal models of schizophrenia show that stimulation of the maternal immune system by viral agents leads to typical symptoms in the offspring. Evidence for pre- or perinatal exposure to infections as a risk factor for schizophrenia has been obtained not only from animal models, but also from studies with various viruses in humans. Increased risk for schizophrenia in the offspring was also observed after respiratory infections or genital or reproductive tract infections. *T. gondii* infection in mothers was also described to be a risk factor. Interestingly, recent animal research showed that stressful events in later stages of life (during puberty, an especially vulnerable phase in life) unmask latent neuropathological consequences of prenatal immune activation [84]. This animal model might explain the delay between an early inflammation and the onset of schizophrenia years later.

Both infections before birth and infections, particularly of the CNS, during later stages of brain development increase the risk for later schizophrenia. Antibody titers against viruses have been examined in the sera of people with schizophrenia for many years, but the results have been inconsistent due to reasons such as interfering factors not being controlled for. Antibody levels are associated with the medication state, a finding which partly explains earlier controversial results. In one of our own studies, people with schizophrenia had higher titers of different pathogens than controls, a phenomenon that we call the 'infectious index'.

Prenatal immune activation – regardless of whether it is triggered by infection – is an important risk factor for schizophrenia. In humans, increased maternal levels of the proinflammatory cytokine IL-8 during pregnancy were shown to increase the risk for schizophrenia in the offspring, whatever the reason for the increase in IL-8. Moreover, increased maternal IL-8 levels in pregnancy were also significantly related to decreased brain volume, leading to lower volumes of the right posterior cingulum and the left entorhinal cortex, and higher volumes of the ventricles in the offspring with schizophrenia (fig. 2).

Cyclooxygenase-2 Inhibition as an Example of an Anti-Inflammatory Therapeutic Approach in Schizophrenia and Major Depression

An immune-based therapeutic approach for psychiatric disorders was first proposed decades ago when the Nobel laureate Julius Wagner von Jauregg developed a vaccination therapy for psychoses [85]. He treated patients successfully with vaccines derived from attenuated *Mycobacterium tuberculosis*, *Plasmodium malariae* or *Salmonella* Typhi, all of which stimulate a type 1 immune response [86]. This therapy showed the best results in syphilis infection, but Wagner von Jauregg also administered the vaccination therapy for other psychiatric disorders. After the introduction of penicillin and as a consequence of the overwhelming success of the neurotransmitter approach in psychiatry, the therapeutic vaccination approach was not pursued further. In the past decade, the

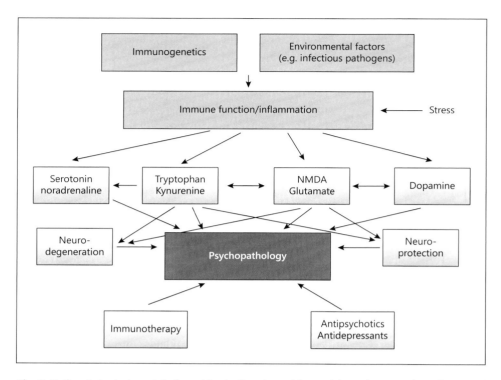

Fig. 2. Pathoetiological model of psychiatric disorders with special emphasis on the influence of infections, inflammation and the immune system. Besides other environmental factors such as stress (chronic stress depletes the immune response), pathogens are an important factor. Immune genes are involved in psychiatric disorders. The activation or inhibition of the immune response influences the noradrenergic, serotonergic, dopaminergic and glutamatergic neurotransmission and the (neuroprotective and/or neurotoxic) tryptophan/kynurenine system, and through these mechanisms contributes to the psychopathology of psychiatric disorders. Anti-inflammatory drugs show beneficial effects in disorders such as schizophrenia or major depression.

emerging limitations of the neurotransmitter approach for pathogenetic research have resulted in increased interest in other therapeutic approaches, including the possible use of modern anti-inflammatory agents in schizophrenia [87]. The cyclooxygenase-2 (COX-2) inhibitor celecoxib was studied as an add-on to risperidone in a prospective, randomized, double-blind study of acute exacerbation of schizophrenia; patients receiving celecoxib had a statistically significant better outcome and showed an increase in the type 1 immune response [88]. The clinical effects of COX-2 inhibition in schizophrenia are especially pro-

nounced in cognition [89]. The efficacy of therapy with a COX-2 inhibitor seems most pronounced in the first years of the schizophrenia disease process [90, 91]. A recent study also found a beneficial effect of acetylsalicylic acid in schizophrenia spectrum disorders [92]. A recent meta-analysis on the use of nonsteroidal anti-inflammatory drugs in schizophrenia found a significant benefit of add-on treatment with nonsteroidal anti-inflammatory drugs on positive and negative symptoms and on the total symptomatology over all studies [93]. A second meta-analysis on the same topic, but based on a broader database, found a benefit only in the early stages of the disease, in particular in first manifestations of schizophrenia [94].

COX-2 inhibitors also showed interesting effects in animal models of depression. Treatment with the COX-2 inhibitor celecoxib, but not with a COX-1 inhibitor, prevented the dysregulation of the hypothalamic-pituitary-adrenal axis, in particular the increase of cortisol, one of the key biological features associated with depression [95, 96]. This effect was expected because prostaglandin E_2, which stimulates the hypothalamic-pituitary-adrenal axis in the CNS [97], is inhibited by COX-2 inhibition. The functional effects of IL-1 in the CNS, which include sickness behavior, were also shown to be antagonized by treatment with a selective COX-2 inhibitor [98].

COX-2 inhibitors also affect the CNS serotonergic system, either directly or via CNS immune mechanisms. In a rat model, treatment with rofecoxib was followed by an increase of serotonin in the frontal and temporoparietal cortex [99]. COX-2 inhibitors would be expected to show a clinical antidepressant effect since a lack of serotonin is one of the main factors in the pathophysiology of depression. The antidepressant action of COX-2 inhibitors may be mediated through inhibition of IL-1 and IL-6 release. In the depression model of bulbectomized rats, a decrease in hypothalamus cytokine levels and a change in behavior have been observed after chronic celecoxib treatment [100]. In another animal model of depression, however, the mixed COX-1/COX-2 inhibitor acetylsalicylic acid showed an additional antidepressant effect by accelerating the antidepressant effect of fluoxetine [101]. In an open-label pilot study in humans, acetylsalicylic acid also accelerated the antidepressant effect of fluoxetine and increased the response rate to monotherapy with fluoxetine in depressed nonresponders [102]. A significant therapeutic effect of the COX-2 inhibitor celecoxib in major depression was also found in a randomized, double-blind pilot add-on study [103]. Another randomized, double-blind study

in 50 patients with major depression also showed a significantly better outcome with the COX-2 inhibitor celecoxib plus fluoxetine than with fluoxetine alone [104]. A similar result was obtained with a celecoxib add-on approach to sertraline in major depression [105, 106]. A meta-analysis on the use of COX-2 inhibitors in major depression found an overall benefit of celecoxib add-on therapy [107].

Interestingly, etanercept, which blocks the interaction of TNF-α with the TNF-α cell surface receptors, showed a highly significant antidepressant effect [108]. A study with another TNF-α receptor blocker, infliximab, found no overall benefit in treatment-resistant patients with major depression, but did find a benefit in those with higher levels of inflammatory markers, such as CRP, TNF-α or soluble TNF receptors [106].

Although those preliminary data have to be interpreted cautiously and further research is needed to evaluate the therapeutic effects of COX-2 inhibitors in major depression, the results are encouraging for further studies on the inflammatory hypothesis of depression and the pathogenesis, course and therapy of the disease.

Childhood Infections: A Common Cause for Mental Disorders?

Maternal infection during pregnancy and childhood infections are risk factors for later schizophrenia, especially in combination with stress during puberty [84, 109]. Furthermore, infections in later life are risk factors for both major depression [52] and schizophrenia [110]. In major depression, an inflammatory process seems to play a role in a subgroup of patients, but no specific infectious pathogens have been described. Stress and other environmental factors may contribute to the proinflammatory state. For example, animal models indicate that early life separation is associated with increased cytokine levels and passive behavior [111] and that early childhood stress disrupts the regulation of innate immune resistance to a challenge (lipopolysaccharide, viral infection), resulting in enhanced immunological and behavioral responses to immune activation in animals [112]. In people with depression, early-life stress is associated with enhanced inflammatory responsiveness to stress [113]. Moreover, a relationship between early childhood stress, inflammatory markers and depression in adult patients has been described [114, 115]. Overall, studies indicate that stress and adverse events in childhood seem to be risk factors for an inflammatory state in adulthood.

The Concepts of Pediatric Autoimmune Neuropsychiatric Disorder Associated with Streptococcal Infections, Pediatric Infection-Triggered Autoimmune Neuropsychiatric Disorder and Pediatric Acute-Onset Neuropsychiatric Syndrome as Infectious Disorders Presenting as (Neuro-) Psychiatric Symptoms

There are further examples for the involvement of infections in psychiatric disorders. Pediatric autoimmune neuropsychiatric disorder associated with streptococcal infections (PANDAS) manifests with tics, Tourette's syndrome and/or obsessive-compulsive symptoms [116], and is a consequence of streptococcal infection. However, not only *Streptococcus* but also other infectious agents such as *Borrelia burgdorferi* [117] or *Mycoplasma pneumoniae* [118, 119] may directly or indirectly cause this syndrome. Therefore, the concept of pediatric infection-triggered autoimmune neuropsychiatric disorder, a postinfectious syndrome not restricted to streptococcal infection, was introduced [116, 120]. The broader concepts of pediatric acute-onset neuropsychiatric syndrome [121] and childhood acute neuropsychiatric syndromes, which define a much broader clinical spectrum encompassing etiologically diverse entities, were recently proposed to overcome the criticism that the postinfectious syndrome might present with behavioral symptoms or comorbidities other than tics and obsessive-compulsive symptoms. Exploratory studies aiming to identify clinical or cognitive features that could discriminate PANDAS from other pediatric obsessive-compulsive and tic disorders have presented methodological limitations and are therefore inconclusive. Given the uncertainties regarding the clinical definition of PANDAS, it is not surprising that the evidence for a postinfectious, immune-mediated pathophysiology has to be further elucidated and specified [122]. However, therapeutic studies based on the PANDAS concept have shown that immunomodulating therapies, such as intravenous γ-immunoglobulin or plasmapheresis, have highly significant advantages compared to placebo [123].

The conceptual and terminological heterogeneity discussed above reflects the difficulties not only of postinfectious (auto-)immune syndromes, but also of infection- and immune-mediated disorders in psychiatry in general: the pathophysiological process is not fully elucidated, specific mechanisms still need to be explored and further scientific efforts are necessary. On the other hand, similar to the neurotransmitter-centered biological approach in psychiatry in which therapies were developed first and biological explanations came later, effective therapeutic approaches are on the way and may provide post hoc validation of the discussed concepts.

Conclusions

The possible influences of infection and immune processes on the pathogenesis of major psychiatric disorders resulting in inflammation have long been neglected. Increasing evidence for a role of proinflammatory cytokines in major depression and schizophrenia, the strong influence of pro- and anti-inflammatory cytokines on the tryptophan/kynurenine metabolism and – related to that mechanism – the influence of cytokines on the glutamatergic neurotransmission support the view that infection, psychoneuroimmunology and inflammation rightly should be a focus of psychiatric research. This view is fostered by the results of (immuno-) genetic findings and the exhibited therapeutic effects of anti-inflammatory drugs in schizophrenia and major depression. On the other hand, it is possible that immunological research in patients may be susceptible to artefacts; interfering variables such as medication, smoking, stress, sleep and others play an important role and cannot always been controlled. This can be shown by the example of stress: stress is not only – according to the 'vulnerability-stress-model' of schizophrenia – a condition sine qua non in schizophrenia, it is also a confounding factor for research of the immune system and inflammatory processes.

These considerations show that further research is needed to clarify the role of infection and of the immune system in psychiatric disorders. Recent results encourage placing further emphasis on this fascinating field. Therapeutic studies, including meta-analyses, support the view that therapeutic progress based on anti-inflammatory and/or immunomodulating approaches are not only of theoretical interest, but may have an important clinical impact and might lead to a paradigm change in psychiatric therapy.

References

1 O'Neill LA: How frustration leads to inflammation. Science 2008;320:619–620.
2 Kraepelin E: Über Psychosen nach Influenza. Dtsch Med Wochenschr 1890;11:209–212.
3 Kraepelin E: Ziele und Wege der Psychiatrischen Forschung. Z Ges Neurol Psychiatrie 1918;42:169–205.
4 Steinberg H, Himmerich H: Emil Kraepelin's habilitation and his thesis: a pioneer work for modern systematic reviews, psychoimmunological research and categories of psychiatric diseases. World J Biol Psychiatry 2013;14:248–257.
5 Anderson G, Berk M, Dodd S, Bechter K, Altamura AC, Dell'osso B, Kanba S, Monji A, Fatemi SH, Buckley P, Debnath M, Das UN, Meyer U, Muller N, Kanchanatawan B, Maes M: Immuno-inflammatory, oxidative and nitrosative stress, and neuroprogressive pathways in the etiology, course and treatment of schizophrenia. Prog Neuropsychopharmacol Biol Psychiatry 2013;42:1–4.
6 Felgenhauer K: Psychiatric disorders in the encephalitic form of multiple sclerosis. J Neurol 1990;237:11–18.
7 Chiveri L, Sciacco M, Prelle A: Schizophreniform disorder with cerebrospinal fluid PCR positivity for herpes simplex virus type 1. Eur Neurol 2003;50:182–183.
8 Oommen KJ, Johnson PC, Ray CG: Herpes simplex type 2 virus encephalitis presenting as psychosis. Am J Med 1982;73:445–448.
9 Fazekas C, Enzinger C, Wallner M, Kischka U, Greimel E, Kapeller P, Stix P, Pieringer W, Fazekas F: Depressive symptoms following herpes simplex encephalitis – an underestimated phenomenon? Gen Hosp Psychiatry 2006;28:403–407.
10 Hiroshi H, Seiji K, Toshihiro K, Nobuo K: An adult case suspected of recurrent measles encephalitis with psychiatric symptoms (in Japanese). Seishin Shinkeigaku Zasshi 2003;105:1239–1246.
11 Mercadante MT, Busatto GF, Lombroso PJ, Prado L, Rosario-Campos MC, do VR, Marques-Dias MJ, Kiss MH, Leckman JF, Miguel EC: The psychiatric symptoms of rheumatic fever. Am J Psychiatry 2000;157:2036–2038.
12 Teixeira AL Jr, Maia DP, Cardoso F: Psychosis following acute Sydenham's chorea. Eur Child Adolesc Psychiatry 2007;16:67–69.
13 Kerbeshian J, Burd L, Tait A: Chain reaction or time bomb: a neuropsychiatric-developmental/neurodevelopmental formulation of tourettisms, pervasive developmental disorder, and schizophreniform symptomatology associated with PANDAS. World J Biol Psychiatry 2007;8:201–207.
14 Bechter K, Bindl A, Horn M, Schreiner V: Therapy-resistant depression with fatigue. A case of presumed streptococcal-associated autoimmune disorder (in German). Nervenarzt 2007;78:338, 340–341.
15 Müller N, Gizycki-Nienhaus B, Günther W, Meurer M: Depression as a cerebral manifestation of scleroderma: immunological findings in serum and cerebrospinal fluid. Biol Psychiatry 1992;31:1151–1156.
16 Müller N, Gizycki-Nienhaus B, Botschev C, Meurer M: Cerebral involvement of scleroderma presenting as schizophrenia-like psychosis. Schizophr Res 1993;10:179–181.
17 van Dam AP: Diagnosis and pathogenesis of CNS lupus. Rheumatol Int 1991;11:1–11.
18 Nikolich-Zugich J: Ageing and life-long maintenance of T-cell subsets in the face of latent persistent infections. Nat Rev Immunol 2008;8:512–522.
19 Bechter K: Mild encephalitis underlying psychiatric disorders – a reconsideration and hypothesis exemplified on Borna disease. Neurol Psychiatry Brain Res 2001;9:55–70.
20 American Psychiatric Association Diagnostic Criteria from DSM-IV. Washington, American Psychiatric Association, 1994.

21 Dantzer R: Cytokine-induced sickness behavior: where do we stand? Brain Behav Immun 2001;15:7–24.

22 Dantzer R, O'Connor JC, Freund GG, Johnson RW, Kelley KW: From inflammation to sickness and depression: when the immune system subjugates the brain. Nat Rev Neurosci 2008;9:46–56.

23 Reichenberg A, Yirmiya R, Schuld A, Kraus T, Haack M, Morag A, Pollmacher T: Cytokine-associated emotional and cognitive disturbances in humans. Arch Gen Psychiatry 2001;58:445–452.

24 Reichenberg A, Kraus T, Haack M, Schuld A, Pollmacher T, Yirmiya R: Endotoxin-induced changes in food consumption in healthy volunteers are associated with TNF-alpha and IL-6 secretion. Psychoneuroendocrinology 2002;27:945–956.

25 Raison CL, Miller AH: Do cytokines really sing the blues? Cerebrum 2013; 2013:10.

26 Raison CL, Miller AH: The evolutionary significance of depression in pathogen host defense (PATHOS-D). Mol Psychiatry 2013;18:15–37.

27 Mills CD, Kincaid K, Alt JM, Heilman MJ, Hill AM: M-1/M-2 macrophages and the Th1/Th2 paradigm. J Immunol 2000;164:6166–6173.

28 Lanquillon S, Krieg JC, Bening-Abu-Shach U, Vedder H: Cytokine production and treatment response in major depressive disorder. Neuropsychopharmacology 2000;22:370–379.

29 Häfner S, Baghai TC, Eser D, Schüle C, Rupprecht R, Bondy B, Bedarida G, von Schacky C: C-reactive protein is associated with polymorphisms of the angiotensin-converting enzyme gene in major depressed patients. J Psychiatr Res 2008; 42:163–165.

30 Danner M, Kasl SV, Abramson JL, Vaccarino V: Association between depression and elevated C-reactive protein. Psychosom Med 2003;65:347–356.

31 Ford DE, Erlinger TP: Depression and C-reactive protein in US adults: data from the Third National Health and Nutrition Examination Survey. Arch Intern Med 2004;164:1010–1014.

32 Kling MA, Alesci S, Csako G, Costello R, Luckenbaugh DA, Bonne O, Duncko R, Drevets WC, Manji HK, Charney DS, Gold PW, Neumeister A: Sustained low-grade pro-inflammatory state in unmedicated, remitted women with major depressive disorder as evidenced by elevated serum levels of the acute phase proteins C-reactive protein and serum amyloid A. Biol Psychiatry 2007;62:309–313.

33 Cizza G, Eskandari F, Coyle M, Krishnamurthy P, Wright EC, Mistry S, Csako G: Plasma CRP levels in premenopausal women with major depression: a 12-month controlled study. Horm Metab Res 2009;41:641–648.

34 Gimeno D, Marmot MG, Singh-Manoux A: Inflammatory markers and cognitive function in middle-aged adults: the Whitehall II study. Psychoneuroendocrinology 2008;33:1322–1334.

35 Müller N, Hofschuster E, Ackenheil M, Mempel W, Eckstein R: Investigations of the cellular immunity during depression and the free interval: evidence for an immune activation in affective psychosis. Prog Neuropsychopharmacol Biol Psychiatry 1993;17:713–730.

36 Maes M, Meltzer HY, Bosmans E, Bergmans R, Vandoolaeghe E, Ranjan R, Desnyder R: Increased plasma concentrations of interleukin-6, soluble interleukin-6, soluble interleukin-2 and transferrin receptor in major depression. J Affect Disord 1995;34:301–309.

37 Maes M, Meltzer HY, Buckley P, Bosmans E: Plasma-soluble interleukin-2 and transferrin receptor in schizophrenia and major depression. Eur Arch Psychiatry Clin Neurosci 1995;244:325–329.

38 Irwin M: Immune correlates of depression. Adv Exp Med Biol 1999;461:1–24.

39 Nunes SO, Reiche EMV, Morimoto HK, Matsuo T, Itano EN, Xavier EC, Yamashita CM, Vieira VR, Menoli AV, Silva SS, Costa FB, Reiche FV, Silva FL, Kaminami MS: Immune and hormonal activity in adults suffering from depression. Braz J Med Biol Res 2002;35:581–587.

40 Müller N, Schwarz MJ: Immunology in anxiety and depression; in Kasper S, den Boer JA, Sitsen JMA (eds): Handbook of Depression and Anxiety. New York, Marcel Dekker, 2002, pp 267–288.

41 Mikova O, Yakimova R, Bosmans E, Kenis G, Maes M: Increased serum tumor necrosis factor alpha concentrations in major depression and multiple sclerosis. Eur Neuropsychopharmacol 2001;11:203–208.

42 Friebe A, Horn M, Schmidt F, Janssen G, Schmid-Wendtner MH, Volkenandt M, Hauschild A, Goldsmith CH, Schaefer M: Dose-dependent development of depressive symptoms during adjuvant interferon-{alpha} treatment of patients with malignant melanoma. Psychosomatics 2010;51:466–473.

43 Herbert TB, Cohen S: Depression and immunity: a meta-analytic review. Psychol Bull 1993;113:472–486.

44 Seidel A, Arolt V, Hunstiger M, Rink L, Behnisch A, Kirchner H: Major depressive disorder is associated with elevated monocyte counts. Acta Psychiatr Scand 1996;94:198–204.

45 Rothermundt M, Arolt V, Fenker J, Gutbrodt H, Peters M, Kirchner H: Different immune patterns in melancholic and non-melancholic major depression. Eur Arch Psychiatry Clin Neurosci 2001;251: 90–97.

46 Duch DS, Woolf JH, Nichol CA, Davidson JR, Garbutt JC: Urinary excretion of biopterin and neopterin in psychiatric disorders. Psychiatry Res 1984;11:83–89.

47 Dunbar PR, Hill J, Neale TJ, Mellsop GW: Neopterin measurement provides evidence of altered cell-mediated immunity in patients with depression, but not with schizophrenia. Psychol Med 1992; 22:1051–1057.

48 Maes M, Scharpe S, Meltzer HY, Okayli G, Bosmans E, D'Hondt P, Vanden Bossche BV, Cosyns P: Increased neopterin and interferon-gamma secretion and lower availability of L-tryptophan in major depression: further evidence for an immune response. Psychiatry Res 1994;54:143–160.

49 Bonaccorso S, Lin AH, Verkerk R, Van Hunsel F, Libbrecht I, Scharpe S, DeClerck L, Biondi M, Janca A, Maes M: Immune markers in fibromyalgia: comparison with major depressed patients and normal volunteers. J Affect Disord 1998;48:75–82.

50 Müller N, Myint AM, Schwarz MJ: Inflammatory biomarkers and depression. Neurotox Res 2011;19:308–318.

51 Maes M: Depression is an inflammatory disease, but cell-mediated immune activation is the key component of depression. Prog Neuropsychopharmacol Biol Psychiatry 2011;35:664–675.

52 Benros ME, Waltoft BL, Nordentoft M, Ostergaard SD, Eaton WW, Krogh J, Mortensen PB: Autoimmune diseases and severe infections as risk factors for mood disorders: a nationwide study. JAMA Psychiatry 2013;70:812–820.

53 Körschenhausen DA, Hampel HJ, Ackenheil M, Penning R, Müller N: Fibrin degradation products in post mortem brain tissue of schizophrenics: a possible marker for underlying inflammatory processes. Schizophr Res 1996;19:103–109.

54 Wildenauer DB, Körschenhausen D, Hoechtlen W, Ackenheil M, Kehl M, Lottspeich F: Analysis of cerebrospinal fluid from patients with psychiatric and neurological disorders by two-dimensional electrophoresis: identification of disease-associated polypeptides as fibrin fragments. Electrophoresis 1991;12:487–492.

55 Schwarz MJ, Müller N, Riedel M, Ackenheil M: The Th2-hypothesis of schizophrenia: a strategy to identify a subgroup of schizophrenia caused by immune mechanisms. Med Hypotheses 2001;56:483–486.

56 Müller N, Schwarz MJ: Immune system and schizophrenia. Curr Immunol Rev 2010;6:213–220.

57 Potvin S, Stip E, Sepehry AA, Gendron A, Bah R, Kouassi E: Inflammatory cytokine alterations in schizophrenia: a systematic quantitative review. Biol Psychiatry 2008;63:801–808.

58 Carlsson A: The current status of the dopamine hypothesis of schizophrenia. Neuropsychopharmacology 1988;1:179–186.

59 Ling ZD, Potter ED, Lipton JW, Carvey PM: Differentiation of mesencephalic progenitor cells into dopaminergic neurons by cytokines. Exp Neurol 1998;149:411–423.

60 Kabiersch A, Furukawa H, del RA, Besedovsky HO: Administration of interleukin-1 at birth affects dopaminergic neurons in adult mice. Ann NY Acad Sci 1998;840:123–127.

61 Potter ED, Ling ZD, Carvey PM: Cytokine-induced conversion of mesencephalic-derived progenitor cells into dopamine neurons. Cell Tissue Res 1999;296:235–246.

62 Jarskog LF, Xiao H, Wilkie MB, Lauder JM, Gilmore JH: Cytokine regulation of embryonic rat dopamine and serotonin neuronal survival in vitro. Int J Dev Neurosci 1997;15:711–716.

63 Winter C, Djodari-Irani A, Sohr R, Morgenstern R, Feldon J, Juckel G, Meyer U: Prenatal immune activation leads to multiple changes in basal neurotransmitter levels in the adult brain: implications for brain disorders of neurodevelopmental origin such as schizophrenia. Int J Neuropsychopharmacol 2009;12:513–524.

64 Rouse BT, Sehrawat S: Immunity and immunopathology to viruses: what decides the outcome? Nat Rev Immunol 2010;10:514–526.

65 Müller N, Schwarz MJ: The immunological basis of glutamatergic disturbance in schizophrenia: towards an integrated view. J Neural Transm 2007;suppl 72:269–280.

66 Stone TW: Neuropharmacology of quinolinic and kynurenic acids. Pharmacol Rev 1993;45:309–379.

67 Müller N, Myint AM, Schwarz MJ: Kynurenine pathway in schizophrenia: pathophysiological and therapeutic aspects. Curr Pharm Des 2011;17:130–136.

68 Erhardt S, Blennow K, Nordin C, Skogh E, Lindstrom LH, Engberg G: Kynurenic acid levels are elevated in the cerebrospinal fluid of patients with schizophrenia. Neurosci Lett 2001;313:96–98.

69 Nilsson LK, Linderholm KR, Engberg G, Paulson L, Blennow K, Lindstrom LH, Nordin C, Karanti A, Persson P, Erhardt S: Elevated levels of kynurenic acid in the cerebrospinal fluid of male patients with schizophrenia. Schizophr Res 2005;80:315–322.

70 Linderholm KR, Skogh E, Olsson SK, Dahl ML, Holtze M, Engberg G, Samuelsson M, Erhardt S: Increased levels of kynurenine and kynurenic acid in the CSF of patients with schizophrenia. Schizophr Bull 2012;38:426–432.

71 Schwarcz R, Rassoulpour A, Wu HQ, Medoff D, Tamminga CA, Roberts RC: Increased cortical kynurenate content in schizophrenia. Biol Psychiatry 2001;50:521–530.

72 Sathyasaikumar KV, Stachowski EK, Wonodi I, Roberts RC, Rassoulpour A, McMahon RP, Schwarcz R: Impaired kynurenine pathway metabolism in the prefrontal cortex of individuals with schizophrenia. Schizophr Bull 2011;37:1147–1156.

73 Olsson SK, Andersson AS, Linderholm KR, Holtze M, Nilsson-Todd LK, Schwieler L, Olsson E, Larsson K, Engberg G, Erhardt S: Elevated levels of kynurenic acid change the dopaminergic response to amphetamine: implications for schizophrenia. Int J Neuropsychopharmacol 2009;12:501–512.

74 Condray R, Dougherty GG, Keshavan MS, Reddy RD, Haas GL, Montrose DM, Matson WR, McEvoy J, Kaddurah-Daouk R, Yao JK: 3-Hydroxykynurenine and clinical symptoms in first-episode neuroleptic-naive patients with schizophrenia. Int J Neuropsychopharmacol 2011;14:756–767.

75 Myint AM, Schwarz MJ, Verkerk R, Mueller HH, Zach J, Scharpe S, Steinbusch HW, Leonard BE, Kim YK: Reversal of imbalance between kynurenic acid and 3-hydroxykynurenine by antipsychotics in medication-naive and medication-free schizophrenic patients. Brain Behav Immun 2011;25:1576–1581.

76 Kuehne LK, Reiber H, Bechter K, Hagberg L, Fuchs D: Cerebrospinal fluid neopterin is brain-derived and not associated with blood CSF barrier dysfunction in non-inflammatory affective and schizophrenic spectrum disorders. J Psychiatr Res 2013;47:1417–1422.

77 Ceresoli-Borroni G, Rassoulpour A, Wu HQ, Guidetti P, Schwarcz R: Chronic neuroleptic treatment reduces endogenous kynurenic acid levels in rat brain. J Neural Transm 2006;113:1355–1365.

78 Hare EH, Price JS, Slater E: Schizophrenia and season of birth. Br J Psychiatry 1972;120:124–125.

79 Machon RA, Mednick SA, Schulsinger F: The interaction of seasonality, place of birth, genetic risk and subsequent schizophrenia in a high risk sample. Br J Psychiatry 1983;143:383–388.

80 Wright P, Takei N, Rifkin L, Murray RM: Maternal influenza, obstetric complications, and schizophrenia. Am J Psychiatry 1995;152:1714–1720.

81 Brown AS: Prenatal infection as a risk factor for schizophrenia. Schizophr Bull 2006;32:200–202.

82 Torrey EF, Leweke MF, Schwarz MJ, Mueller N, Bachmann S, Schroeder J, Dickerson F, Yolken RH: Cytomegalovirus and schizophrenia. CNS Drugs 2006;20:879–885.

83 Caroff SN, Mann SC, McCarthy M, Naser J, Rynn M, Morrison M: Acute infectious encephalitis complicated by neuroleptic malignant syndrome. J Clin Psychopharmacol 1998;18:349–351.

84 Giovanoli S, Engler H, Engler A, Richetto J, Voget M, Willi R, Winter C, Riva MA, Mortensen PB, Schedlowski M, Meyer U: Stress in puberty unmasks latent neuropathological consequences of prenatal immune activation in mice. Science 2013;339:1095–1099.

85 Wagner von Jauregg J: Fieberbehandlung bei Psychosen. Wien Med Wochenschr 1926;76:79–82.

86 Müller N, Schwarz MJ, Riedel M: COX-2 inhibition in schizophrenia: focus on clinical effects of celecoxib therapy and the role of TNF-alpha; in Eaton WW (ed): Medical and Psychiatric Comorbidity over the Course of Life. Washington, American Psychiatric Publishing, 2005, pp 265–276.

87 Fond G, Hamdani N, Kapczinski F, Boukouaci W, Drancourt N, Dargel A, Oliveira J, Le GE, Marlinge E, Tamouza R, Leboyer M: Effectiveness and tolerance of anti-inflammatory drugs' add-on therapy in major mental disorders: a systematic qualitative review. Acta Psychiatr Scand 2014;129:163–179.

88 Müller N, Riedel M, Scheppach C, Brandstätter B, Sokullu S, Krampe K, Ulmschneider M, Engel RR, Möller HJ, Schwarz MJ: Beneficial antipsychotic effects of celecoxib add-on therapy compared to risperidone alone in schizophrenia. Am J Psychiatry 2002;159:1029–1034.

89 Müller N, Riedel M, Schwarz MJ, Engel RR: Clinical effects of COX-2 inhibitors on cognition in schizophrenia. Eur Arch Psychiatry Clin Neurosci 2005;255:149–151.

90 Müller N: COX-2 inhibitors as antidepressants and antipsychotics: clinical evidence. Curr Opin Investig Drugs 2010;11:31–42.

91 Müller N, Krause D, Dehning S, Musil R, Schennach-Wolff R, Obermeier M, Möller HJ, Klauss V, Schwarz MJ, Riedel M: Celecoxib treatment in an early stage of schizophrenia: results of a randomized, double-blind, placebo-controlled trial of celecoxib augmentation of amisulpride treatment. Schizophr Res 2010; 121:119–124.

92 Laan W, Grobbee DE, Selten JP, Heijnen CJ, Kahn RS, Burger H: Adjuvant aspirin therapy reduces symptoms of schizophrenia spectrum disorders: results from a randomized, double-blind, placebo-controlled trial. J Clin Psychiatry 2010;71:520–527.

93 Sommer IE, de WL, Begemann M, Kahn RS: Nonsteroidal anti-inflammatory drugs in schizophrenia: ready for practice or a good start? A meta-analysis. J Clin Psychiatry 2012;73:414–419.

94 Nitta M, Kishimoto T, Müller N, Weiser M, Davidson M, Kane JM, Correll CU: Adjunctive use of nonsteroidal anti-inflammatory drugs for schizophrenia: a meta-analytic investigation of randomized controlled trials. Schizophr Bull 2013;39:1230–1241.

95 Casolini P, Catalani A, Zuena AR, Angelucci L: Inhibition of COX-2 reduces the age-dependent increase of hippocampal inflammatory markers, corticosterone secretion, and behavioral impairments in the rat. J Neurosci Res 2002;68:337–343.

96 Hu F, Wang X, Pace TW, Wu H, Miller AH: Inhibition of COX-2 by celecoxib enhances glucocorticoid receptor function. Mol Psychiatry 2005;10:426–428.

97 Song C, Leonard BE: Fundamentals of psychoneuroimmunology. Chicester, J Wiley and Sons, 2000.

98 Cao C, Matsumura K, Ozaki M, Watanabe Y: Lipopolysaccharide injected into the cerebral ventricle evokes fever through induction of cyclooxygenase-2 in brain endothelial cells. J Neurosci 1999;19:716–725.

99 Sandrini M, Vitale G, Pini LA: Effect of rofecoxib on nociception and the serotonin system in the rat brain. Inflamm Res 2002;51:154–159.

100 Myint AM, Steinbusch HW, Goeghegan L, Luchtman D, Kim YK, Leonard BE: Effect of the COX-2 inhibitor celecoxib on behavioural and immune changes in an olfactory bulbectomised rat model of depression. Neuroimmunomodulation 2007;14:65–71.

101 Brunello N, Alboni S, Capone G, Benatti C, Blom JM, Tascedda F, Kriwin P, Mendlewicz J: Acetylsalicylic acid accelerates the antidepressant effect of fluoxetine in the chronic escape deficit model of depression. Int Clin Psychopharmacol 2006;21:219–225.

102 Mendlewicz J, Kriwin P, Oswald P, Souery D, Alboni S, Brunello N: Shortened onset of action of antidepressants in major depression using acetylsalicylic acid augmentation: a pilot open-label study. Int Clin Psychopharmacol 2006;21:227–231.

103 Müller N, Schwarz MJ, Dehning S, Douhet A, Cerovecki A, Goldstein-Müller B, Spellmann I, Hetzel G, Maino K, Kleindienst N, Möller HJ, Arolt V, Riedel M: The cyclooxygenase-2 inhibitor celecoxib has therapeutic effects in major depression: results of a double-blind, randomized, placebo controlled, add-on pilot study to reboxetine. Mol Psychiatry 2006;11:680–684.

104 Akhondzadeh S, Jafari S, Raisi F, Nasehi AA, Ghoreishi A, Salehi B, Mohebbi-Rasa S, Raznahan M, Kamalipour A: Clinical trial of adjunctive celecoxib treatment in patients with major depression: a double blind and placebo controlled trial. Depress Anxiety 2009; 26:607–611.

105 Abbasi SH, Hosseini F, Modabbernia A, Ashrafi M, Akhondzadeh S: Effect of celecoxib add-on treatment on symptoms and serum IL-6 concentrations in patients with major depressive disorder: randomized double-blind placebo-controlled study. J Affect Disord 2012; 141:308–314.

106 Raison CL, Rutherford RE, Woolwine BJ, Shuo C, Schettler P, Drake DF, Haroon E, Miller AH: A randomized controlled trial of the tumor necrosis factor antagonist infliximab for treatment-resistant depression: the role of baseline inflammatory biomarkers. JAMA Psychiatry 2013;70:31–41.

107 Na KS, Lee KJ, Lee JS, Cho YS, Jung HY: Efficacy of adjunctive celecoxib treatment for patients with major depressive disorder: a meta-analysis. Prog Neuropsychopharmacol Biol Psychiatry 2014;48:79–85.

108 Tyring S, Gottlieb A, Papp K, Gordon K, Leonardi C, Wang A, Lalla D, Woolley M, Jahreis A, Zitnik R, Cella D, Krishnan R: Etanercept and clinical outcomes, fatigue, and depression in psoriasis: double-blind placebo-controlled randomised phase III trial. Lancet 2006;367:29–35.

109 Meyer U, Schwarz MJ, Müller N: Inflammatory processes in schizophrenia: a promising neuroimmunological target for the treatment of negative/cognitive symptoms and beyond. Pharmacol Ther 2011;132:96–110.

110 Benros ME, Mortensen PB, Eaton WW: Autoimmune diseases and infections as risk factors for schizophrenia. Ann NY Acad Sci 2012;1262:56–66.

111 Hennessy MB, Schiml-Webb PA, Miller EE, Maken DS, Bullinger KL, Deak T: Anti-inflammatory agents attenuate the passive responses of guinea pig pups: evidence for stress-induced sickness behavior during maternal separation. Psychoneuroendocrinology 2007;32:508–515.

112 Avitsur R, Sheridan JF: Neonatal stress modulates sickness behavior. Brain Behav Immun 2009;23:977–985.

113 Pace TW, Mletzko TC, Alagbe O, Musselman DL, Nemeroff CB, Miller AH, Heim CM: Increased stress-induced inflammatory responses in male patients with major depression and increased early life stress. Am J Psychiatry 2006;163:1630–1633.

114 Zeugmann S, Quante A, Heuser I, Schwarzer R, Anghelescu I: Inflammatory biomarkers in 70 depressed inpatients with and without the metabolic syndrome. J Clin Psychiatry 2010;71:1007–1016.

115 Zeugmann S, Quante A, Popova-Zeugmann L, Kossler W, Heuser I, Anghelescu I: Pathways linking early life stress, metabolic syndrome, and the inflammatory marker fibrinogen in depressed inpatients. Psychiatr Danub 2012;24:57–65.

116 Swedo SE, Leonard HL, Garvey M, Mittleman B, Allen AJ, Perlmutter S, Dow S, Zamkoff J, Dubbert BK, Lougee L: Pediatric autoimmune neuropsychiatric disorders associated with streptococcal infections: clinical description of the first 50 cases. Am J Psychiatry 1998;155:264–271.

117 Riedel M, Straube A, Schwarz MJ, Wilske B, Müller N: Lyme disease presenting as Tourette's syndrome. Lancet 1998;351:418–419.

118 Müller N, Riedel M, Forderreuther S, Blendinger C, Abele-Horn M: Tourette's syndrome and mycoplasma pneumoniae infection. Am J Psychiatry 2000;157:481–482.

119 Müller N, Riedel M, Blendinger C, Oberle K, Jacobs E, Abele-Horn M: Mycoplasma pneumoniae infection and Tourette's syndrome. Psychiatry Res 2004;129:119–125.

120 Allen AJ, Leonard HL, Swedo SE: Case study: a new infection-triggered, autoimmune subtype of pediatric OCD and Tourette's syndrome. J Am Acad Child Adolesc Psychiatry 1995;34:307–311.

121 Macerollo A, Martino D: Pediatric autoimmune neuropsychiatric disorders associated with streptococcal infections (PANDAS): an evolving concept. Tremor Other Hyperkinet Mov (N Y). 2013 Sep 25;3. pii: tre-03-167-4158-7.

122 Macerollo A, Martino D: Pediatric autoimmune neuropsychiatric disorders associated with streptococcal infections (PANDAS): an evolving concept. Tremor Other Hyperkinet Mov (N Y) 2013;3: pii: tre-03-167-4158-7.

123 Perlmutter SJ, Leitman SF, Garvey MA, Hamburger S, Feldman E, Leonard HL, Swedo SE: Therapeutic plasma exchange and intravenous immunoglobulin for obsessive-compulsive disorder and tic disorders in childhood. Lancet 1999;354:1153–1158.

124 Maes M, Bosmans E, Calabrese J, Smith R, Meltzer HY: Interleukin-2 and interleukin-6 in schizophrenia and mania: effects of neuroleptics and mood stabilizers. J Psychiatr Res 1995;29:141–152.

125 Hestad KA, Tonseth S, Stoen CD, Ueland T, Aukrust P: Raised plasma levels of tumor necrosis factor alpha in patients with depression: normalization during electroconvulsive therapy. J ECT 2003;19:183–188.

126 Müller N, Schwarz MJ, Riedel M: COX-2 inhibition in schizophrenia; in Eaton WW (ed): Medical and Psychiatric Comorbidity over the Course of Life. Washington, American Psychiatric Publishing, 2006, pp 265–276.

127 Benros ME, Nielsen PR, Nordentoft M, Eaton WW, Dalton SO, Mortensen PB: Autoimmune diseases and severe infections as risk factors for schizophrenia: a 30-year population-based register study. Am J Psychiatry 2011;168:1303–1310.

Prof. Dr. med. Dipl.-Psych. Norbert Müller
Department of Psychiatry and Psychotherapy
Ludwig-Maximilian University
Nussbaumstrasse 7, DE–80336 Munich (Germany)
E-Mail Norbert.Mueller@med.uni-muenchen.de

Sartorius N, Holt RIG, Maj M (eds): Comorbidity of Mental and Physical Disorders.
Key Issues Ment Health. Basel, Karger, 2015, vol 179, pp 114–128 (DOI: 10.1159/000365543)

Physical Diseases and Addictive Disorders: Associations and Implications

Adam J. Gordon[a–c] · James W. Conley[a, b] · Joanne M. Gordon[d]

[a]Center for Health Equity Research and Promotion (CHERP) and [b]Mental Illness Research, Education, and Clinical Center (MIRECC), VA Pittsburgh Healthcare System, [c]Division of General Internal Medicine, University of Pittsburgh School of Medicine, Pittsburgh, Pa., and [d]Biomedical Sciences, Missouri State University, Springfield, Mo., USA

Abstract

Increasingly, the identification, assessment and treatment of unhealthy use of alcohol and other drugs often occur within general medical settings. Within this climate, there is a growing awareness of the physical effects connected to acute or chronic use of substances of abuse. By examining these associations and their purported biological causative mechanisms, greater clinical attention – in the form of screening, identification and treatment – to co-occurring medical conditions as well as to the use of illicit substances itself may be possible. In this review, we examine recent peer-reviewed literature regarding three substances of abuse (cocaine, marijuana and opioids) and their direct associations with physical disorders. We group the association of diseases based on organ systems and critically examine the literature regarding the evidence to supporting those associations and causative mechanisms. There is good evidence to support the association of cocaine, marijuana and opioid use with a variety of physical health conditions. Unfortunately, while the causative evidence of these associations is preliminary, we could conclude that the use of these substances can incite a host of medical illnesses or complicate their treatment. When combined with societal, mental health and public health harms associated with the use of illicit substances, co-occurring or incident physical health conditions associated with substance use may present a substantial healthcare cost to the individual as well as to the healthcare system at large, resulting in a debilitating strain on often limited time and resources.

© 2015 S. Karger AG, Basel

Alcohol and illicit drug use and related use disorders impact mental, physical and environmental health. Identification and treatment of addictive disorders are the responsibility of all healthcare providers. Currently, the education and training of healthcare professionals to address co-occurring physical and mental health conditions associated with alcohol and illicit drug use and related use disorders may not be a focus of medical education and training. Because they have not been exposed to sufficient undergraduate or graduate medical education regarding screening, assessment, and treatment of alcohol and illicit drug use, providers may feel inadequately equipped to engage the complex intersection between mental and physical health presented by ongoing alcohol and substance use. In some countries, a concerted effort has been undertaken in primary care to educate generalist healthcare providers about addiction and alcohol and illicit drug-related physical and medical health disorders [1–4]. While much attention has been devoted to physical conditions resulting from alcohol use [5–8], less attention has been directed to the associations between physical conditions and other illicit drug use [9, 10].

A pressing need exists for better understanding among healthcare providers of the serious health and healthcare implications of illicit substance abuse, particularly for physical health conditions. The purpose of this review is to examine the co-occurring and comorbid relationships between major drugs of abuse and physical illness. Similar to previous efforts, we examined the recent peer-reviewed literature regarding evidence of the associations of illicit substance use on physical health conditions [9, 10]. We investigated the literature to detail physical health issues associated with the use of three of the most common substances of abuse (cocaine, marijuana and opioids). While physical illnesses associated with use of other broad categories of drugs of abuse, such as stimulants and hallucinogens, may mirror the health effects of cocaine (stimulants) or marijuana (hallucinogens), for simplicity and brevity we concentrated our review on only cocaine, marijuana and opioids. Although each substance may invite risk of physical illness due to the nature of taking the substance (e.g. injection or inhalation), or social and environmental problems associated with use (e.g. risky sexual practices, trauma or other criminal activity), we concentrated our review on the direct associations between the substance in question and physical health. For many of these associations, we examined purported pathophysiological reasons for the association with physical ill-health. Thus, we provide a brief description of physical health conditions related to use of these three substances, organized according to generalized bodily systems.

Immune System

Cocaine

An increasing body of evidence, both from clinical epidemiological and laboratory studies, points to an association between cocaine use and an altered innate immune response that involves a decrease in monocyte expression of several cytokines [11]. As a weak agonist for sigma receptors, cocaine has also been found to alter cytokine release from both proinflammatory and anti-inflammatory T cells [12]. These studies suggest that cocaine use can have a direct effect on the innate immune system and thus increase the likelihood of greater risk for infectious diseases. Adulterants in cocaine, specifically levamisole, which is found in more than half of the cocaine in the USA [13], has a direct effect on the immune system. Leukopenia (especially neutropenia), agranulocytosis and vasculitis have been associated with levamisole.

Marijuana

Despite strong evidence that cannabinoid type 2 receptors are found predominantly on cells involved in immunity and inflammation and can decrease activity of immune cells [14], no link has been shown between marijuana use and hematopoietic or lymphatic disorders.

Opioids

Some of the opioids, including fentanyl, methadone, loperamide and β-endorphin, have been found to increase the levels of interleukin-4 (IL-4) in human type 2 T cells while other opioids, such as morphine and buprenorphine decrease the levels of IL-4 [15]. However, a study of male long-term daily opium users in Iran did not show a change in IL-4 levels compared to controls [16], although there were higher levels of other cytokines associated with either cellular or humoral immunity (interferon-γ, IL-10 and IL-17), indicating that some opioids have an effect on the immune response and the ability to react to infectious agents.

Infection

Cocaine

Besides the effect of cocaine on the innate immune system, cocaine use can increase the risk of infections through risky behavior associated with drug use, e.g. unprotected sex, multiple sexual partners, needle sharing and contaminated drug paraphernalia. Unhealthy living conditions and malnutrition can also influence the risk for infections.

Marijuana

Marijuana users may be more vulnerable to infection than the general public. Combined with cannabinoids' suppression of the inflammatory response and natural immunity [17], marijuana use may promote greater susceptibility and decreased resistance to a wide array of infections. The common practice of shared or communal use of bongs, pipes and marijuana cigarettes may further promote transmission of airborne and fluid-based diseases, such as tuberculosis [18, 19]. Among other diseases for which marijuana use has been correlated with infection are *Neisseria meningitidis* [20, 21], oral candidiasis [22, 23] and sexually transmitted disease [24]. As well, marijuana users with chronic hepatitis C may be at greater risk of developing steatosis and fibrosis in the liver [25, 26].

Opioids

Use of opioids is often associated with risky behavior, thus increasing the likelihood of being infected by human immunodeficiency virus (HIV), hepatitis B and C, and other sexually transmitted pathogens. Intravenous use of opioids can increase the risk of cellulitis and endocarditis.

Cancers

Cocaine

There appears to be an increased risk of developing non-Hodgkin's lymphoma in frequent users of cocaine compared to those who used amphetamines, lysergic acid diethylamide (LSD) or methaqualone [27].

Marijuana

There appears to be a link between marijuana use and some cancers in long-term users. However, many studies are hampered by selection bias, small sample size, lack of adjustment for concurrent tobacco use and other problems. Marijuana use has been linked to bladder cancer [28], cancer of the head and neck [29, 30], and lung cancer [31–33]. Marijuana use has also been associated with testicular germ cell tumors [34–36]. Smoked marijuana tar contains carcinogens similar to those found in cigarettes [37], and while studies are still inconclusive, it is reasonable to suspect that marijuana smoking may contribute to other cancers as well, including oral and pharyngeal cancer.

Hematopoietic Disorders

Cocaine

Cocaine has a role in coagulopathy. Recent research has found that use of cocaine increases von Willebrand factor release from the endothelium [38]. An increase in plasma von Willebrand factor can enhance platelet aggregation and thrombus formation, leading to increased risk for systemic thrombi in large and small vessels. Cocaine use is associated with thrombi formation in coronary stents [39] and atherosclerotic lesions and total thrombus occlusion in the main coronary arteries in long-term cocaine users [40].

Marijuana

A determination has yet to be made regarding whether cannabis arteritis is a distinct and separate disease from the thromboangiitis obliterans seen in cigarette smokers. Over 50 cases of cannabis arteritis have been reported since 1960 in marijuana users who did not smoke tobacco [41], and cases of arteritis have been described in regular marijuana users who were moderate users of tobacco [42]. Cannabis arteritis may contribute to juvenile peripheral obstructive arterial disease [41]. In addition, arteriographic studies have found distal abnormalities similar to thromboangiitis obliterans, with changes in the architecture of the vasa nervorum [42].

Cardiovascular Disease

Cocaine
The surge of catecholamines in the plasma soon after use of cocaine can cause significant diffuse and focal coronary vasospasm. Additionally, the increase in heart contractility and heart rate and resultant high blood pressure can cause cardiac ischemia, vasospasm and infarction. Cocaine-related endothelin-1 release from the endothelium and alterations in platelet aggregation and formation of vessel thrombi can contribute to the increased risk of acute myocardial infarction in cocaine users. Young cocaine users may experience chest pain, ischemia, arrhythmias and acute myocardial infarction. Atherosclerotic lesions are not primarily associated with cocaine-related infarcts [43]. However, myonecrosis and coronary stenosis is often found in cocaine users with previous infarctions. Asymptomatic cocaine users may have significant cardiac disease (myocardial dysfunction, tissue edema or fibrosis) [44] and cocaine-users may have a higher risk than nonusers in developing silent acute myocardial infarction. The young age of cocaine users may be a survival benefit for those who experience a resuscitated cardiac arrest [45]. Compared to noncocaine users, cocaine users often survive the arrest without neurological sequelae. However, the likelihood of young cocaine users experiencing a nonfatal acute myocardial infarction was higher than those who were not cocaine users. Twenty-five percent of nonfatal acute myocardial infarction in 18- to 45-year-olds has been at-tributed to cocaine use. Cocaine users may also be more susceptible to developing coronary artery aneurysm [46]. Compared to a control group of individuals with similar cardiovascular risk, 30.4% of cocaine users (mean age 44 years) had coronary artery aneurysms, compared to only 7.6% in a control group. Although rare, postpartum coronary artery dissection has been reported in a 25-year-old woman who had been using cocaine [47]. Arrhythmias, in addition to tachycardia, may occur in cocaine users and have been attributed to ischemia and electrolyte imbalance. However, cocaine sequestration in myocytes may interfere with calcium storage and release and normal excitation and contraction, thus predisposing the heart to lethal arrhythmias [48]. Oxidative stress and direct myocardial toxicity has been suggested as another reason for the myocardial cell death associated with ischemia and acute myocardial infarction in cocaine users [49]. Cardiac oxidative stress occurs soon after cocaine enters the vascular system, leading to myocyte dysfunction and an increase in the number of inflammatory cells in the heart.

Marijuana
Marijuana use has already been associated with some clinical cardiovascular issues, specifically heart palpitations, orthostatic hypotension and acute increase in heart rate [50, 51]. Long-term users may experience an increase in heart rate, potentially resulting in cardiac ischemia and the arrhythmic effects of the catecholamines [52]. These users may delay pursuing medical help in response to the pain normally associated with ischemia because of marijuana's effect as an analgesic and dissociative agent, further exacerbating damage over time. There are competing data regarding marijuana and mortality risk with acute myocardial infarction. While marijuana has been shown to increase the risk of acute myocardial infarction within an hour of use when compared to nonsmokers [53], a longitudinal study taken over the course of 15 years did not find an increased

risk of acute myocardial infarction in users [54]. Furthermore, no statistically significant association has yet been found between marijuana use and general mortality [55]. It should be noted that marijuana users often have other cardiovascular risk factors, such as higher alcohol and overall caloric intake, which increase postmyocardial infarction mortality in those individuals with coronary heart disease [56].

Opioids

Cardiovascular effects of opioids include some risk of infective endocarditis (associated with intravenous opiate use) and cardiac arrhythmias, especially long QT syndrome and torsades de pointes. Long QT syndrome is a condition associated with an abnormal gene coding for a protein component of myocardial cell potassium-voltage gated channels that is important in repolarization, resulting in a lengthening of the depolarization/repolarization cycle [57]. Other risks for long QT syndrome include hypokalemia. Long QT syndrome can lead to the development of torsades de pointes, a potentially lethal ventricular arrhythmia. In a randomized trial comparing the rate-adjusted QT length (QTc) in opioid-dependent subjects, the QTc increased in those subjects treated with the opioids levomethadyl (21%) and methadone (12%), but not in those treated with buprenorphine [58]. Significant risk factors for the development of a prolonged QTc in individuals on methadone maintenance therapy include the presence of congestive heart failure and other cardiac disease, elevated HbA_{1c} and use of cocaine [59]. Congestive heart failure and poor glycemic control increase the risk for mortality.

Oral, Ear, Nose and Throat Disorders

Cocaine

Midline nasal and oral destructive lesions are significant complications of insufflation of cocaine [60]. Lesions can include ischemic and necrotic changes to the mucosa, perichondrium, nasal septum (including perforation), hard and soft palate, and sinuses. Lacrimal duct obstruction and destruction of the nasal turbinates may also be seen. Because similar lesions may be seen in patients with granulomatosis, sarcoidosis and lymphoma, diagnosis can be difficult, particularly since antineutrophil cytoplasmic antibody tests may be positive in all of these conditions. Sniffling, nasal crusts, nosebleeds and sinus problems are common problems in cocaine users who may also have burns to their upper airway. Depressed hearing and diminished sense of smell have also been reported.

Marijuana

Similar to tobacco, marijuana smoking increases the risk of a number of oral diseases and disorders, including xerostomia, tooth decay, periodontitis, severe gingivitis and mucosal abnormalities [23], as well as leukoedema and traumatic ulcers of the mouth [61]. It should be noted that it is not yet clear whether the higher incidence of caries and periodontal disease in marijuana smokers is a direct effect of use or a byproduct of attendant poor hygiene [62].

Opioids

A recent article suggests that nasal mucosal necrosis found in a small number of patients is related to heroin snorting [63].

Respiratory Disease

Cocaine

Bronchial and lung dysfunction in cocaine users include cough, black sputum, hemoptysis and chest pain [9]. Some studies have reported an exacerbation of asthma symptoms in those who smoke crack cocaine [64] and a higher incidence of out-of-hospital asthma deaths [65].

Although crack cocaine users are less likely to have hemoptysis, respiratory distress and abnormal pulmonary function tests than those participants who use tobacco [66], cocaine users are more likely to have an increase in alveolar macrophages and endothelin-1 (a potent vasoconstrictor) in bronchial alveolar lavage samples, suggesting that microvascular injury is associated with heavy crack cocaine smoking.

Marijuana
Studies suggest that marijuana users are at an elevated risk of experiencing increased mucus production as well as symptoms of chronic bronchitis [67–70]. Cannabis may also be an allergen for some [71]. A recent report found that forensic laboratory workers handling hashish or marijuana for 16–25 years developed marijuana hypersensitivity [72]. Others may be at risk for developing an allergy to the drug.

Opioids
Respiratory depression is a major adverse effect of many of the opioids and can cause death in users. As many as 58% of the deaths related to drug abuse in Ontario, Canada, between 2006 and 2008 were related to opioid use, with over one third of these associated with oxycodone use [73]. Respiratory depression and death may also occur with opioid use in neonates, the elderly and obese, and those with cardiopulmonary disease. Opioid respiratory depression has also been reported in noncancer patients using methadone or transdermal fentanyl for chronic pain [74]. Other opioid-related respiratory conditions have also been reported. Use of methadone was found to be associated with sleep apnea in a study of 392 patients using the opioid for chronic pain [75, 76]. Exacerbation of asthma symptoms can occur in heroin users [77, 78], possibly associated with histamine release by the opioid. Aspiration pneumonia is also associated with opiate use. Chest wall rigidity in adults [79] and

infants [80] can occur with fentanyl use in procedural events, but can also occur with illegitimate use of the drug.

Gastrointestinal Disorders

Cocaine
Cocaine use has been implicated in ischemic disease of the digestive system, with ischemia and/or infarction being reported in the mesentery vessels [81], and occlusive disease of the small and large bowel [82]. Frequently, the onset of abdominal pain is in temporal proximity to use of either crack or intravenous cocaine. The mortality rate associated with ischemic colitis has been found to be higher in cocaine users than noncocaine users [83].

Marijuana
A number of articles, including a case series [84], have been published on cases of chronic marijuana users who were diagnosed with cannabinoid hyperemesis, characterized by cyclical, chronic vomiting and severe abdominal pain, and often accompanied by a compulsion to take hot baths or showers. The authors report that discontinuing marijuana use causes symptoms to dissipate and further assert that the illness is often underdiagnosed and underreported.

Hepatobiliary Disease

Cocaine
Hepatotoxicity in cocaine users is likely the result of direct toxicity mediated by oxidative stress and mitochondrial dysfunction occurring during metabolism of cocaine [85]. It is likely that cocaine-induced oxidative cell stress leads to cell damage, fibrosis and abnormal liver function. This mechanism also occurs in the kidney and many body systems, including the cardiovascular, central nervous, immune and reproductive systems [86].

Metabolic, Nutritional and Endocrine Disorders

Marijuana

Although some research has shown that overactivity of cannabinoid receptors may lead to abdominal obesity, dyslipidemia and hyperglycemia [87], there is little clinical evidence that marijuana use is associated with development of diabetes mellitus or hyperlipidemia.

Cocaine

While cocaine use has not been found to have an effect on the development of diabetes mellitus, cocaine use has been shown to increase the risk of diabetic ketoacidosis and for hospitalization of recurrent diabetic ketoacidosis [88]. Noncompliance with the therapeutic regimen is thought to be a contributing factor in diabetic ketoacidosis.

Renal and Male Urogenital Disorders

Cocaine

The risk for rhabdomyolysis and acute renal failure is significant for those who use cocaine. Cocaine has direct toxic effects on skeletal muscle and, along with severe vasoconstriction, can cause muscle ischemia and release of myoglobin and other cell contents from damaged cells [89]. Myoglobin is freely filterable in glomeruli, but accumulates in the distal tubules, resulting in obstruction. The effect of vasoconstriction on the renal vessels by cocaine, and a possible direct toxic effect of cocaine and myoglobin on renal tissue, contributes to the development of acute renal failure. However, with aggressive therapy, almost 80% of the individuals survive and most recover adequate renal function.

Genital ulcer disease found in male cocaine users is generally related to unprotected sex and contact with partners with sexually transmitted diseases and immune dysfunction associated with cocaine use.

Marijuana

Glomerular, interstitial and renal vascular disease may all be associated with marijuana use [90], though that link is not definite [91]. Marijuana may contribute to male infertility [92], decrease spermatogenesis and circulating testosterone levels [93], and has been linked to inhibited orgasm and painful sex [94].

Opioids

A recent study found that morphine use can accelerate chronic kidney disease [95]. Glomerular podocytes appear to be affected by morphine-induced oxidative stress, leading to albuminuria and renal dysfunction.

Female Reproductive System

Cocaine

Genital ulcer disease and pelvic inflammatory disease have been reported in women who use cocaine. Both conditions are likely due to sexually transmitted diseases associated with risky behavior and unprotected sex, as well as immune dysfunction.

Marijuana

There is a potential link between female infertility and marijuana, either as a lone agent or in concert with other illicit substances [96]. A case control study found that women who used marijuana within 1 year of attempting to conceive were not likely to become pregnant [97]. Additionally, marijuana users are six times more likely to develop *Trichomonas vaginalis* infections than nonusers [98].

Pregnancy

Cocaine

A comparison of 18 studies describing pregnancy complications found increased risk for preterm labor, placenta abruptio, fetal death, placenta previa and spontaneous abortion [9]. Infants of cocaine-using mothers are more at risk for decreased weight and length than infants of noncocaine users. Infants of cocaine-using mothers were also found to be more at risk for transient atrial and ventricular arrhythmias than infants of noncocaine-using mothers [99]. At birth, neonates may experience some autonomic dysregulation, but withdrawal symptoms are generally minimal [100]. Cocaine is not likely to be a direct fetal teratogen, although some evidence exists for alteration of cerebral development [101].

Marijuana
Young women using marijuana during pregnancy may often have infants with low birth weight and decreased length. However, a direct link to these consequences as a result of marijuana use is unclear. Often lack of prenatal care, social problems or poor economic conditions may be associated with these infant outcomes.

Opioids
As seen with other drugs of abuse, use of opioids during pregnancy can have detrimental effects on newborns, including low birth weight and length. Often, infants are exposed in utero to a number of drugs, including cocaine, heroin, cannabinoids and benzodiazepines, and their related side effects. Newborns of opioid-using mothers are particularly at risk for neonatal abstinence syndrome, which typically occurs within the first 3 days of life [102]. Methadone and buprenorphine have both been used to manage opioid dependence in pregnant women. In the newborn, buprenorphine appears to be less likely to alter cardiac function and produces fewer severe side effects than methadone [103].

Dermatologic Disorders

Cocaine
Cutaneous vasculopathy is a dermatologic condition seen in cocaine users, especially in women [104]. Retiform rashes with purpuric plaques are found predominantly on the lower extremities, but can also develop on the face and ears. Leukopenia and neutropenia may be seen, and laboratory tests for antineutrophil cytoplasmic antibodies can be positive, suggesting an immune reaction. Thrombotic vasculopathy and small-vessel vasculitis may be found on skin biopsies. Levamisole contamination in cocaine often contributes to the development of these skin lesions.

Neurological Disorders

Cocaine
The major harms associated with cocaine abuse of the nervous system are related to cerebrovascular disease. Cocaine users are at risk for development of subarachnoid hemorrhage associated with ruptured aneurysms, ischemic stroke and hemorrhagic stroke [105]. Compared to nonusers, cocaine users are more likely to experience an aneurysm rupture and less likely to survive subarachnoid hemorrhage than nonusers. Ischemic strokes are also seen in cocaine users and may be associated with hypertension, vasospasm, arteritis and increased platelet aggregation [106]. Cocaine users with ischemic stroke are often younger than nonusers and are more likely to smoke tobacco. Morbidity and mortality are similar in both cocaine users and nonusers. Seizures may also occur after cocaine use, especially in women, when high doses are used, with chronic use of cocaine, and in users previously experiencing seizures [107].

Marijuana
Use of marijuana has been associated with vascular disease in the central nervous system, with several cases of ischemic strokes documented in recent literature [108–110], including a study finding increased risk of stroke in marijuana users [111]. Marijuana use may increase the risk of the movement disorder tardive dyskinesia [112]. In a study of the incidence of tardive dyskinesia in

a group of people with chronic schizophrenia, women and older patients who smoked marijuana while taking antipsychotic drugs were more likely to develop repetitive and involuntary movements than other patients. Links between marijuana and transient amnesia [113], ataxia [114], propriospinal myoclonus [115] and spasticity [116] have yet to be fully explored.

Opioids

Opioids are often abused because of their stimulatory effects on the nervous system. However, in large doses, opioids can have a detrimental effect on the central nervous system and can lead to delirium and coma. Hydromorphone, on the other hand, can cause neuroexcitation, as reported in a study of 156 hospice patients receiving the drug while in an inpatient setting [117]. An increased risk of hydromorphone-induced neuroexcitation was associated with large doses and longer duration of drug use, increased age of the patient, and increased serum creatinine. Symptoms often associated with hydromorphone-induced neuroexcitation include tremor, myoclonus and agitation. Cognitive dysfunction is also commonly seen [118]. Spongiform leukoencephalopathy is a rare sequela of inhalation of heated heroin smoke. In one study, postmortem findings in 4 patients with spongiform leukoencephalopathy showed significantly higher numbers of apoptotic cells in both the cerebellum and corpus callosum [119]. Cerebral vacuolar degeneration was also found, particularly around microvessels. Sequelae include hydrocephalus and cerebellar swelling [120]. Although rare or possibly underreported, seizures can occur with opioid use, including generalized tonic-clonic seizures and status epilepticus [121].

Musculoskeletal Disease

Cocaine

As previously mentioned, two musculoskeletal conditions, rhabdomyolysis with acute renal failure and midline destructive lesions of the face and oral cavity, are strongly associated with cocaine use. Although no other significant musculoskeletal disorders have been reported with cocaine use, the inclusion of levamisole in cocaine has the potential of leading to untoward rheumatic consequences [122].

Conclusion

In this review, we relate the recent literature regarding the physical health associations of the use of three drugs of abuse (cocaine, marijuana and opioids) and a variety of physical illnesses (table 1). The use of cocaine, marijuana and opioids has been shown to impart a plethora of physical illnesses, many with purported and examined pathophysiological mechanisms. While associations of these conditions are known, the causative rationales for these conditions are less known. More research is certainly needed to examine causation of these drugs with physical illness. It may be that when more people use certain drugs (e.g. legalization of marijuana and increase in opioid prescription drug misuse), their related physical health conditions will become more readily apparent.

For the clinician, our findings that use of illicit substances, namely cocaine, marijuana and opioids, have some evidence in the peer-reviewed literature of physical health consequences may not be a surprise. Clinicians often treat patients who use illicit substances and often appreciate the deleterious social and environmental harms associated with this use. Often, patients who use illicit substances have co-occurring mental health conditions and these are readily appreciated by clinicians. However, what may be less known are the physical health conditions that may be directly attributable to use of illicit substances. Certainly, we found that significant evidence exists of a myriad of physical health conditions that may be directly attributable to illicit substance use.

Table 1. Conditions clinicians are likely to see with use of three commonly abused substances

System	Cocaine	Marijuana	Opioids
Immune system	altered cytokine release leading to increased risk of infections; leukopenia, agranulocytosis, vasculitis associated with additive levamisole	no association with altered immunity, inflammation	altered cytokine function; increased risk of altered cellular, humoral immune response
Infection	increased due to risky behavior, unhealthy living conditions, malnutrition	higher risk for *Neisseria*, *Candida*, sexually transmitted diseases, chronic hepatitis C with liver steatosis, fibrosis	increased risky behavior associated with HIV, hepatitis B and C, other sexually transmitted disease; intravenous use and increased cellulitis, endocarditis
Cancer	increased risk of non-Hodgkin's lymphoma	increase risk of bladder cancer, cancer of head and neck, lung; testicular germ cell cancer; oral and pharyngeal cancer	
Hematopoietic disorders	increased risk of coagulopathy (VWF), thrombus formation; atherosclerotic lesions, thrombi in systemic, main coronary arteries	cannabis arteritis (thromboangiitis obliterans); peripheral obstructive arterial disease	
Cardiovascular disease	high blood pressure, cardiac ischemia, vasospasm, infarction; increased systemic vessel thrombi, AMI, silent infarct; arrhythmias; coronary aneurysms	cardiac palpitations, orthostatic hypotension, tachycardia; increased risk of silent AMI and infarct soon after use; coexisting cardiac risk factors	infective endocarditis; arrhythmias including long QT-syndrome, torsades de pointes; congestive heart failure
Oral, ear, nose, throat disorders	midline nasal, oral destructive lesions with insufflation, positive ANCA test; sinus disease; upper airway burns	xerostomia, periodontitis, gingivitis, mucosal lesions, ulcers	mucosal necrosis in heroin snorters
Respiratory disease	bronchial, lung dysfunction, cough, hemoptysis, chest pain; exacerbation of asthma symptoms; increased microvascular injury	increased mucus production, signs and symptoms of chronic bronchitis; increased risk for marijuana allergy	respiratory depression and death (oxycodone), particularly in neonates, elderly, obese, those with cardiopulmonary disease; increased sleep apnea; exacerbation of asthma symptoms (heroin); aspiration pneumonia; chest wall rigidity
Gastrointestinal disorders	mesenteric ischemia, infarction, occlusive disease of small and large bowel; increased risk of death from ischemic colitis	cannabinoid hyperemesis, often associated with compulsion for hot bath or shower	
Hepatobiliary disease	liver fibrosis, abnormal liver function secondary to oxidative stress		
Metabolic, nutritional, endocrine disorders	increased risk of diabetic ketoacidosis secondary to noncompliance to treatment regime	possible abdominal obesity, dyslipidemia, hyperglycemia	

Table 1. Continued

System	Cocaine	Marijuana	Opioids
Renal, male urogenital disorders	increased risk of rhabdomyolysis, acute renal failure; genital ulcer disease secondary to unprotected sex	glomerular, interstitial, renal vascular disease; possible infertility with decreased spermatogenesis and testosterone; erectile dysfunction	acceleration of chronic renal disease associated with oxidative stress
Female reproductive system	genital ulcer disease, pelvic inflammatory disease	infertility; increased risk of *Trichomonas* infection	
Pregnancy	increased risk of preterm labor, placenta abruptio, fetal death, placenta previa, spontaneous abortion; transient atrial and ventricular arrhythmias; decreased birth length and weight	decreased birth length and weight	decreased birth length and weight; high risk for neonatal abstinence syndrome
Dermatologic disorders	cutaneous vasculopathy (retiform rash, purpuric plagues); leukopenia, neutropenia; small vessel disease; positive ANCA test; thrombic vasculopathy		
Neurological disease	cerebrovascular disease (ischemic, hemorrhagic stroke); aneurysm rupture, subarachnoid hemorrhage; seizures	cerebrovascular disease (ischemic stroke); increased risk for tardive dyskinesia; transient amnesia; ataxia; propriospinal myoclonus, spasticity	delirium, coma; neuro-excitation (hydromorphone); cognitive dysfunction; spongiform leukoencephalopathy (heated heroin smoke); seizures
Musculoskeletal disease	rhabdomyolysis with acute renal failure; midline destructive lesions (face, oral cavity); rheumatoid findings with levamisole		

AMI = Acute myocardial infarction; ANCA = antineutrophil cytoplasmic antibody; VWF = von Willebrand factor.

Clinicians, particularly general practitioners or primary care providers, should screen and assess for illicit substances among their patients. If they identify a patient who uses an illicit substance, our review of literature relates that they should consider evaluating for physical health conditions associated with that use. Even mental health providers should consider assessing for these physical health conditions, as patients with illicit substances may not seek care with a general practitioner or primary care provider. A proactive approach for assessing and treating these physical health conditions associated with illicit use may be valuable, as patients who use illicit substances may not seek medical care, and certainly may not establish longitudinal healthcare services, such as a general practitioner or primary care provider. In addition, attention in healthcare professional schools and training programs regarding the association of illicit substances and physical health may be warranted. In sum, physical health conditions associated with use of illicit drugs is a significant concern for all patients who use illicit substances and should be a concern for their healthcare providers as well as healthcare provider educators.

This review has significant limitations related to our approach which should temper overreaching or generalizing our findings. We reviewed only the recent (over the last 2 decades) peer-reviewed literature, and only that which was published in English. It may be that some published studies remained undiscovered in the process of our electronic review. We did not cover other illicit drugs of abuse, but much of the literature on amphetamines is similar to the literature on cocaine and much of the literature on hallucinogens is similar to the literature on marijuana. We did not examine the behavioral, mental health, social and environmental problems that afflict persons who use substances of abuse, and we did not concentrate this review on the associations made through the route of drug administration (e.g. increase in hepatitis C and HIV through injections of illicit drugs) as these were not direct drug associations to physical illness, but due to the route of exposure. While we critically examined the literature, much of the literature examines associations rather than causations, or exists in the form of case reports, case series or descriptive studies. Conclusions regarding the specificity and strength of the association with drugs of abuse and physical illness should be tempered unless there is evidence of biological mechanisms to support the association.

Despite these limitations, drugs of abuse unquestionably cause physical health effects. Some of the diseases connected to cocaine, marijuana and opioid use possess strong evidence of disease association. These diseases are often serious, resulting in a significant burden on healthcare systems to finance, treat or support long-term management of these conditions. All healthcare providers should be aware of these associations and discuss these associations with patients who use these substances. By doing so, illicit use, as well as the physical harm and diseases associated with that use, may be diminished or even eliminated.

References

1 Gordon AJ, Sullivan LE, Alford DP, Arnsten JH, Gourevitch MN, Kertesz SG, Kunins HV, Merrill JO, Samet JH, Fiellin DA: Update in addiction medicine for the generalist. J Gen Intern Med 2007; 22:1190–1194.
2 Gordon AJ, Fiellin DA, Friedmann PD, Gourevitch MN, Kraemer KL, Arnsten JH, Saitz R: Update in addiction medicine for the primary care clinician. J Gen Intern Med 2008;23:2112–2116.
3 Gordon AJ, Kunins HV, Rastegar DA, Tetrault JM, Walley AY: Update in addiction medicine for the generalist. J Gen Intern Med 2011;26:77–82.
4 Rastegar DA, Kunins HV, Tetrault JM, Walley AY, Gordon AJ: 2012 Update in addiction medicine for the generalist. Addict Sci Clin Pract 2013;8:6.
5 Gordon AJ, Gordon JM, Broyles LM: Medical consequences of unhealthy alcohol use; in Saitz R (ed): Addressing Unhealthy Alcohol Use in Primary Care. Ames, Springer, 2013, pp 107–118.

6 Brick J: Handbook of the Medical Consequences of Alcohol and Drug Abuse. New York, Haworth, 2004.
7 Frances RJ, Miller SI, Mack AH: Clinical Textbook of Addictive Disorders, ed 3. New York, Guilford, 2005.
8 Rastegar DA, Fingerhood MI: Addiction Medicine: An Evidence-Based Handbook. Philadelphia, Lippincott, Williams & Wilkins, 2005.
9 Gordon AJ, Gordon JM, Carl K, Hilton MT, Striebel J, Maher M: Physical Illness and Drugs of Abuse: A Review of the Evidence. Cambridge, Cambridge University Press, 2010.
10 Gordon AJ, Conley JW, Gordon JM: Medical consequences of marijuana use: a review of current literature. Curr Psychiatry Rep 2013;15:419.

11 Irwin MR, Olmos L, Wang M, Valladares EM, Motivala SJ, Fong T, Newton T, Butch A, Olmstead R, Cole SW: Cocaine dependence and acute cocaine induce decreases of monocyte proinflammatory cytokine expression across the diurnal period: autonomic mechanisms. J Pharmacol Exp Ther 2007;320:507–515.
12 Cabral GA: Drugs of abuse, immune modulation, and AIDS. J Neuroimmune Pharmacol 2006;1:280–295.
13 Larocque A, Hoffman RS: Levamisole in cocaine: unexpected news from an old acquaintance. Clin Toxicol (Phila) 2012; 50:231–241.
14 Friedman H, Pross S, Klein TW: Addictive drugs and their relationship with infectious diseases. FEMS Immunol Med Microbiol 2006;47:330–342.
15 Borner C, Lanciotti S, Koch T, Hollt V, Kraus J: Mu opioid receptor agonist-selective regulation of interleukin-4 in T lymphocytes. J Neuroimmunol 2013; 263:35–42.

16 Ghazavi A, Solhi H, Moazzeni SM, Rafiei M, Mosayebi G: Cytokine profiles in long-term smokers of opium (Taryak). J Addict Med 2013;7:200–203.

17 Klein TW, Friedman H, Specter S: Marijuana, immunity and infection. J Neuroimmunol 1998;83:102–115.

18 Munckhof WJ, Konstantinos A, Wamsley M, Mortlock M, Gilpin C: A cluster of tuberculosis associated with use of a marijuana water pipe. Int J Tuberc Lung Dis 2003;7:860–865.

19 Oeltmann JE, Oren E, Haddad MB, Lake LK, Harrington TA, Ijaz K, Narita M: Tuberculosis outbreak in marijuana users, Seattle, Washington, 2004. Emerg Infect Dis 2006;12:1156.

20 Krause G, Blackmore C, Wiersma S, Lesneski C, Woods CW, Rosenstein NE, Hopkins RS: Marijuana use and social networks in a community outbreak of meningococcal disease. South Med J 2001;94:482–485.

21 Finn R, Groves C, Coe M, Pass M, Harrison LH: Cluster of serogroup C meningococcal disease associated with attendance at a party. South Med J 2001;94:1192–1194.

22 Darling MR, Arendorf TM, Coldrey NA: Effect of cannabis use on oral candidal carriage. J Oral Pathol Med 1990;19:319–321.

23 Darling MR, Arendorf TM: Review of the effects of cannabis smoking on oral health. Int Dent J 1992;42:19–22.

24 Liau A, Diclemente RJ, Wingood GM, Crosby RA, Williams KM, Harrington K, Davies SL, Hook EW III, Oh MK: Associations between biologically confirmed marijuana use and laboratory-confirmed sexually transmitted diseases among African American adolescent females. Sex Transm Dis 2002;29:387–390.

25 Hezode C, Zafrani ES, Roudot-Thoraval F, Costentin C, Hessami A, Bouvier-Alias M, Medkour F, Pawlostky JM, Lotersztajn S, Mallat A: Daily cannabis use: a novel risk factor of steatosis severity in patients with chronic hepatitis C. Gastroenterology 2008;134:432–439.

26 Ishida JH, Peters MG, Jin C, Louie K, Tan V, Bacchetti P, Terrault NA: Influence of cannabis use on severity of hepatitis C disease. Clin Gastroenterol Hepatol 2008;6:69–75.

27 Nelson RA, Levine AM, Marks G, Bernstein L: Alcohol, tobacco and recreational drug use and the risk of non-Hodgkin's lymphoma. Br J Cancer 1997;76:1532–1537.

28 Nieder AM, Lipke MC, Madjar S: Transitional cell carcinoma associated with marijuana: case report and review of the literature. Urology 2006;67:200.

29 Berthiller J, Lee YC, Boffetta P, Wei Q, Sturgis EM, Greenland S, et al: Marijuana smoking and the risk of head and neck cancer: pooled analysis in the INHANCE consortium. Cancer Epidemiol Biomarkers Prev 2009;18:1544–1551.

30 Aldington S, Harwood M, Cox B, Weatherall M, Beckert L, Hansell A, Pritchard A, Robinson G, Beasley R: Cannabis use and cancer of the head and neck: case-control study. Otolaryngol Head Neck Surg 2008;138:374–380.

31 Voirin N, Berthiller J, Benhaim-Luzon V, Boniol M, Straif K, Ayoub WB, Ayed FB, Sasco AJ: Risk of lung cancer and past use of cannabis in Tunisia. J Thorac Oncol 2006;1:577–579.

32 Aldington S, Harwood M, Cox B, Weatherall M, Beckert L, Hansell A, Pritchard A, Robinson G, Beasley R: Cannabis use and risk of lung cancer: a case-control study. Eur Respir J 2008;31:280–286.

33 Taylor FM III: Marijuana as a potential respiratory tract carcinogen: a retrospective analysis of a community hospital population. South Med J 1988;81:1213–1216.

34 Daling JR, Doody DR, Sun X, Trabert BL, Weiss NS, Chen C, Biggs ML, Starr JR, Dey SK, Schwartz SM: Association of marijuana use and the incidence of testicular germ cell tumors. Cancer 2009;115:1215–1223.

35 Trabert B, Sigurdson AJ, Sweeney AM, Strom SS, McGlynn KA: Marijuana use and testicular germ cell tumors. Cancer 2011;117:848–853.

36 Lacson JC, Carroll JD, Tuazon E, Castelao EJ, Bernstein L, Cortessis VK: Population-based case-control study of recreational drug use and testis cancer risk confirms an association between marijuana use and nonseminoma risk. Cancer 2012;118:5374–5383.

37 Hashibe M, Ford DE, Zhang ZF: Marijuana smoking and head and neck cancer. J Clin Pharmacol 2002;42(11 suppl):103S–107S.

38 Hobbs WE, Moore EE, Penkala RA, Bolgiano DD, Lopez JA: Cocaine and specific cocaine metabolites induce von Willebrand factor release from endothelial cells in a tissue-specific manner. Arterioscler Thromb Vasc Biol 2013;33:1230–1237.

39 McKee SA, Applegate RJ, Hoyle JR, Sacrinty MT, Kutcher MA, Sane DC: Cocaine use is associated with an increased risk of stent thrombosis after percutaneous coronary intervention. Am Heart J 2007;154:159–164.

40 Kolodgie FD, Virmani R, Cornhill JF, Herderick EE, Smialek J: Increase in atherosclerosis and adventitial mast cells in cocaine abusers: an alternative mechanism of cocaine-associated coronary vasospasm and thrombosis. J Am Coll Cardiol 1991;17:1553–1560.

41 Peyrot I, Garsaud AM, Saint-Cyr I, Quitman O, Sanchez B, Quist D: Cannabis arteritis: a new case report and a review of literature. J Eur Acad Dermatol Venereol 2007;21:388–391.

42 Disdier P, Granel B, Serratrice J, Constans J, Michon-Pasturel U, Hachulla E, Conri C, Devulder B, Swiader L, Piquet P, Branchereau A, Jouglard J, Moulin G, Weiller PJ: Cannabis arteritis revisited – ten new case reports. Angiology 2001;52:1–5.

43 Kontos MC, Jesse RL, Tatum JL, Ornato JP: Coronary angiographic findings in patients with cocaine-associated chest pain. J Emerg Med 2003;24:9–13.

44 Aquaro GD, Gabutti A, Meini M, Prontera C, Pasanisi E, Passino C, Emdin M, Lombardi M: Silent myocardial damage in cocaine addicts. Heart 2011;97:2056–2062.

45 Qureshi AI, Suri MF, Guterman LR, Hopkins LN: Cocaine use and the likelihood of nonfatal myocardial infarction and stroke: data from the Third National Health and Nutrition Examination Survey. Circulation 2001;103:502–506.

46 Satran A, Bart BA, Henry CR, Murad MB, Talukdar S, Satran D, Henry TD: Increased prevalence of coronary artery aneurysms among cocaine users. Circulation 2005;111:2424–2429.

47 Katikaneni PK, Akkus NI, Tandon N, Modi K: Cocaine-induced postpartum coronary artery dissection: a case report and 80-year review of literature. J Invasive Cardiol 2013;25:E163–E166.

48 Sanchez EJ, Hayes RP, Barr JT, Lewis KM, Webb BN, Subramanian AK, Nissen MS, Jones JP, Shelden EA, Sorg BA, Fill M, Schenk JO, Kang C: Potential role of cardiac calsequestrin in the lethal arrhythmic effects of cocaine. Drug Alcohol Depend 2013;133:344–351.

49 Cerretani D, Fineschi V, Bello S, Riezzo I, Turillazzi E, Neri M: Role of oxidative stress in cocaine-induced cardiotoxicity and cocaine-related death. Curr Med Chem 2012;19:5619–5623.

50 Sidney S: Cardiovascular consequences of marijuana use. J Clin Pharmacol 2002;42(11 suppl):64S–70S.

51 Aryana A, Williams MA: Marijuana as a trigger of cardiovascular events: speculation or scientific certainty? Int J Cardiol 2007;118:141–144.

52 Malinowska B, Baranowska-Kuczko M, Schlicker E: Triphasic blood pressure responses to cannabinoids: do we understand the mechanism? Br J Pharmacol 2012;165:2073–2088.

53 Mittleman MA, Lewis RA, Maclure M, Sherwood JB, Muller JE: Triggering myocardial infarction by marijuana. Circulation 2001;103:2805–2809.

54 Rodondi N, Pletcher MJ, Liu K, Hulley SB, Sidney S: Marijuana use, diet, body mass index, and cardiovascular risk factors (from the CARDIA study). Am J Cardiol 2006;98:478–484.

55 Frost L, Mostofsky E, Rosenbloom JI, Mukamal KJ, Mittleman MA: Marijuana use and long-term mortality among survivors of acute myocardial infarction. Am Heart J 2013;165:170–175.

56 Mukamal KJ, Maclure M, Muller JE, Mittleman MA: An exploratory prospective study of marijuana use and mortality following acute myocardial infarction. Am Heart J 2008;155:465–470.

57 Stringer J, Welsh C, Tommasello A: Methadone-associated Q-T interval prolongation and torsades de pointes. Am J Health Syst Pharm 2009;66:825–833.

58 Wedam EF, Bigelow GE, Johnson RE, Nuzzo PA, Haigney MC: QT-interval effects of methadone, levomethadyl, and buprenorphine in a randomized trial. Arch Intern Med 2007;167:2469–2475.

59 Fareed A, Vayalapalli S, Scheinberg K, Gale R, Casarella J, Drexler K: QTc interval prolongation for patients in methadone maintenance treatment: a five years follow-up study. Am J Drug Alcohol Abuse 2013;39:235–240.

60 Trimarchi M, Bussi M, Sinico RA, Meroni P, Specks U: Cocaine-induced midline destructive lesions – an autoimmune disease? Autoimmun Rev 2012;12:496–500.

61 Darling MR, Arendorf TM: Effects of cannabis smoking on oral soft tissues. Community Dent Oral Epidemiol 1993; 21:78–81.

62 Cho CM, Hirsch R, Johnstone S: General and oral health implications of cannabis use. Aust Dent J 2005;50:70–74.

63 Peyriere H, Leglise Y, Rousseau A, Cartier C, Gibaja V, Galland P: Necrosis of the intranasal structures and soft palate as a result of heroin snorting: a case series. Subst Abus 2013;34:409–414.

64 Osborn HH, Tang M, Bradley K, Duncan BR: New-onset bronchospasm or recrudescence of asthma associated with cocaine abuse. Acad Emerg Med 1997;4:689–692.

65 Greenberger PA, Miller TP, Lifschultz B: Circumstances surrounding deaths from asthma in Cook County (Chicago) Illinois. Allergy Proc 1993;14:321–326.

66 Baldwin GC, Choi R, Roth MD, Shay AH, Kleerup EC, Simmons MS, Tashkin DP: Evidence of chronic damage to the pulmonary microcirculation in habitual users of alkaloidal ('crack') cocaine. Chest 2002;121:1231–1238.

67 Polen MR, Sidney S, Tekawa IS, Sadler M, Friedman GD: Health care use by frequent marijuana smokers who do not smoke tobacco. West J Med 1993;158:596–601.

68 Taylor DR, Poulton R, Moffitt TE, Ramankutty P, Sears MR: The respiratory effects of cannabis dependence in young adults. Addiction 2000;95:1669–1677.

69 Moore BA, Augustson EM, Moser RP, Budney AJ: Respiratory effects of marijuana and tobacco use in a U.S. sample. J Gen Intern Med 2005;20:33–37.

70 Taylor DR, Fergusson DM, Milne BJ, Horwood LJ, Moffitt TE, Sears MR, Poulton R: A longitudinal study of the effects of tobacco and cannabis exposure on lung function in young adults. Addiction 2002;97:1055–1061.

71 Stokes JR, Hartel R, Ford LB, Casale TB: Cannabis (hemp) positive skin tests and respiratory symptoms. Ann Allergy Asthma Immunol 2000;85:238–240.

72 Herzinger T, Schopf P, Przybilla B, Rueff F: IgE-mediated hypersensitivity reactions to cannabis in laboratory personnel. Int Arch Allergy Immunol 2011; 156:423–426.

73 Madadi P, Hildebrandt D, Lauwers AE, Koren G: Characteristics of opioid-users whose death was related to opioid-toxicity: a population-based study in Ontario, Canada. PLoS One 2013;8:e60600.

74 Dahan A, Overdyk F, Smith T, Aarts L, Niesters M: Pharmacovigilance: a review of opioid-induced respiratory depression in chronic pain patients. Pain Physician 2013;16:E85–E94.

75 Webster LR, Choi Y, Desai H, Webster L, Grant BJ: Sleep-disordered breathing and chronic opioid therapy. Pain Med 2008;9:425–432.

76 Ankichetty S, Wong J, Chung F: A systematic review of the effects of sedatives and anesthetics in patients with obstructive sleep apnea. J Anaesthesiol Clini Pharmacol 2011;27:447.

77 Elia D, Marinou A, Chetta A: Life-threatening asthma after heroin inhalation. A case report and a review of the literature. Acta Biomed 2010;81:63–67.

78 Krantz AJ, Hershow RC, Prachand N, Hayden DM, Franklin C, Hryhorczuk DO: Heroin insufflation as a trigger for patients with life-threatening asthma. Chest 2003;123:510–517.

79 Coruh B, Tonelli MR, Park DR: Fentanyl-induced chest wall rigidity. Chest 2013;143:1145–1146.

80 Dewhirst E, Naguib A, Tobias JD: Chest wall rigidity in two infants after low-dose fentanyl administration. Pediatr Emerg Care 2012;28:465–468.

81 Byard RW: Acute mesenteric ischaemia and unexpected death. J Forensic Leg Med 2012;19:185–190.

82 Osorio J, Farreras N, Ortiz De Zarate L, Bachs E: Cocaine-induced mesenteric ischaemia. Digest Surg 2001;17:648–651.

83 Elramah M, Einstein M, Mori N, Vakil N: High mortality of cocaine-related ischemic colitis: a hybrid cohort/case-control study. Gastrointest Endosc 2012; 75:1226–1232.

84 Simonetto DA, Oxentenko AS, Herman ML, Szostek JH: Cannabinoid hyperemesis: a case series of 98 patients. Mayo Clin Proc 2012;87:114–119.

85 Valente MJ, Carvalho F, Bastos M, de Pinho PG, Carvalho M: Contribution of oxidative metabolism to cocaine-induced liver and kidney damage. Cur Med Chem 2012;19:5601–5606.

86 Riezzo I, Fiore C, De Carlo D, Pascale N, Neri M, Turillazzi E, Fineschi V: Side effects of cocaine abuse: multiorgan toxicity and pathological consequences. Curr Med Chem 2012;19:5624–5646.

87 Matias I, Di Marzo V: Endocannabinoids and the control of energy balance. Trends Endocrinol Metab 2007;18:27–37.

88 Nyenwe EA, Loganathan RS, Blum S, Ezuteh DO, Erani DM, Wan JY, Palace MR, Kitabchi AE: Active use of cocaine: an independent risk factor for recurrent diabetic ketoacidosis in a city hospital. Endocr Pract 2007;13:22–29.

89 Nemiroff L, Cormier S, LeBlanc C, Murphy N: Don't you forget about me: considering acute rhabdomyolysis in ED patients with cocaine ingestion. Can Fam Physician 2012;58:750–754.

90 Crowe AV, Howse M, Bell GM, Henry JA: Substance abuse and the kidney. QJM 2000;93:147–152.

91 Vupputuri S, Batuman V, Muntner P, Bazzano LA, Lefante JJ, Whelton PK, He J: The risk for mild kidney function decline associated with illicit drug use among hypertensive men. Am J Kidney Dis 2004;43:629–635.

92 Thompson ST: Preventable causes of male infertility. World J Urol 1993;11: 111–119.

93 Ramos JA, Bianco FJ: The role of cannabinoids in prostate cancer: basic science perspective and potential clinical applications. Indian J Urol 2012;28:9–14.

94 Johnson SD, Phelps DL, Cottler LB: The association of sexual dysfunction and substance use among a community epidemiological sample. Arch Sex Behav 2004;33:55–63.

95 Lan X, Rai P, Chandel N, Cheng K, Lederman R, Saleem MA, Mathieson PW, Husain M, Crosson JT, Gupta K: Morphine induces albuminuria by compromising podocyte integrity. PloS One 2013;8:e55748.

96 Buck GM, Sever LE, Batt RE, Mendola P: Life-style factors and female infertility. Epidemiology 1997;8:435–441.

97 Mueller BA, Daling JR, Weiss NS, Moore DE: Recreational drug use and the risk of primary infertility. Epidemiology 1990;1:195–200.

98 Crosby R, DiClemente RJ, Wingood GM, Harrington K, Davies SL, Hook EW III, Oh MK: Predictors of infection with *Trichomonas vaginalis*: a prospective study of low income African-American adolescent females. Sex Transm Infect 2002;78:360–364.

99 Frassica JJ, Orav EJ, Walsh EP, Lipshultz SE: Arrhythmias in children prenatally exposed to cocaine. Arch Pediat Adol Med 1994;148:1163.

100 Eyler FD, Behnke M, Garvan CW, Woods NS, Wobie K, Conlon M: Newborn evaluations of toxicity and withdrawal related to prenatal cocaine exposure. Neurotoxicol Teratol 2001;23: 399–411.

101 Dow-Edwards D: Translational issues for prenatal cocaine studies and the role of environment. Neurotoxicol Teratol 2011;33:9–16.

102 Bhatt-Mehta V, Ng CM, Schumacher RE: Effectiveness of a clinical pathway with methadone treatment protocol for treatment of neonatal abstinence syndrome following in utero drug exposure to substances of abuse. Pediatr Crit Care Med 2014;15:162–169.

103 Finnegan LP, Kaltenbach K: Methadone and buprenorphine for the management of opioid dependence in pregnancy. Drugs 2012;72:747–757.

104 Arora NP: Cutaneous vasculopathy and neutropenia associated with levamisole-adulterated cocaine. Am J Med Sci 2013;345:45–51.

105 Chang TR, Kowalski RG, Caserta F, Carhuapoma JR, Tamargo RJ, Naval NS: Impact of acute cocaine use on aneurysmal subarachnoid hemorrhage. Stroke 2013;44:1825–1829.

106 Bhattacharya P, Taraman S, Shankar L, Chaturvedi S, Madhavan R: Clinical profiles, complications, and disability in cocaine-related ischemic stroke. J Stroke Cerebrovasc Dis 2011;20:443–449.

107 Dhuna A, Pascual-Leone A, Langendorf F, Anderson DC: Epileptogenic properties of cocaine in humans. Neurotoxicology 1990;12:621–626.

108 Zachariah SB: Stroke after heavy marijuana smoking. Stroke 1991;22:406–409.

109 Geller T, Loftis L, Brink DS: Cerebellar infarction in adolescent males associated with acute marijuana use. Pediatrics 2004;113:e365–e370.

110 Finsterer J, Christian P, Wolfgang K: Occipital stroke shortly after cannabis consumption. Clin Neurol Neurosurg 2004;106:305–308.

111 Herning RI, Better WE, Tate K, Cadet JL: Marijuana abusers are at increased risk for stroke. Preliminary evidence from cerebrovascular perfusion data. Ann NY Acad Sci 2001;939:413–415.

112 Zaretsky A, Rector NA, Seeman MV, Fornazzari X: Current cannabis use and tardive dyskinesia. Schizophr Res 1993;11:3–8.

113 Stracciari A, Guarino M, Crespi C, Pazzaglia P: Transient amnesia triggered by acute marijuana intoxication. Eur J Neurol 1999;6:521–523.

114 Bonkowsky JL, Sarco D, Pomeroy SL: Ataxia and shaking in a 2-year-old girl: acute marijuana intoxication presenting as seizure. Pediatr Emerg Care 2005;21:527–528.

115 Lozsadi DA, Forster A, Fletcher NA: Cannabis-induced propriospinal myoclonus. Mov Disord 2004;19:708–709.

116 Malec J, Harvey RF, Cayner JJ: Cannabis effect on spasticity in spinal cord injury. Arch Phys Med Rehabil 1982; 63:116–118.

117 Kullgren J, Le V, Wheeler W: Incidence of hydromorphone-induced neuroexcitation in hospice patients. J Palliat Med 2013;16:1205–1209.

118 Paramanandam G, Prommer E, Schwenke DC: Adverse effects in hospice patients with chronic kidney disease receiving hydromorphone. J Palliat Med 2011;14:1029–1033.

119 Yin R, Lu C, Chen Q, Fan J, Lu J: Microvascular damage is involved in the pathogenesis of heroin induced spongiform leukoencephalopathy. Int J Med Sci 2013;10:299.

120 Bach AG, Jordan B, Wegener NA, Rusner C, Kornhuber M, Abbas J, Surov A: Heroin spongiform leukoencephalopathy (HSLE). Clin Neuroradiol 2012;22: 345–349.

121 Jovanovic-Cupic V, Martinovic Z, Nesic N: Seizures associated with intoxication and abuse of tramadol. Clin Toxicol (Phila) 2006;44:143–146.

122 Graf J: Rheumatic manifestations of cocaine use. Curr Opin Rheumatol 2013;25:50–55.

Adam J. Gordon, MD, MPH
Center for Health Equity Research and Promotion, CHERP: 151-C, VA Pittsburgh Healthcare System
University of Pittsburgh School of Medicine
University Drive C
Pittsburgh, PA 15240-1001 (USA)
E-Mail gordona@medschool.pitt.edu

Sartorius N, Holt RIG, Maj M (eds): Comorbidity of Mental and Physical Disorders.
Key Issues Ment Health. Basel, Karger, 2015, vol 179, pp 129–136 (DOI: 10.1159/000365544)

The Role of General Practitioners and Family Physicians in the Management of Multimorbidity

P. Boeckxstaens[a, c, d] · J. De Maeseneer[a, c, d] · A. De Sutter[b–d]

[a]Community Health Centre 'Botermarkt' and [b]Community Health Centre 'Rabot', [c]Department of Family Medicine and Primary Health Care and [d]International Center for PHC and Family Medicine, Ghent University, Ghent, Belgium

Abstract

The rising prevalence of chronic conditions also implies a rise in multimorbidity. Comorbid diseases are important because they influence the diagnostic process, the therapeutic approach, the effect of the treatment and ultimately the patient's outcome. Most studies on chronic diseases have focused on patients with a single condition and the evidence on how to manage coexisting chronic diseases is lacking. Moreover, most health systems have been developed to tackle diseases through vertical disease-oriented programs. This chapter discusses the challenges of multimorbidity (including mental illness) from a primary care perspective and the role of family physicians or general practitioners in the management of multimorbidity. Strong primary care systems can enable a comprehensive approach to multimorbidity, shifting the paradigm from 'disease orientation' towards 'goal orientation'.

© 2015 S. Karger AG, Basel

The Epidemiological Transition towards People with Multiple Chronic Conditions

Due to the aging of the population and the rising prevalence of chronic diseases, the number of people suffering from more than one disease will continuously increase. Anderson et al. [1] have reported that in the general population, 50% of those aged over 65 years have at least 3 chronic conditions, and 20% of those aged over 65 years have at least 5 chronic conditions. The lack of comparability between studies precludes giving an overall estimate on the prevalence of multimorbidity since this is very dependent on the way multimorbidity is measured [2, 3]. However, regardless of the measure used, the prevalence of multimorbidity is high and will rise further. This is especially the case in older persons, where multimorbidity will become the rule rather than the exception in clinical care. The comorbidity of mental and physical disorders is the least well researched, with many studies excluding patients with psychiatric comorbidity, despite the mental comorbidity creating important challenges for clinical management.

General Practice: From a Comorbidity to a Multimorbidity Perspective

In the 1980s and 1990s, the focus of chronic care was on single diseases. Comorbidity was included as a MeSH term for the first time in 1989. Most research on the coexistence of chronic diseases originated from fundamental research and focused on the underlying mechanisms of comorbidities. In the case of chronic obstructive pulmonary disease (COPD), abundant comorbidity research has indicated that selected comorbidities, such as atherosclerotic disease, depression, chronic kidney disease and cognitive impairment, are found more frequently among people with COPD [4–7]. The same applies for diabetes, rheumatoid arthritis and many other diseases for which comorbidities have been documented.

The term 'multimorbidity' was introduced in the 1990s and is not yet a MeSH term. It is important to distinguish the concepts of comorbidity and multimorbidity [8]. Comorbidity always implies an index disease, whereas multimorbidity is defined as any co-occurrence of medical conditions within a person. From the perspective of primary healthcare, the construct of multimorbidity is particularly relevant because general practitioners deal with the broad spectrum of diseases affecting these patients and do not necessarily put one disease or body system at the forefront. When it comes to mental illness, Gunn et al. [9] clearly demonstrated that the number of (physical) chronic conditions is directly related to the presence of depressive symptoms [9]. Moreover, as is the case for most chronic conditions, in patients with multimorbidity there is a clear social

gradient for every age group, with multimorbidity being more prevalent in the most deprived groups [10], while deprivation is frequently linked to depressive symptoms.

Moreover, from the patients' perspective, the distinction between index diseases and comorbid diseases is often irrelevant because the impact of diseases on their lives crosses the boundaries of individual diseases. In fact, as indicated in one of the latest reviews on COPD and comorbidities [4], whatever the underlying mechanism of comorbidities, the personal, clinical, prognostic and therapeutic impact on the patient asks for a shift from comorbidity to multimorbidity.

How Does the Health System Address Patients with (Several) Chronic Conditions Today?

In recent years, not only Western countries, but also developing countries, have started 'chronic disease management programs' [11, 12] in order to improve care for long-term chronic conditions. A recent survey of 'chronic disease management' in 10 European countries illustrated that disease-management programs in most countries are organized around a single chronic condition, e.g. diabetes, sometimes focusing on subgroups within a specific chronic disease, e.g. disease-management programs that only include people with type 2 diabetes [12]. Incentives have been defined in order to stimulate both patients and providers to adhere to guidelines. This development has led to important results, e.g. in process and (biomedical) outcome indicators defined by the UK Quality and Outcomes Framework [13]. Moreover, the 'chronic disease management' approach has led to an acceleration of task-shifting from physicians to nurses, dieticians and health educators.

Disease-management programs also have increased the attention given to interventions that improve the knowledge and skills of patients in dealing with their chronic condition, e.g. self-management of diabetes. Despite some criticism regarding equity [14, 15], the sustainability of the quality of improvement and comprehensiveness versus a reductionist nature of the programs [16], these programs in general have received positive feedback from providers, patients and politicians. However, the continuous development of single-disease programs may also entail a growing mismatch between the needs of people living with multimorbidity and the resources offered by a health system that increasingly focuses on disease-defined care.

Why Primary Care?

Although much has been learned from vertical disease-oriented programs, better outcomes could be reached by addressing diseases through an integrated approach in a strong primary care system. An example is Brazil, where therapeutic coverage for HIV/AIDS reaches almost 100%, which is far higher than HIV/AIDS programs in other countries with less robust primary care. Vertical disease-oriented programs for HIV/AIDS, malaria, tuberculosis and other infectious diseases encourage duplication and the inefficient use of resources. They produce gaps in the care of patients with multimorbidity [17, 18] and cause inequity for patients who do not have the 'right' disease [19]. Horizontal primary care provides the opportunity for integration and addresses the problem of inequity, providing access to the care for all health problems, thereby avoiding 'inequity by disease' [20].

The Case of Jennifer

Jennifer is 75 years old. Fifteen years ago she lost her husband. She has been a patient at the practice for 15 years now. She has been through a difficult medical history: hip replacement surgery for osteoarthritis, hypertension, type 2 diabetes, COPD and episodes of depression.

According to the guidelines, Jennifer is faced with a lot of tasks: joint protection, aerobic exercise, muscle strengthening, a range of motion exercising, self-monitoring of blood glucose, avoiding environmental exposure that might exacerbate COPD, wearing appropriate foot wear, limiting intake of alcohol and maintaining body weight. She has to receive patient education regarding diabetes self-management, foot care, osteoarthritis and the COPD medication delivery system training. Her medication schedule includes 11 different drugs, with a total of 20 administrations a day. The clinical tasks for the general practitioner in relation to this patient include vaccination, blood pressure control at all clinical visits, evaluation of self-monitoring of blood glucose, foot examination, laboratory tests, and psychological assessment and support in episodes of depression. Moreover, referrals are needed for physiotherapy, retinal examination, pulmonary rehabilitation and psychotherapy.

Jennifer lives independently at home, with some help from her youngest daughter, Elisabeth. I visit her regularly and each time she starts by saying: 'Doctor, you must help me'. Then a succession of complaints and unwell feeling follows. Sometimes it has to do with her heart, another time with lungs, then the hip and sometimes depression. Each time I suggest – according to the guidelines – all sorts of examinations that do not improve her condition. Her requests become more and more explicit, while my feelings of powerlessness, inadequacy and irritation increase. Moreover, I have to cope with guidelines that are contradictory: for COPD she sometimes needs corticosteroids, which always worsens her diabetes control. The adaptation of the medication for the blood pressure (once too high, once too low) does not meet with her approval, nor does my interest in her HbA_{1C} and lung function test results.

How Can We Build an Evidence Base for Multimorbidity?

Clinical decisions must be based on adequate knowledge of diseases (medical evidence), but at the same time they must take into account patient-specific aspects of medical care (contextual evidence) and efficiency and equity (policy evidence) [21]. As far as medical evidence is concerned, in primary healthcare we are confronted with the tension between the results of actual clinical research on the one hand and the needs of daily clinical practice on the other hand. As the case of Jennifer illustrates, questions arise about which evidence to follow in the case of multimorbidity. Treatment according to the guidelines for one condition (corticosteroids for COPD) may interfere with the guidelines for another (glycemic control in type 2 diabetes). There is a lot of evidence available on the management of COPD and type 2 diabetes for people younger than 75 years and without comorbidity, but there is little, if any, evidence about how to treat a 75-year-old woman who has both disorders.

This problem implies a need for research on the effectiveness of diagnostic and therapeutic interventions that take into account these aspects of patients in primary care. The challenge of multimorbidity illustrates the lack of appropriate evidence. Most available evidence to treat chronic diseases has been collected in single-disease trials, often excluding patients with comorbid diseases. A possible solution to tackle the evidence gap for multimorbidity may be to engage in the development of randomized clinical trials or guidelines on patients with specific combinations of diseases [22, 23]. However, a practice-based cross-sectional analysis of the medical records of 543 patients aged over 65 years in primary care has shown that patients with multimorbidity have complex and unique combinations of problems [24].

The low prevalence of disease combinations at the practice level will hamper the usefulness of randomized trials and guidelines for providers. Moreover, many of the strongest associations show a contribution of a psychiatric problem or a social problem which demands a tailored approach. Luijks et al. [25] showed that general practitioners agreed on the need to adapt management of multimorbidity to the personal circumstances of these patients, such as vitality, personal preferences and socioeconomic conditions. They stressed the importance of tailoring care to the individual and trying to understand the meaning of illness for a person. A personal patient-doctor relationship and continuity of care were considered major facilitators in the management of multimorbidity, and the presence of mental health problems was regarded as a complicating factor. In order to build a useful and relevant evidence base for multimorbidity, there is a need to explore new generic ways and paradigms to approach patients with multimorbidity which allow tailoring care to focus on the needs, goals and expectations of each individual patient [26–28].

From Problem-Oriented Towards Goal-Oriented Care

Jennifer eventually said, 'Doctor, I want to tell you what really matters to me. On Tuesday and Thursday, I want to visit my friends in the neighborhood and play cards with them. On Saturday, I want to go the supermarket with my daughter. And for the rest of the week, I want to be left in peace. I do not want to continually change the therapy anymore, especially not having to do this and to do that'. In the conversation that followed, it became clear to me how Jennifer had formulated the goals for her life. At the same time I felt challenged to identify how the guidelines could contribute to the achievement of Jennifer's goals. I have enjoyed visiting Jennifer ever since. I know what she wants and how much I can (merely) contribute to her life.

Jennifer's case clearly illustrates the need for a paradigm-shift for chronic care: from problem oriented to goal oriented. In 1991, Mold et al. [27] recognized that the problem-oriented model, which focuses on the eradication of disease and the prevention of death, is not well suited to the management of chronic illness. Therefore, they proposed a goal-oriented approach that encourages each individual to achieve the highest possible level of health, which is defined by the individual instead of the health system. This represents a more positive approach to healthcare, characterized by a greater emphasis on individual strengths and resources. What really matters for patients is their ability to function (functional status) and social participation. Goal-oriented care assists an individual in achieving their maximum individual health potential in line with their individually defined goals. Exploring the goals of patients will require adequate communication with patients to allow providers to explore and elicit personal goals. At a practice level, providers should increasingly pay attention to goal-oriented care and provide an atmosphere of open communication attentive and supportive to patients who should be encouraged to introduce their own goals in clinical decision-making.

The Need for New Types of Evidence

In order to understand the goals of the patients better, new research frameworks and research disciplines will be needed. This will require input from disciplines that contribute to the understanding of provider-patient interaction such as medical philosophy, sociology and anthropology. Research methods will have to shift from purely quantitative (randomized clinical trials) towards qualitative approaches looking at understanding through in-depth interviews and focus groups. We will have to look for research tools and approaches that explore subjective determinants of well-being, and not only biomedical measurements. In the new research designs, patients with multimorbidity will be the rule (instead of an exclusion criterion) and complexity will be embraced instead of avoided [29].

The International Classification of Functioning (ICF) [30] might become as important as the International Classification of Diseases (ICD), as it draws a conceptual framework in which different domains of human functioning are defined. These domains are classified from an eco-, bio- and psychosocial viewpoint by means of a list of body functions and structures, and a list of domains of activity and participation. As an individual's functioning and disability depends on the context, the ICF includes a list of environmental factors and the concept of personal factors in its framework. The ICF is part of the 'Family of International Classifications' (FIC) and meets the standards for health-related classifications as defined by the World Health Organization (WHO). Although the ICD has a dominating role in healthcare data management, the WHO aims to reach the same level with the ICF, a classification that defines functional status irrespective of the underlying health condition.

Implications for the Health System

At a policy level, healthcare systems should become more attentive to goal-oriented care and support providers to engage in the labor-intensive process of goal-oriented care. This will require both a fundamental reflection on time management, task delegation and payment systems. Family physicians should be encouraged to provide less and longer proactive patient contacts instead of more and shorter reactive consultations. Practice nurses and other primary care providers should be increasingly encouraged to engage in chronic care. Moreover, taking into account the social gradient, with deprived patients being more prone to multimorbidity [31, 32], social workers should be included in the team approach. The current focus on fee for (technical) services does not seem well suited to a goal-oriented approach in healthcare.

Multimorbidity, Goal-Oriented Care and Equity

When implementing goal-oriented care, there may be a threat to equity, as the way goals are formulated by patients might be determined by a number of factors including social class. Moreover, integrating the patient's context implies the risk of taking the context for granted; people living in poverty will generally have been obliged to take on lower expectations in terms of quantity and quality of life than well-educated people. Therefore, 'goal-oriented medical care' could contribute to an increase in social inequities in health. Therefore, the primary care team should engage in an approach of intersectoral action for health (interacting with sectors like employment, housing and education) and address the social determinants and 'upstream causes' of ill health.

The Role of the General Practitioner in the Management of Patients with Multimorbidity

The role of the general practitioner in the management of multimorbidity is situated at different levels. The general practitioner is the provider with a comprehensive view on both the biomedical and personal health status of the patient. They are in the frontline to detect the evolution from 'single disease' to 'comorbidity' and 'multimorbidity' in individual patients, and are able to integrate disease-specific guidelines to the personal situation of the patient. They are able to define medical priorities and integrate them with the personal goals and preferences of the patient, thereby supporting a timely shift from 'problem orientation' to 'goal orientation'. The general practitioner can be involved in the facilitation of 'goal definition' by the patients and is well placed to integrate these goals in clinical decision-making for multimorbidity and

build an individual care plan together with the patient. Through continuity of care, the general practitioner can be attentive to the fact that goals of patients can change over time as the context changes. This approach will, however, require more focus on the individual patient-provider interaction and on appropriate communication skills to facilitate goal definition and patient empowerment.

Other primary care providers, such as nurses, physiotherapists, occupational therapists, social workers, dieticians and others, also have invaluable insights into the patients' situation, which should be integrated in the care for the patient. Shared decision-making, starting with patient goals and involving the patient and other care providers, will avoid gaps in the process and encourage empowerment of the patient. Especially in a context of multimorbidity, there is a need for a shift from 'chronic disease management' towards 'participatory patient management', with the patient at the center of the process. Moreover, as definition of 'goals' may often be related to values, the providers in the primary care team will have to act as reflective practitioners that contribute to reconcile individual and community health requirements. It is clear that this process will require more time investment at first, e.g. to engage in a goal-setting encounter with the patient; however, in the long term, goal-oriented care might prove to be more relevant, effective and efficient, and require less time spent on targets not of interest to that individual patient.

At the meso-level, general practitioners may have an important 'signaling' role in order to document and draw attention to problems of inequity. Institutions for health professionals' education are challenged to train providers that are not only 'experts', or excellent 'professionals', but also 'change agents' [33] who continuously improve the health system and question the relevance of knowledge and care. General practitioner education will have to provide the needed support and training of providers and the coordination of the different primary care organizations. General practitioners should be able to reflect on the equitable distribution of resources, taking into account social determinants, on the organization of the healthcare services and the features of the health system in order to tailor care to this growing group of complex patients.

At the macro-level, this will also require dialogue and communication methodologies between the health sector and persons in need of healthcare as well as with other stakeholders within the society involved in healthcare at the practice, research and policy levels in order to guarantee the essential characteristics of an effective health system including relevance, equity, quality, cost-effectiveness, sustainability, people-centeredness and innovation.

References

1   Anderson G, et al: Chronic Conditions: Making the Case for Ongoing Care. Baltimore, Partnership for Solutions, 2002.
2   Fortin M, Stewart M, Poitras ME, et al: A systematic review of prevalence studies on multimorbidity: toward a more uniform methodology. Ann Fam Med 2012;10:142–151.
3   Salive ME: Multimorbidity in older adults: prevalence and implications. Epidemiol Rev 2013;35:75–83.
4   Corsonello A, Antonelli Incalzi R, Pistelli R, et al: Comorbidities of chronic obstructive pulmonary disease. Curr Opin Pulm Med 2011;17(suppl 1):S21–S28.
5   Incalzi RA, Corsonello A, Pedone C, et al: Chronic renal failure: a neglected comorbidity of COPD. Chest 2010;137: 831–837.
6   Casanova C, de Torres JP, Navarro J, et al: Microalbuminuria and hypoxemia in patients with chronic obstructive pulmonary disease. Am J Respir Crit Care Med 2010;182:1004–1010.
7   Ionescu AA, Schoon E: Osteoporosis in chronic obstructive pulmonary disease. Eur Respir J Suppl 2003;46:64s–75s.
8   van den Akker M, Buntinx F, Knottnerus JA: Comorbidity or multimorbidity. What's in a name? A review of literature. Eur J Gen Pract 1996;2: 65–70.
9   Gunn JM, Ayton DR, Densley K: The association between chronic illness, multimorbidity and depressive symptoms in an Australian primary care cohort. Soc Psychiatr Epidemiol 2012;47: 175–184.

10   Barnett K, Mercer SW, Norbury M, et al: Epidemiology of multimorbidity and implications for health care, research, and medical education: a cross-sectional study. Lancet 2012;380:37–43.
11   Bodenheimer T, Wagner EH, Grumbach K: Improving primary care for patients with chronic illness: the chronic care model, part 2. JAMA 2002;288:1909–1914.
12   Rijken PM, Bekkema N: Chronic Disease Management Matrix 2010: Results of a Survey in Ten European Countries. Utrecht, NIVEL, 2011.
13   Gillam S, Siriwardena AN (eds): The Quality and Outcomes Framework. QOF-Transforming General Practice. Oxford, Radcliffe, 2011.
14   Boeckxstaens P, Smedt DD, Maeseneer JD, et al: The equity dimension in evaluations of the quality and outcomes framework: a systematic review. BMC Health Serv Res 2011;11:209.
15   Norbury M, Fawkes N, Guthrie B: Impact of the GP contract on inequalities associated with influenza immunisation: a retrospective population-database analysis. Br J Gen Pract 2011;61:e379–e385.
16   Chew-Graham CA, Hunter C, Langer S, et al: How QOF is shaping primary care review consultations: a longitudinal qualitative study. BMC Fam Pract 2013; 14:103.
17   De Maeseneer J, van Weel C, Egilman D, et al: Funding for primary health care in developing countries. BMJ 2008;336: 518–519.

18   Boyd CM, Darer J, Boult C, Fried LP, Boult L, Wu AW: Clinical practice guidelines and quality of care for older patients with multiple comorbid diseases: implications for pay for performance. JAMA 2005;294:716–724.
19   De Maeseneer J, Roberts RG, Demarzo M, et al: Tackling NCDs: a different approach is needed. Lancet 2012;379: 1860–1861.
20   Starfield B: The hidden inequity in health care. Int J Equity Health 2011;10: 15.
21   De Maeseneer JM, van Driel ML, Green LA, et al: The need for research in primary care. Lancet 2003;362:1314–1319.
22   Fabbri LM, Luppi F, Beghe B, et al: Complex chronic comorbidities of COPD. Eur Respir J 2008;31:204–212.
23   Schafer I, von Leitner EC, Schon G, et al: Multimorbidity patterns in the elderly: a new approach of disease clustering identifies complex interrelations between chronic conditions. PloS One 2010;5: e15941.
24   Boeckxstaens P, Peersman W, Ghali S, Goubin G, De Maeseneer J, Brusselle G, De Sutter A: Practice-based analysis of combinations of diseases in patients aged 65 or older in primary care. BMC family practice, in press.
25   Luijks HD, Loeffen MJ, Lagro-Janssen AL, et al: GPs' considerations in multimorbidity management: a qualitative study. Br J Gen Pract 2012;62:e503–e510.
26   Dawes M: Co-morbidity: we need a guideline for each patient not a guideline for each disease. Fam Pract 2010;27: 1–2.

27 Mold JW, Blake GH, Becker LA: Goal-oriented medical care. Fam Med 1991; 23:46–51.

28 De Maeseneer J, Boeckxstaens P: James Mackenzie Lecture 2011: multimorbidity, goal-oriented care, and equity. Br J Gen Pract 2012;62:e522–e524.

29 Heath I, Rubinstein A, Stange KC, et al: Quality in primary health care: a multidimensional approach to complexity. BMJ 2009;338:b1242.

30 International Classification of Functioning and Disability in Health (ICF). Geneva, WHO, 2001.

31 Macleod U, Mitchell E, Black M, et al: Comorbidity and socioeconomic deprivation: an observational study of the prevalence of comorbidity in general practice. Eur J Gen Pract 2004;10:24–26.

32 Salisbury C, Johnson L, Purdy S, et al: Epidemiology and impact of multimorbidity in primary care: a retrospective cohort study. Br J Gen Pract 2011; 61:e12–e21.

33 Frenk J, Chen L, Bhutta ZA, et al: Health professionals for a new century: transforming education to strengthen health systems in an interdependent world. Lancet 2010;376:1923–1958.

J. De Maeseneer, MD, PhD
Department of Family Medicine and Primary Health Care
Ghent University, UZ-6K3
De Pintelaan, 185
BE–9000 Ghent (Belgium)
E-Mail Jan.DeMaeseneer@UGent.be

Sartorius N, Holt RIG, Maj M (eds): Comorbidity of Mental and Physical Disorders.
Key Issues Ment Health. Basel, Karger, 2015, vol 179, pp 137–147 (DOI: 10.1159/000365598)

Training Physicians at Undergraduate and Postgraduate Levels about Comorbidity

Annie Cushing[a] · Sandra Evans[b]

[a]Clinical and Communication Skills Unit, Institute of Health Sciences Education, and [b]Department of Psychiatry, Barts and The London School of Medicine and Dentistry, St. Bartholomew's Hospital, Queen Mary, University of London, London, UK

Abstract

This chapter addresses the importance of training on comorbidity and the principles of learning. It covers the methods and structuring of such training, the content on which it is based, and what is known in the field. It includes illness versus disease management, holistic approaches, patient and doctor roles regarding shared decision-making, adherence and self-management, polypharmacy, interprofessional and team communication, and effective consultation and communication skills. We highlight methods which are learner-centred, aiming at active engagement in a collaborative endeavour with the trainer. We emphasise the need to recognise the broader systems' factors which support or undermine integration of learning into everyday practice. Training should address cognitive (knowledge), emotional and motivational (attitudes), and behavioural (skills) elements of learning. Whilst undergraduates will need more didactic elements and proscribed activities, postgraduate training benefits from flexibility to the learners' working context. Training the trainers is an important component of an education strategy so that teachers use a learner-centred approach consistent with the patient-centred consultation model needed to manage comorbidity.   © 2015 S. Karger AG, Basel

Physical and mental comorbidity has not been well addressed in medical education, especially in systems-based curriculum designs. Increasing specialisation of healthcare delivery also threatens integrated managemant. Training is important for a commitment to understanding comorbidity from the start of clinical training about patient care. For clinical practice to develop, it requires active engagement, adjustments in daily working and broader support from the healthcare system [1] (fig. 1).

The crowded curriculum in medicine puts each discipline in competition with one another over what is most important for the first-year medical student, foundation trainee or intern to know. The only way to cover the material adequately *and* ensure an appropriate attitude towards patient care is to work cooperatively and in an interdisciplinary manner. From the outset, we need to model ways of integrating mental and physical health care knowledge so that students will see their patients in a way which allows them to feel confident in both spheres.

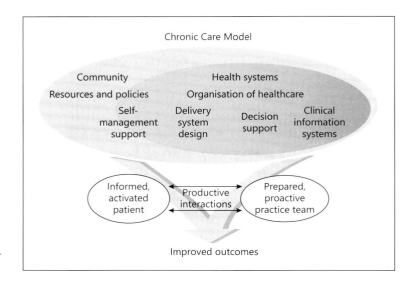

Fig. 1. A model for managing long-term conditions [42].

Our students and trainees are embarked upon a trajectory of life-long learning. We describe how this occurs, including brief coverage of theories of adult learning and how these inform training design and techniques. Examples of model programmes, including the use of communication skills training and other forms of active experiential learning, are included. All learners have to be convinced that their efforts are worthwhile, realistic and manageable, and will bring about desired outcomes. Good practice demonstrated by excellent teachers and practitioners is a strong positive influence. Clinicians and lecturers need to model respect for the psychological aspects of illness. The power of the role model in learning is well documented and so engagement of faculty by training the trainers and postgraduate education is essential for transformative learning and incorporation into clinical practice. Not surprisingly therefore, the shift from paternalism to partnership in the doctor-patient relationship is best mirrored by a shift to a more collaborative trainer-trainee relationship. Training and new skills/approaches must be supported and reinforced by the clinical environment, otherwise formalised learning is not sustained [2, 3].

Educational Theories, Principles and Implications for Training

Important and influential educationalists of our time, including Kolb [4], Schon [5], Dewey [6] and Vygotsky [7], have addressed conditions of effective learning. Kolb's learning cycle explains how learning takes place when (1) having a concrete experience, followed by (2) observation of and reflection on that experience leads to (3) formation of abstract concepts (analysis) and general principles (conclusions) which are then (4) used to test hypotheses in future situations. All four stages are needed, although one can enter at different points and no one stage is an effective learning procedure on its own. Schon's work on the reflective practitioner powerfully shows that learners need to be processing information and feelings while developing insight and responding to changing situations.

Dewey [6] emphasised the importance of the emotional element in learning. Negative emotions, such as extreme anxiety, will act as barriers to engagement in learning. Trainers must establish a supportive, whilst appropriately 'challenging', approach to the educational event. Feedback

Table 1. Examples of learners' needs

Pass the assessment
Manage time in consultation – get there quicker
Be able to deal with the situation if they 'take the lid off it'
Helpful strategies, skills, examples of questions and phrasing
A good history and diagnosis
Not miss pathology
Develop a management plan
Work without all the information and 'mine for data'
Manage uncertainty
Patient safety
Satisfied patient
Connect patients to other healthcare professionals/refer/support

should always be linked to what one is trying to achieve, so goals of the consultation need to be clarified and agreed [8, 9]. Feedback framed in terms of what is effective and examples of any missed opportunities are conducive to useful learning. Emotional involvement is a key feature of learning. The feedback conversation is central and includes checking how the learner is feeling, preferably in a small, supportive group setting [10]. Learners then need to set goals for implementing their learning, based on a collaborative evaluation of the importance of and confidence in being able to apply the new knowledge and behaviour. Vygotsky highlights: 'the distance between the actual developmental level as determined by independent problem solving and the level of potential development as determined through problem solving under adult guidance…' [7, p. 86].

Designing learning activity pitched at a level in order to challenge without overwhelming the learner should:

(1) Consider the learners' agenda (table 1), the patients' agenda ('what I want doctors to help me with'), the trainers' agenda (evidence-based practice) and the service agenda (the pragmatic approach)

(2) Make it real by designing training characterised by relevance, experience, activity and learner-centredness [11]

(3) Pitch training to the level and context of the learner

(4) Ensure feedback and include follow-up action plans

Undergraduates have limited clinical experience and will benefit from an approach which involves more teaching, coaching and real patients or problem-based learning scenarios incorporating comorbidity. Involving the 'patient's voice' and expert patients in education is memorable and helps students and trainees understand patients' particular expertise [12]. Students are strongly motivated by assessment rather than seemingly distant clinical practice; therefore, assessments such as objective structured clinical examinations should incorporate identification of comorbidity. Online resources with case studies, video clips and principles of practice help the novice develop an understanding [13]. Early years' experience of meeting patients and carers using reflective learning assignments and progressing to role-play utilising actors, particularly for more complex consultations, provides a vertical integration in a curriculum.

Postgraduate learners bring their own clinical experience. Incorporating their particular situations maximises relevance and engages motivation. From their own reflections in identifying

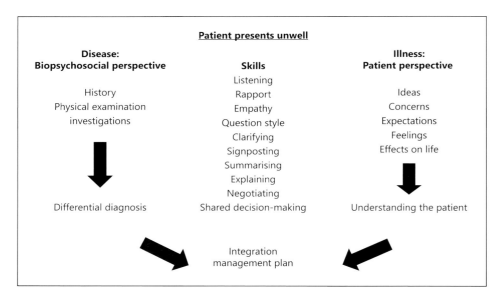

Fig. 2. Disease-illness framework and patient-centred communication. Adapted from McWhinney [15].

the challenges of these interactions, they can practice new strategies in role-play and receive constructive feedback. Good postgraduate training programmes develop skills for working in partnership by involving patients with long-term conditions as co-facilitators alongside trainers [14].

Training Goals

Training needs to incorporate some explanation of comorbidity and the potentially dangerous implications of not identifying it within the consultation. As it will inevitably require more effort initially on the clinician's part to explore comorbidity, conviction and skills are needed. Training outcomes include (1) acceptance of the biopsychosocial model of health and awareness of issues in comorbidity, (2) knowledge of what to manage and how, and what to refer, and (3) communication and interpersonal skills.

The Biopsychosocial Disease-Illness Model and Patient-Centred Care
In 1989, McWhinney [15] described the disease-illness framework and the need to explore both biomedical and psychosocial information to understand the patient and his/her situation (fig. 2). The patient's experience and beliefs are hugely significant, although historically often neglected because a patient's views and expectations will affect adherence to medications and the actions he/she takes regarding lifestyle changes. Discussing raised glycated haemoglobin levels with a patient distracted by depression about having diabetes is unhelpful. Engaging patient understanding and managing his/her healthcare in collaboration with the physician will have better outcomes [16].

As one patient explained, 'You're always hoping there will be a cure, which is why you end up being so depressed, when there isn't one… . Within secondary care in particular, there's still too much emphasis on treatment rather than self-management' (Shani Evans, 2008) [14]. Students need to recognise that partnership between patients and clinicians in a co-creating health relationship is essential both for patients' well-being and tackling escalating costs of care [17].

Issues in Comorbidity: The Dialectic between the Physical and the Mental
The curriculum needs to include the following six themes which should cover the basic understanding of comorbidity for students and junior trainees.

(1) The Interdependence of Mind and Body: How the Psychological Can Impact the Physical and Vice Versa
A psychological understanding and a framework of illness and the emotional responses to it are vital to a well-functioning and quality health service. This perspective becomes increasingly pertinent as survival from disorders that used to be life-threatening becomes more commonplace. Diabetes, HIV and renal disease are a few examples of diseases that cannot be cured but can be managed; and yet the psychological effect of a long-term disorder that will change lives and impoverish expectations is also important. Students must learn the goals after survival include reducing suffering, increasing emotional well-being, pain control, functional ability and vitality. A clinician teacher's role includes sharing awareness of common psychiatric comorbidities and how to manage them in a patient-centred way.

(2) Presentations of Illness That Can Confound Diagnosis
Medical students and young doctors have to struggle with large amounts of new knowledge and tend to prefer clear facts that are easy to digest. As their learning progresses they will be able to recognise when patients' presentations do not follow the usual pattern of a disease profile. Discrepancies in symptoms or repeat presentations by the same person who is not getting better may suggest a misdiagnosis and even the possibility of medically unexplained symptoms.

Physical manifestations of psychological distress are well understood, such as dry mouth or tachycardia when anxious. Some symptoms are less obviously associated with a trauma. They may convey meaning unknown to the sufferer and require more careful history taking to elucidate.

Medically unexplained symptoms are not so easy to understand on the surface, but may be simpler to demonstrate clinically. In a simulated clinical setting, for example, by exploring psychosocial information students can easily be encouraged to divine the likely association of headaches in a person whose partner has just died of a brain tumour, or one who complains of memory problems when stressed and exhausted from looking after their elderly mother who has Alzheimer's disease. The common factor here is encouraging students' curiosity and getting them to ask appropriate questions. Exploring a symptom can be likened to detective work.

How can we engage students and trainees fully in the current governmental commitment to offer 'parity of esteem' as in the USA for mental health issues as for physical ones [18]? We need medical schools to collaborate with psychiatry and psychology departments in order to ensure that the psychological perspective becomes part of teaching all systems and permeates across most aspects of training. Psychiatry is not just a discipline like medicine or surgery: it is also a way of understanding pathological processes that engages the medical model, but also views patients from their own psychological and social perspective. Especially valuable can be educational methods bringing together specialists from different fields of medicine and surgery (gastroenterology, cardiology, gynaecology, primary care, psychologists, psychiatrists) in clinical forums to discuss patients, encouraging the skills needed to communicate effectively and manage care [19]. Similar methods in undergraduate teaching from multispecialist groups are needed to prevent development of negative attitudes towards patients with medically unexplained symptoms [20].

(3) Risk Factors for Mental Health Difficulties in Physical Illness: Particularly Long-Term Conditions

Some physical health conditions often go hand in hand with a psychiatric morbidity. A common example is one of anxiety and depression experienced with severe breathing problems [21]. Students starting their clinical attachments will often come across such patients who may be the subject of their first clerking. In a medical school focused on clinical skills and listening and attending to a patient's agenda, the student may be struck by the worries and concerns of patients with asthma or bronchitis. Their task may be to take a history and then examine the patient physically. They will also ask about the impact of illness on the person's life. They will understand that work may be limited, exercise impossible and enjoyment curtailed. Managing long-term conditions holistically can have a significant positive effect on patients' mental health and quality of life. If psychiatry is integrated into teaching from the outset (including how to perform a mental state examination), students may feel able to ask about mood symptoms as a result and even enquire about suicidal thoughts. Fostering an understanding of these principles and supporting learners who are commonly anxious about asking such potentially upsetting questions is a key goal of educators. Students adjust to knowing that patients with psychiatric symptoms *can be on medical wards* and not just in a psychiatry setting. They also learn that psychiatric symptoms are commonplace, associated with physical conditions and treatable if recognised.

The importance of understanding the interrelationship of conditions and the medications used to treat them are also crucial. Patients dispensed medications from multiple providers are at greater risk of an adverse drug reaction and are more likely to suffer from the prescribing cascade [22]. Medication for physical illness can cause mental health symptoms and conversely drugs taken for mental health problems may cause physical symptoms and predispose to physical disease. How students will be guided to consider these issues and how to approach them requires teaching faculty who are committed to an integrated way of viewing health.

(4) Learners' Own Physical and Mental Health: Knowing One's Self and Being Aware of Assumptions and Judgments

Being aware of one's own views and reactions to other people's misfortunes is essential to enable learners to behave in a non-partisan, professional manner that does not seek to judge but merely to inform. Knowing something about the nature and management of addictions is also enormously important when deciding on the best course of action in the treatment of physical problems in people with substance misuse, alcoholism or addiction (e.g. liver failure). Religious and cultural diversity among patients and students will influence understanding, personal attitudes and communication.

Mental health problems may remain uncovered for patients whose doctors do not explore this aspect of the patient's psychosocial history [23]. Whilst patients may drop cues from demeanour or language, they are less likely to raise these worries directly. Doctors commonly use distancing tactics such as focusing only on biomedical facts, premature reassurance or jollying patients along rather than pursue cues, and thus miss significant mental health problems. Key communication skills are associated with increased disclosure. Teaching learners to observe demeanour, note speech quality, listen, allow silence and express empathy are particularly important. Skills training helps the healthcare professional to engage the patient and discuss with them their ideas, concerns and expectations in conjunction with addressing biomedical facts [24].

Mental illness carries stigma. Those most at risk of this way of thinking are the medical students and doctors themselves. Students often fear a mental health diagnosis because of ignorance, stigma and a belief that it will prevent their qualifying as a doctor [25]. Stress, one of our biggest difficulties in busy, demanding and responsible jobs, can cause much physical and mental ill health. Sometimes alleviated by alcohol use, which may become a problem in itself, it is more dangerous when we fail to recognise it in ourselves.

Students and trainees can experience distressing situations in their own lives as well as in clinical practice. A curriculum which includes teaching about stress, its impact on doctors and the available support services enables students and trainees to recognize when this may be an issue and where to get help.

Experiential learning is also powerful. For example, clinical skills training combining the ability to 'break bad news' sensitively while attempting to understand the unique perspective of the person with a particular physical or indeed 'mental illness' diagnosis is one learning strategy that is used [26]. Role-playing the clinician can be very helpful in that one is exposed to a range of affects from the simulated patient and one learns how to manage each. If students are asked to play the patient as well as the doctor, this adds a power to the scenario, but can be challenging. These methods can really assist medical students and trainees to empathise. Exercises such as having a conversation whilst breathing through a straw to simulate the experience of someone with chronic obstructive pulmonary disease (COPD) [Kim C, pers. commun., 2013] and the 'hearing voices' audiotaped exercise used to illustrate the experience of patients with psychosis [27] help learners imagine the lived experience of disability and appreciate of the patients' suffering. By being in the patients' 'shoes', the potential consequences of a doctor choosing to listen attentively or maintaining distance can be understood. Train-

ers must be skilled in facilitating such situations and be prepared to listen and support students who are upset or having difficulties. Preferably they will have received training in role-play methods using ground rules for safety.

(5) Risk Factors for Physical Health Difficulties in People with Mental Illness

Depressed people are less likely to be able to manage their illness, medications or lifestyle changes [16, 17]. Difficulties exercising and keeping fit are often associated with feeling unmotivated, anxious about facing the world or being indifferent to one's own future. Drugs used in treating psychotic disorders often cause weight gain, induce diabetes mellitus and risk heart disease. Enabling students to discover these issues early on in their training through talking to patients with chronic mental health problems, and their families, also encourages a more compassionate and thoughtful view of the complexity of psychiatric disorder. Interestingly, there is some evidence that although the coexistence of depression and multiple physical conditions is associated with increased illness burden, such patients benefit most from the Chronic Disease Self-Management Programs, and students and trainees should learn about these approaches [28].

(6) Consultation Skills to Identify and Plan Management for Comorbidity

Goals for the consultation include an open, respectful, empathic, accurate and constructive consultation based on both the patient's and doctor's agenda, focussing on gathering relevant biomedical and psychosocial information and shared decision-making. The very important therapeutic function of the consultation, in and of itself, is well known.

To operationalise the disease/illness and shared decision/partnership care, a number of consultation guides for skills training have been developed [29–31]. These frameworks define the skills that, when used in context, are known to be helpful. Particularly important are listening (and silence), observing non-verbal cues, listening to quality of speech and responding to cues using empathic reflection.

Training Issues

Barriers to Identifying Comorbidity
Whilst clinicians may be aware of comorbidity, they can also feel time pressured and powerless to manage the problems, as well as lack confidence or strategies to deal with all the issues, and thus act to avoid being overwhelmed by a variety of patient needs. Training must take account of the fact that clinicians may control and limit the interview as a way of avoiding emotional difficulties [32].

Comorbidity may mean that patients are already seeing, or will need to see, other members of the healthcare team. Accessing and transferring patient information between healthcare providers is not easy where multiple information systems of patients' data exist. If clinicians see only problems and no ways of efficiently dealing with these, they may be reticent to explore comorbidity and may focus narrowly or exclusively on the primary presenting problem. Similarly, students and trainees need to have a strategy of how to respond. These can include listening attentively, acknowledgement of the problem and advocacy by offering, with the patient's permission, to talk to the doctor or attending physician. Trainees may in addition be able to offer simple advice, help patients to problem solve, book a longer appointment and refer to colleagues. Without plans for what to do next, students and trainees will likely not ask about comorbidity. Training should incorporate strategies for the next steps.

Skills for Patients and Clinicians to Understand Each Other
The doctor-patient interaction is recognised as one of unequal power which brings with it a number of challenges for open communication. Patients frequently hint rather than say what their problems are. If the doctor overly controls the nature of information gained and the type of information the patient gives, an inadequate problem definition may occur. Skills are needed to pick up on cues, create trust and gain an accurate comprehensive history, and these skills can be taught [33].

Teaching Consultation and Communication Skills

Communication skills training promoting patient-centred approaches in clinical consultations is best designed on a blended learning skills-based and attitude development approach with incorporation of peer support using a variety of training techniques [32, 34–36]. Group problem-solving discussions on how to respond to comorbidity and practical management planning addresses learners' concerns about 'taking the lid off' problems and not having confidence or strategies to tackle them. Without this, application in practice will be compromised [36]. Case studies, such as those below can be used to discuss goals for a consultation, practical management strategies and to practice communication skills.

Case Study 1
Mr. Peters, 58 years of age, was admitted through the accident and emergency department with acute shortness of breath, and is now on intravenous antibiotics. He has a 5-year history of COPD and has had three chest infections already this year. Mr. Peters had smoked 20 cigarettes a day for 40 years, but has now cut down. COPD is significantly affecting his life.

The patient's ideas: 'My lungs are damaged from working on the buses, exhaust fumes in the garage and stress. I know smoking is bad but helps with stress and I've cut down but not quit.'

The patient's concerns: 'My breathing is bad and I can't do much or go far. I retired early on health grounds and miss my mates. I'm worried about all the hospital admissions, but staff are wonderful, I feel safer in hospital and enjoy the company.'

The patient's expectations: 'I want the doctor to give me a stronger drug to help breathing. He'll probably "have a go at me" again about quitting smoking.'

Two years later, Mr. Peters, has become increasingly isolated, rarely goes out, is now having panic attacks about his COPD, cannot sleep and often wakes in the night to use his nebulizer. When he cannot breathe his wife phones an ambulance. He is scared he is dying and his wife feels distraught and does not know how to cope.

Case Study 2

Erica Johnson is a 31-year-old woman of African-Caribbean parentage. She developed schizophrenia in her mid-20s. Although compliant with treatment, a depot antipsychotic medication for the past 3 years and no hospital admissions, her general health is suffering. She has gained a lot of weight and is now morbidly obese, has developed type II diabetes and has raised blood pressure. Her self-esteem is at an all-time low and she feels depressed. Her general practitioner notices that recent blood tests suggest her diabetes is not well controlled.

The general practitioner is mainly concerned about her diabetes. He sees that Erica is overweight but is unsure whether there is enough time to tackle this problem today and feels unsure about the potential impact on her mental health.

Erica is desperately unhappy about her weight. She feels low and miserable, is lonely, and feels unattractive. She wants a family, but has no confidence to find herself a boyfriend. Erica wants to give up the injections which she feels are the cause of her problems.

Summary

Role-play provides a powerful and effective teaching tool. The participant has space for self-reflection and comment followed by feedback from the actor and facilitator. Using video, a recording can be played back so that particular points in the interaction can be identified. Feedback is vital with the opportunity to then repeat any aspects since an experience of success in doing something differently consolidates learning.

Training Course Designs

Intensive experiential postgraduate courses consisting of a 2- or 3-day programmes with a group size of no more than 8 participants, involving videoing and delivered by expert facilitators, are most successful [24, 35, 37]. More pragmatic courses include three consecutive small group sessions of 3–4 h each, a week or more apart, with practice between sessions [38]. As with patients, changing clinicians' habits is difficult and has to start with a belief in the importance and achievability of the changes. Action plans for implementation in practice, subsequent review of success and troubleshooting closes the training loop [4].

New Models of Learning

Some educationalists have called for a broadening of concepts of education, away from the conventional pedagogy in medicine where learning is an individual enterprise, to a collective activity [39, 40]. Clinicians do not work alone and their actions are determined by many external factors. Just as patients have a psychosocial world, so do clinicians, and the influence it has on working practice should be recognised. The whole culture and materiality of the workplace environment affects the daily interactions and practice patterns [1, 41]. An electronic record, for example, that includes or does not include a section on whether comorbidity has been screened for will affect practitioners' behaviour and should be included in training about consultations. Such systems' enablers and barriers need to be recognised for training to be real and credible. Observing practice 'in situ' strengthens both learners' and teachers' abilities to engage with performance in practice. As communication within teams is essential and liaison and referrals are important, team learning is to be promoted.

Conclusions

This chapter has addressed the importance of training for patient-centred consultations on comorbidity and principles of learning to guide the methods and structuring of such training. A spiral curriculum is advocated with interdisciplinary teaching, using a variety of educational methods and incorporating identification and management of comorbidity into summative assessments.

Training the trainers is an important component of an education strategy so that teachers use a learner-centred approach consistent with the holistic patient-centred consultation model. With training that addresses issues of comorbidity, communication skills and the ability to plan management in a shared decision-making approach, our students and trainees will be better prepared for the reality of high-quality, modern practice in whichever field they work.

References

1 Wagner EH, Austin BT, Davis C, Hindmarsh M, Schaefer J, Bonomi A: Improving chronic illness care: translating evidence into action. Health Aff (Millwood) 2001;20:64–78.
2 Heaven C, Clegg J, Maguire P: Transfer of communication skills training from workshop to workplace: the impact of clinical supervision. Patient Educ Couns 2006;60:313–325.
3 Brown J: Transferring clinical communication skills from the classroom to the clinical environment: perceptions of a group of medical students in the UK. Acad Med 2010;85:1052–1059.
4 Kolb D: Experiential Learning. Englewood Cliffs, Prentice Hall, 1984.
5 Schon D: The Reflective Practitioner: How Professionals Think in Action. New York, Basic Books, 1983.
6 Dewey J: Human Nature and Conduct: An Introduction to Social Psychology. New York, Holt, 1922.
7 Vygotsky L: Interaction between learning and development; in: Mind in Society. Cambridge, Harvard University Press 1978, pp 79–91.
8 Hewson MG, Little ML: Giving feedback in medical education. Verification of recommended techniques. J Gen Intern Med 1998;13:111–116.
9 Silverman JD, Kurtz SM, Draper J: The Calgary-Cambridge approach to communication skills teaching. Agenda-led, outcome-based analysis of the consultation. J Educ Gen Pract 1996;7:288–299.
10 Sargeant J, Mann K, Sinclair D, van der Vleuten C, Metsemakers J: Understanding the influence of emotions and reflection upon multi-source feedback acceptance and use. Adv Health Sciences Educ 2008;13:275–288.
11 Morris C: Learning and Teaching; in McKimm J, Forrest K (eds): Professional Practice for Foundation Doctors. Exeter, Learning Matters Ltd, 2011, pp 223–238.
12 Towle A, Bainbridge L, Godolphin W, Katz A, Kline C, Lown B, Madularu I, Solomon P, Thistlethwaite J: Active patient involvement in the education of health professionals. Med Educ 2010;44:64–74.
13 UK Council of Clinical Communication in Undergraduate Medical Education e-learning resource. http://www.ukccc.org.uk/consultationse-learning.
14 Health Foundation: Co-creating health: building partnerships. Briefing May 2008. http://www.health.org.uk/publications/co-creating-health-briefing-paper.
15 McWhinney I: The need for a transformed clinical method; in Stewart M, Roter D (eds): Communicating with Medical Patients. London, Sage Publications, 1989, p 25.
16 World Health Organization: Adherence to Long-Term Therapies. Evidence for Action. Geneva, WHO, 2003.
17 Naylor C, Parsonage M, McDaid D, Knapp M, Fossey M, Galea A: Long-Term Conditions and Mental Health: The Cost of Co-Morbidity. London, The Kings Fund and Centre for Mental Health, 2012, pp 12–15.
18 The Mental Health Parity and Addiction Equity Act of 2008 (MHPAEA). Washington, US Department of Labor Employee Benefits Security Administration, 2008.
19 Weiland A, Blankenstein AH, Willems MH, Van Saase JL, Van der Molen HT, Van Dulmen AM, Arends LR: Postgraduate education for medical specialists focused on patients with medically unexplained physical symptoms; development of a communication skills training programme. Patient Educ Couns 2013;92:355–360.
20 Shattock L, Williamson H, Caldwell K, Anderson K, Peters S: 'They've just got symptoms without science': medical trainees' acquisition of negative attitudes towards patients with medically unexplained symptoms. Patient Educ Couns 2013;91:249–254.
21 Evans S, Katona C: Epidemiology of depressive symptoms in elderly primary care attenders. Dementia 1993;4:327–333.
22 Rochon P, Gurwitz J: Optimising drug treatment for elderly people: the prescribing cascade. Br Med J 1997;315:1096.
23 Fallowfield L, Ratcliffe D, Jenkins V, Saul J: Psychiatric morbidity and its recognition by doctors in patients with cancer. Br J Cancer 2001;84:1011–1015.
24 Wilkinson S, Perry R, Blanchard K: Effectiveness of a three day communications skills programme in changing nurses' communication skills with cancer/palliative care patients: a randomised control trial. Palliat Med 2008;22:365–375.
25 Korszun A, Dinos S, Ahmed K, Bhui K: Medical student attitudes about mental illness: does medical-school education reduce stigma? Acad Psychiatry 2012;36:197–204.
26 Cushing AM, Jones A: Evaluation of a breaking bad news course for medical students. Med Educ 1995;29:430–435.

27 Deegan P: Hearing Voices Curriculum: Complete Training and Curriculum Package. http://www.power2u.org/mm5.

28 Harrison M, Reeves D, Harkness E, Valderas J, Kennedy A, Rogers A, Hann M, Bower P: A secondary analysis of the moderating effects of depression and multimorbidity on the effectiveness of a chronic disease self-management programme. Patient Educ Couns 2012;87:67–73.

29 Boon H, Stewart M: Patient-physician communication assessment instruments: 1986 to 1996 in review. Patient Educ Couns 1998;35:161–176.

30 Kurtz SM, Silverman JD: The Calgary-Cambridge Referenced Observation Guides: an aid to defining the curriculum and organising the teaching in communication training programmes. Med Educ 1996;30:83–89.

31 Makoul G: Essential elements of communication in medical encounters: the Kalamazoo consensus statement. Acad Med 2001;76:390–393.

32 Parle M, Maguire P, Heaven CM: The development of a training model to improve health professionals' skills, self-efficacy and outcome expectancies when communicating with cancer patients. Soc Sci Med 1997;44:231–240.

33 Silverman J, Kurtz S, Draper J: Skills for Communicating with Patients, ed 3. Abingdon, Radcliffe Medical Press Ltd, 2013.

34 Gask LL, Usherwood T, Thompson H, Williams B: Evaluation of a training package in the assessment and management of depression in primary care. Med Educ 1998;32:190–198.

35 Moore P, Mercado SR, Artigues MG, Lawrie TA: Communication skills training for healthcare professionals working with people who have cancer. Cochrane Database Syst Rev 2013;3:CD003751.

36 Fallowfield L, Jenkins V, Farewell V, Solis-Trapala I: Enduring impact of communication skills training: results of a 12-month follow-up. Br J Cancer 2003;89:1445–1449.

37 Connected; National Advanced Communication Skills Training, NHS. https://www.connectedonlinebookings.co.uk/training.php http://www.royalmarsden.nhs.uk/education/school/courses/Pages/connected.aspx (accessed December 2013).

38 Health Foundation: Co-creating health. http:// www.health.org.uk/areas-of-work/programmes/co-creating-health/about/ (accessed February 21, 2014).

39 Bleakley A: Broadening conceptions of learning in medical education: the message from team-working. Med Educ 2006;40:150–157.

40 Frenk J, Chen L, Bhutta ZA, Cohen J, Crisp N, Evans T, Fineberg H, Garcia P, Ke Y, Kelley P, Kistnasamy B, Meleis A, Naylor D, Pablos-Mendez A, Reddy S, Scrimshaw S, Sepulveda J, Serwadda D, Zurayk H: Health professionals for a new century: transforming education to strengthen health systems in an interdependent world. Lancet 2010;376:1923–1958.

41 Fenwick T, Jensen K, Nerland M: Socio-material approaches to conceptualising professional learning and practice. J Educ Work 2012;25:1–13.

42 Wagner EH: Chronic disease management: what will it take to improve care for chronic illness? Eff Clin Pract 1998;1:2–4.

Prof. Annie Cushing, PhD, FDSRCS (Eng), BDS (Hons)
Clinical and Communication Skills Unit, Institute of Health Sciences Education
Barts and The London School of Medicine and Dentistry, St. Bartholomew's Hospital, Queen Mary, University of London
London EC1A 7 BE (UK)
E-Mail a.m.cushing@qmul.ac.uk

Sartorius N, Holt RIG, Maj M (eds): Comorbidity of Mental and Physical Disorders.
Key Issues Ment Health. Basel, Karger, 2015, vol 179, pp 148–156 (DOI: 10.1159/000365599)

The Dialogue on Diabetes and Depression African Nursing Training Programme: A Collaborative Training Initiative to Improve the Recognition and Management of Diabetes and Depression in Sub-Saharan Africa

H.L. Millar[a] · L. Cimino[b] · A.S. van der Merwe[c]

[a]Mental Health Directorate, The Carseview Centre, Dundee, UK; [b]International Center for Intercultural Communication, Indiana University, Indianapolis, Ind., USA; [c]Division of Nursing, Faculty of Medicine and Health Sciences, Stellenbosch University, Stellenbosch, South Africa

Abstract

The Dialogue on Diabetes and Depression (DDD) is an international collaborative effort to address the problems related to the comorbidity of depression and diabetes. The Association for the Improvement of Mental Health Programmes, a Swiss-based NGO, established the DDD to raise awareness, coordinate research, develop training materials, and organise scientific meetings and training courses. The DDD developed the Diabetes and Depression African Nursing Training Programme in collaboration with the International Council of Nurses to address identified needs of nurses in Sub-Saharan Africa to whom the delivery of primary healthcare often devolves. An international faculty of experts delivered the educational programme to nurses from seven countries in Sub-Saharan Africa and involved over 175 participants, most of whom have responsibility for the education or in-service training of nurses. Participants appreciated the programme – especially the opportunity to enhance their knowledge of these two common disorders and to practice new skills to recognise and manage comorbid conditions. This programme is an example of a unique and innovative educational effort regarding comorbidity with a practical clinical approach. It enables nurses to screen, recognise and treat diabetes and depression in Sub-Saharan Africa by promoting a patient-centred collaborative approach model with early recognition and management of these comorbid conditions in order to improve outcomes and life expectancy in this population.

© 2015 S. Karger AG, Basel

The Dialogue on Diabetes and Depression (DDD), established in 2007, is an international collaborative initiative addressing research and healthcare needs related to the comorbidity of diabetes and depression [1]. Together with the International Council of Nurses, the DDD embarked on a capacity-building programme, focussing on nurse training in seven countries in Sub-

Saharan Africa. The programme aimed at 'training the trainers' to increase capacity in frontline healthcare staff to recognise and manage these comorbid conditions and to enhance the ability of nurses to promote and enact educational programmes of this nature within their own healthcare systems.

Background

Thomas Willis, a 17th-century English physician and anatomist described the association between depression and diabetes, noting that diabetes appeared more frequently in those who suffered life traumas or long-term sorrow [2]. Contemporary epidemiological studies suggest that at least one third of this population suffer from depression [3, 4] and up to 45% of those with diabetes have depressive symptoms not amounting to the ICD diagnosis of depressive disorders [5]. Additionally, those suffering from depression are at an increased risk of developing diabetes [6]. Studies now clearly point to a bidirectional relationship between diabetes and depression, which is complex in terms of the pathogenesis, pathophysiology and psychological mechanisms. Evidence from high-income countries suggests that depression with diabetes is associated with socio-economic status, marital status, physical activity and chronic somatic diseases. Psychosocial factors may impact on the relationship between socio-economic status and depression in people with diabetes, including social isolation, poor social support, limited coping ability and burden of work. Overall studies have shown an inverse relationship, i.e. the risk for depression in diabetes is higher with lower socio-economic status. However, the relationship may vary depending on the socio-economic context of the particular country. In low-income countries, a higher socio-economic status is generally associated with higher levels of chronic disease risk factors, whilst the poor often experi-

ence a higher burden of infectious and chronic diseases [7, 8].

Contemporary evidence demonstrates that effective treatment of depression in people with diabetes depends on a multidisciplinary collaborative approach to optimise a comprehensive package of care ensuring the best outcomes in terms of physical and mental well-being [9, 10]. International programmes have been introduced to manage diabetes in a range of settings, most notably those by the International Diabetes Federation (IDF) [11].

Within well-integrated healthcare services, programmes have been developed for the effective treatment of depression. By contrast, holistic programmes to manage people with comorbid depression and diabetes are not yet well established despite the evidence available for treating this specific comorbidity [12]. The quality of various conceptual frameworks varies depending on the personnel available and the resources within the healthcare system. The preparation and training of healthcare professionals to deal with such comorbid conditions is limited, and this situation is probably exacerbated within more deprived and challenging healthcare systems where both financial and human resources are more limited and where deep-rooted layers of stigma and stereotyping exist. As a result, the fragmentation of services with poor accessibility may lead to inadequate care pathways, lack of seamlessness and a delay in any meaningful interventions. This may culminate in more complications and overall a worse prognosis and clinical outcomes for those presenting with these two comorbid conditions [13, 14]. It is often the case that mental healthcare professionals feel unable to provide adequate services for the physical health of the mentally ill population; however, the reverse is also probably true [15] due to training inadequacies and lack of experience.

Another challenge in dealing with the complexity of chronic comorbid conditions is the need for a range of skills and the expertise of a multicondition collaborative care approach by a multidisciplinary team working together across specialities, clinics and distances [10]. The patient with comorbid conditions presents with complex challenges requiring education to enhance engagement in self-care management to achieve optimal outcomes. This is especially important in areas of the world where access to care systems is challenged with limited capacity and skill mix.

To initiate programmes addressing multimorbidity, it was decided to select a commonly occurring comorbidity and to use the experience gained to design other programmes managing multimorbidity in general. Both diabetes and depression are common disorders with increasing incidences and are associated with a high cost burden to society. Both disorders are relatively easy to diagnose and have recognised effective treatments which have had an impact on reducing the stigma associated with them.

Nurses are an essential part of the interdisciplinary team and were selected for this training programme because of their broad reach and potential impact on care for patients with such conditions. Nurses are the largest group of healthcare professionals in most low- and middle-income countries, and are at the critical interface with patients and their carers. This scenario was considered especially pertinent for Africa. Hence, the aim of the programme was to strengthen the nurses' core competencies in the assessment and management of patients with comorbid diabetes and depression. The programme adopted a train-the-trainer approach – empowering nurses to train others and to enact countrywide and local programmes that address healthcare problems related to comorbidity.

Programme Rollout

The African Nurse Training Programme on Diabetes and Depression was a collaborative effort co-ordinated by the DDD and engaged a number of organisations including support from the Lundbeck Institute and the International Council of Nurses, which represents nursing associations from 135 countries and is made up of more than 13 million nurses worldwide. The International Council of Nurses works to ensure high quality in nursing care and the advancement of nursing knowledge, and promotes the nursing profession as a competent workforce worldwide.

A steering group was set up that included representatives from the DDD, the International Council of Nurses, Lundbeck Institute and international experts to support the implementation of the project. The group used a logic model framework to steer the project work within stipulated timeframes. The logic model focuses on achieving planned actual change and has been extensively used in planning, application and evaluation of a range of programmes [16–19]. It forces careful reflection on the relationships between outcomes (short and long term), the rationale and assumptions within the unique context of the programme to be delivered with the necessary actions and resources required to achieve such outcomes. Immediate and direct outputs versus long-term impacts are also outlined.

The steering group provided the leadership for the design and rollout of the DDD African Nurse Training Programme. The first series of training sessions included nurses from five countries in Africa, namely South Africa, Uganda, Botswana, Lesotho and Swaziland. The steering group reconvened after this first set of sessions to review feedback and to further fine-tune the programme to meet the needs of nurses and patients in clinical practice. They then conducted a second set of training sessions in Ethiopia and Kenya. The IDF recommended local diabetes educators from South Africa and Kenya to participate in the workshops to strengthen local knowledge and relevance of the skills and to assist in understanding local attitudes and values.

In planning the educational curriculum, the steering group was mindful of the importance of the context of the African countries and considered political, economic, social and psychological factors when designing the programme. The steering group also considered how the diagnosis and treatment of diabetes or depression, or both, needed to fit into different cultural value systems and social practices. The complex status of the healthcare system and the seemingly poor integration of mental and physical healthcare in many of the countries required careful consideration. It was also recognised that there might be limited integration between primary and secondary care systems as well as a lack of integration between the medical and nursing competency frameworks in such a multiprofessional initiative.

The nurses who participated in the programme were exposed to a total of ten educational modules. Interactive sessions included role-play, interviewing and assessment, self-management, and train-the-trainer guidance to implement the programme and deal with the environment. The International Faculty Steering Group prepared the educational materials in a modular format with each participant receiving a binder containing the programme outline, module outline, narratives, fact sheets, instruments and tools, and evaluation forms. The content used the evidence-based integrated approach to the recognition and management of diabetes and depression with the most up-to-date literature in the field.

The co-ordinators of each of the workshops promoted an interactive and participatory teaching and learning approach including opportunities for role-play, assessment and interviewing under their supervision. The last session in each of the programmes focused on the development of an action plan for the participant to ensure a focus on changes in clinical practice and a commitment by each nurse to meet their goals and expected outcomes from the course. The International Council of Nurses monitors these action plans and the steering group use them for ongoing evaluation of the impact of the programme on the practice of these nurses.

In reflecting on the outcomes as stated by the logic model, the following challenges presented themselves in the designing and planning of the programme.

Develop Core Competencies and Capacity in the Field

Teaching the management of a patient with co-morbid conditions presented a unique educational challenge because the relevant skills and knowledge had to be imparted to groups of nurses who were either from a mental health or a general nursing background. It was important to integrate the new knowledge and skills with the baseline of knowledge and skills that the nurses had in their area of expertise. A questionnaire was sent to prospective participants in advance to establish baseline knowledge and clinical practices. The data from this survey assisted in informing the development of the theoretical and applied content. Comprehensive slide sets, narratives and fact sheets were prepared to provide the necessary documentary support for all participants, and emphasis was placed on interactive teaching and learning practices, such as through the use of case studies and role-plays to strengthen critical thinking and problem-solving skills.

The selection of the participants in the courses was given careful attention because it was expected that the nurses participating in the course would become ambassadors for the programme, drivers of initiatives for better care of patients with comorbid diseases and trainers – using the educational material provided as a resource and basis.

Facilitate Change in the Environment

The steering group considered the rollout of the programme and public involvement as important aspects of the programme. In most cases, a representative of the DDD preceded the arrival of the faculty to the country to meet the organisers from the national nursing association and to make contact with policy makers, patient and family organisations, and key contacts in the media. The DDD representative organised interaction with local government officials and senior healthcare advisors, and considered them as critical to assist in or facilitate policy change. The faculty members also assumed the roles of advocates, participating in local media opportunities (including local radio and television interviews) and discussions with local politicians. Where feasible, the national nursing associations invited important stakeholders and the media to public meetings where patients told their own stories, seamlessly integrating their personal experiences of, for example, stigma, assessment and treatment.

Within the programme, the faculty made participants aware of their own responsibilities working in the field of diabetes and depression. They encouraged them to consider the potential barriers hindering the patients' commitment to changes in lifestyle as well as engagement with self-help and treatment. They advocated reflection on their own clinical practice and the need to embrace evidence-based competencies. The organisation of the workshops with their unique exposure to international experts, well-designed material, and contemporary teaching and learning strategies was intended to make a difference in the lives of all concerned. The sessions promoted networking as a strong conduit to address quality issues by encouraging collaborative work in groups, organisations and within the regional political structures.

Address Issues of Stigma in the Diagnosis of Diabetes and Depression

The course placed particular importance on the recognition of the role of stigma in the management of comorbidity [20]. Although stigmatisation was not addressed in a specific module, the faculty and participants within the group work explored the realities of stigma from avoidance of recognition to management of the comorbid conditions. It was important to discuss the stigmatisation issues within the wider cultural context and how they applied to diabetes and depression. Context-specific strategies were discussed, especially in relation to personal and public campaigns and collaborative actions. It is, however, a challenge to change the way healthcare users with comorbid disease are perceived, assessed and treated. These challenges are even more pronounced in lower income countries, in less-effective healthcare systems and in the presence of stigmatisation and stereotyping.

Workshop Implementation and Evaluation

A total of 175 clinical nurse practitioners and nurse educators were trained in the six workshops held in South Africa, Botswana, Swaziland, Uganda, Ethiopia and Kenya. The DDD, the International Council of Nurses and the Lundbeck Institute provided the logistical support for the identification of participants and organisation of workshops. The International Council of Nurses worked closely with local nursing organisations to identify and select nurses representing a range of educational and healthcare settings. The International Council of Nurses accredited the workshops and provided each participant with a formal certificate of completion. As follow-up, each participant developed an action plan to guide them in the incorporation of the new knowledge and skills into their practice.

The steering group developed an evaluation instrument that addressed the outcomes of each module and items related to the teaching methods. The latter items were kept constant to facilitate ease of use. Participants evaluated each item using a Likert scale with 5 being the highest or best scoring. An opportunity for open-ended responses was also provided for each module and a final part of the evaluation instrument allowed the participants to reflect on the workshop as a whole.

The system of formal participant feedback was explained to participants at the start of the programme. At the time of writing this chapter the first 146 sets of evaluation forms were received, but individual item responses varied from 106 to 146 because of various factors. Survey Monkey software was used to analyse the quantitative data whilst the qualitative responses were transcribed and categorised, and themes developed from the data.

Results

The participants' overall evaluation of the workshop was positive with mean scores not lower than 4.69 of a maximum of 5. Participants especially appreciated the useful exchange of knowledge, values and skills, and considered the public event an important achievement. The qualitative responses echoed these positive results with clear reference to the value of and approach to the workshops. Participants considered the workshops to be 'eye opening' and 'straightforward' – appreciating the presence and approach used by experts throughout. The quality of the organisation was also highlighted.

Within the first rollout, participants made a number of recommendations that resonated well with the experience and expressed opinions of the steering group. These included:

- Provision of further support and monitoring of actions, such as drug fact sheets, conversation maps and the involvement of local multidisciplinary teams in further training
- Introduction of even more interactive work such as role-plays and group work
- Refining some workshop material, the flow of certain modules and time allocation for the modules on diagnosis and assessment of depression in people with diabetes
- Fine-tuning of the workshop evaluation format and the management of post-workshop expectations
- Identification of barriers to change and mechanisms to deal with such; mostly

through new partnerships and community capacity building

It was meaningful that the participants highlighted specific skills and tools in their feedback. The demonstration and introduction of the Patient Health Questionnaire (PHQ9) for the assessment of depression was considered useful for their practical clinical setting [21]. The participants considered the PHQ9 'wonderful and will be embraced'. The nominal group technique [22, 23] as adapted by the educational expert in the steering group was viewed as meaningful for enhancing group participation. Motivational interviewing was considered an essential technique to be included in future nursing curricula.

Discussion

Participants and facilitators considered the first phase of this project as successful and the feedback guided the final phase of the programme that incorporated the above. The integration of training about the two conditions of depression and diabetes within the context of comorbidity was challenging and this series of workshops provided valuable pointers on how to achieve this effectively. It was clear that nurses and most other healthcare professionals still undergo training that emphasises systems-based or disease-oriented models. The comorbidity framework provides new insights and ways of thinking and implementation – both in education and clinical practice [10]. This model encourages multiprofessional working with case management, a structured management plan and enhanced interprofessional communication. There is now growing evidence that collaborative care can successfully improve depression and diabetes outcomes with cognitive behaviour therapy enhancing diabetes self-management, reducing diabetes morbidity, improving stability and treating depression effectively. In addition, other risk factors, such as low-density lipoprotein and cholesterol levels as well as high blood pressure, can be better controlled by adoption of this person-centred collaborative model of care [9]. Rushton et al. [24] confirmed the need for health professionals to rethink how to manage patients with multiple healthcare conditions, given that the care environment itself remains fragmented.

It was clear to the steering group that the selection of participants for such programmes should be more focused and differentiated; for example, there is a need to focus more on nurse educators in future programmes and to provide a variety of modules to meet the needs and backgrounds of different groups at different times. It was also acknowledged that multiprofessional collaboration is critical and that specific sessions and applied exercises are needed to drive home the complexities of comorbid disease assessment and treatment.

Limitations of the Programme

Being the first round of this type of programme, it was considered important to provide participants with an evaluation form for each module and one for the overall workshop. The feedback provided valuable insights to the steering group, but it is acknowledged that data collection instruments of this nature tend to elicit more subjective responses. The Likert scale is relatively easy to use, but suffers from traditional concerns such as participant honesty, interpretation of the scale, feeling-bias and (in this case) a laborious analysis process. It is, however, important to note that the qualitative data provided by participants corresponded well with the Likert-type scale findings.

Next Steps in Comorbidity Training

Organising the delivery of services in such a way that collaborative and coordinated care is possible requires the buy-in of not only the other relevant healthcare professionals, but also those in a position to restructure the health system and delegate responsibilities appropriately. Subsequent skill and knowledge training of other primary and secondary healthcare professionals would be necessary and is recommended as a follow-up to nurse training. Additional resources and the commitment of the trained trainers to cascade the learning from the African Nurse Training Programme to other new and practicing nurses will be essential to the institutionalisation of the concepts and the broad-scale benefits to affected patients.

The International Council of Nurses and the national nursing associations should prioritise the further dissemination of the knowledge and skills from the African Nurse Training Programme by establishing regional centres of excellence to institutionalise the concepts and maximise their adoption in nursing practice.

The programme as designed forms a good baseline to be adapted for other healthcare professionals and multiprofessional groups. Such a rollout would provide further strength to the initiative to better manage and support patients with comorbid conditions. Material would also be coded for use as half day, full day or 2.5 days – depending on participant needs, timeframe and resources available.

To further support this aim, an integrated manual, which will serve as a comprehensive reference, is in process. This manual will also include guidelines for logistical and other arrangements of such a programme, pre-workshop material and action plans. Heuristic hints for the development of good case studies, role-plays and other teaching and learning activities would provide further guidance.

Another action relates to the strengthening of multiprofessional, and especially nursing, research relating to comorbidity within Africa. An example would be PhD and Masters research projects that strengthen care outcomes for patients with comorbid disease.

Conclusions

Using the comorbidity of disease framework as a legitimate springboard for redesigning both formal and informal educational programmes is warranted, feasible and acceptable. The framework rings true to the clinical challenges of medicine in the 21st century, with the increasing prevalence of comorbidity and how patients present in healthcare systems. Stigmatisation remains a serious concern in many cultural contexts, and good research and clinical work that addresses this issue directly and indirectly within a comorbidity of disease framework would contribute to equitable access and better-quality healthcare.

Further follow-up of the participants' progress from the African experience in relation to changes in clinical practice will help to inform and optimise the benefits of such future programmes. Given the positive African experience, the faculty is better equipped and more confident in their ability to deliver such comorbidity programmes in other culturally challenging environments.

Acknowledgements

The authors would like to acknowledge the important contributions and/or support of the following entities and/or persons:

- Expert faculty members: Professor N. Sartorius (President AIMHIP, Switzerland), Professor R. Holt (UK, Endocrinology and Diabetology), Dr. H.L. Millar (UK, Consultant Psychiatrist) and Dr. Tesfamicael Ghebrehiwet (Consultant in Nursing and Health Policy, ICN)
- Expert academic and technical facilitators: Dr. J. Hayes (USA, Psychiatry), Larry Cimino (USA, Programme Director), André Joubert (Director, Lundbeck Institute) and Marianne Helwigh (Operational Manager, Lundbeck Institute)
- Regional experts: Professor S. Rataemane (University of Limpopo, Pretoria, South Africa), Dr. S. Bahendeka (IDF Uganda) and Dr. I. Westmore (Consultant Psychiatrist, South Africa)
- IDF educators: B. Majikela-Dlangamandla (South Africa) and A. Jalang'o (Kenya)
- The International Diabetes Federation (IDF)
- The Dialogue on Diabetes and Depression (DDD)
- The Association for the Improvement of Mental Health Programmes (AIMHP)
- International Council of Nurses (ICN)
- The Lundbeck Institute
- Eli Lilly and Company
- The World Federation for Mental Health (WFMH)
- The University of Southampton Faculty of Medicine
- The School of Nursing, Faculty of Health Sciences, University of the Free State, South Africa
- Democratic Nursing Organisation of South Africa (DENOSA)
- Ethiopian Nurses Association (ENA)
- Lesotho Nursing Association
- National Nursing Association of Kenya (NNAK)
- Nursing Association of Botswana
- Swaziland Nurses Association
- Uganda Nurses and Midwives Union (UNMU)

References

1 Sartorius N, Cimino L: The Dialogue on Diabetes and Depression (DDD): origins and achievements. J Aff Disorder 2012; 142(suppl):S4–S7.
2 Willis T: Pharmaceutice rationalis sive diatriba de medicamentorum operationibus in humano corpore, theatro sheldoniano. Oxford, 1674.
3 Anderson RJ, Freedland KE, Clouse RE, Lustman PJ: The prevalence of co-morbid depression in adults with diabetes. Diabetes Care 2001;6:1069–1078.
4 Barnard K, Skinner T, Peveler R: The prevalence of co-morbid depression in adults with type 1 diabetes: systematic literature review. Diabetes Med 2006;23: 445–448.
5 Hermanns N, Kulzer B, Krichbaum M, et al: How to screen for depression and emotional problems in patients with diabetes: comparison of screening characteristics of depression questionnaires, measurements of diabetes-specific emotional problems and standard clinical assessment. Diabetologia 2006;49:469–477.
6 Pouwer F, Beekman TF, Nijpels G, et al: Rates and risks for comorbid depression in patients with type 2 diabetes mellitus: results from a community-based study. Diabetologia 2003;46:892–898.
7 Lyketsos CG: Depression and diabetes: more on what the relationship might be. Am J Psychiatry 2010;167:496–497.
8 Leone T, Coast E, Narayanan S, et al: Diabetes and depression comorbidity and socio-economic status in low and middle income countries (LMICs): a mapping of the evidence. Global Health 2012;8:39.

9 Coleman M, et al: Treatment implications for comorbid diabetes mellitus and depression. Psychiatric Times 2013;30.

10 Katon WJ, Lin EH, Von Korff M, et al: Collaborative care for patients with depression and chronic illnesses. N Engl J Med 2010;363:2611–2620.

11 International Diabetes Federation Clinical Guideline Task Force. Global Guideline for Type 2 Diabetes. Brussels, International Diabetes Federation, 2005.

12 van der Feltz-Cornelis CM, Nuyen J, Stoop C, et al: Effect of interventions for major depressive symptoms in patients with diabetes mellitus: a systematic review and meta-analysis. Gen Hosp Psychiatry 2010;32:380–395.

13 Goldney RD, Phillips PJ, Fisher LJ, et al: Diabetes, depression, and quality of life: a population study. Diabetes Care 2004; 27:1066–1070.

14 Hislop AL, Fegan PG, Schlaeppi MJ, et al: Prevalence and associations of psychological distress in young adults with type 1 diabetes. Diabet Med 2008;25: 91–96.

15 De Hert M, Cohen D, Bobes J, et al: Physical illness in patients with severe mental disorders. II. Barriers to care, monitoring and treatment guidelines, plus recommendations at the system and individual level. World Psychiatry 2011;10:138–151.

16 Schreirer MA: Getting more bangs for your buck. Am J Eval 2000;21:139–149.

17 Sullivan TM, Ohkubo S, Rinehart W, Storey JD: From research to policy and practice: a logic model to measure impact of knowledge management for health programs. Knowl Manag Dev J 2010;6:53–69.

18 Torghele K, Buyum A, Dubriel N, Augustine J, Houlihan C, Alperim M, Miner KR: Logic model use in developing a survey instrument for program evaluation: emergency preparedness summits for schools of nursing in Georgia. Public Health Nurs 2007;24:472–479.

19 Logic Model Development Guide. Battle Creek, W.K. Kellogg Foundation, 2004. http://www.wkkf.org/knowledge-center/resources/2006/02/WK-Kellogg-Foundation-Logic-Model-Development-Guide.aspx (accessed March 19, 2012).

20 Weiss MG, Ramakrishna J, Somma D: Health-related stigma: rethinking concepts and interventions. Psychol Health Med 2006;11:277–287.

21 Kroenke K, Spitzer RL, Williams JB, et al: The PHQ 9 – validity of a brief depression severity measurement. J Gen Intern Med 2001;16:606–613.

22 Miller LE: Evidence-based instruction: a classroom experiment comparing nominal and brainstorming groups. Organ Manag J 2009;6:229–238.

23 WBI Evaluation Group. 2007. Nominal Group. http://siteresources.worldbank.org/WBI/Resources/213798–1194538727144/7Final-Nominal_Group_Technique.pdf (accessed March 19, 2012).

24 Rushton CA, Satchithananda DK, Kadam UT: Comorbidity in modern nursing: a closer look at heart failure. Br J Nurs 2011;20:280–285.

Dr. H.L. Millar
Mental Health Directorate, The Carseview Centre
4 Tom McDonald Ave
Dundee, Scotland DD2 1NH (UK)
E-Mail hlmillar1@gmail.com

Sartorius N, Holt RIG, Maj M (eds): Comorbidity of Mental and Physical Disorders.
Key Issues Ment Health. Basel, Karger, 2015, vol 179, pp 157–164 (DOI: 10.1159/000365600)

The Challenge of Developing Person-Centred Services to Manage Comorbid Mental and Physical Illness

Linda Gask

Centre for Primary Care, Institute of Population Health, University of Manchester, Manchester, UK

Abstract

This chapter considers the difficulties posed by the direction in which healthcare has developed across the world, in particular problems arising from fragmentation and specialisation of care provision. There has been an increasing recognition of the need for improved systems of primary care; however, there is no universal model of provision, and barriers to the management of physical and mental comorbidity can be identified in primary care settings. Models of collaborative care which derive from the Chronic Care Model have shown some promise in management of comorbidity. In order to improve outcomes for people who present with comorbid and multimorbid health problems, healthcare professionals in all settings will need to acquire a range of specific skills. These include being able to explore the impact of physical and mental health problems on the patient, and the negotiation of patient-centred goals.

© 2015 S. Karger AG, Basel

Other chapters in this book have described the nature and magnitude of the problems facing healthcare in addressing the problem of multimorbidity, and the challenges posed by comorbidity of physical and mental health problems in particular. At the heart of this challenge is the need for us not to lose sight of the needs of the *person* who is seeking help for his/her ailments, from the macro-level of designing healthcare systems to the micro-level of interaction between doctor and patient within the consulting room.

The Fragmentation of Healthcare

Heath systems are increasingly fragmented. Even the British National Health Service, which historically has a strong orientation to primary care, has become less integrated in the way it delivers care. At the organisational level this is reflected in an ever-increasing number of different 'providers' being 'commissioned' to deliver care – some profit-making, some not-for-profit – and each one of them requiring an army of administrative staff (and not a few lawyers) to negotiate the detailed contracts, performance management and financial arrangements that go with them. Hospitals are moving to take over and develop community resources such as services for older people to integrate them 'vertically', but in doing so loosen the 'horizontal' ties they have with other services, the most important of these being primary care. Within primary care, a payment-for-performance system called the 'Quality and Outcomes Framework' rewards doctors according to criteria based on single diseases rather than management of multimorbidity [1].

Take for instance John, who is 58 years old and has multiple health concerns, diabetes, coronary heart disease, arthritis and severe depression following the death of his wife. In the past he went to his general practitioner when he did not feel well, but now he does not know where he should go. There seem to be far more doctors at the practice than there used to be, but he does not seem to know any of them very well, and it seems harder to see the same doctor each time than it once was. According to the practice website, the doctors now have particular expertise in certain diseases (such as diabetes or coronary heart disease). Does that mean he should go and see different doctors for each problem? He is called in for appointments with the practice nurse to review how he is doing with his diabetes as she works her way through the patients on the diabetes register. Next week he may be asked to come in for a different review appointment for his cardiovascular disease, generated by another disease register to meet the needs of reporting in the Quality and Outcomes Framework. John's experience is of being 'under surveillance' and 'monitored' [2] rather than being an active participant in care. The practice has put up a sign saying it is now run by Angel Healthcare Providers for the NHS. Are not they a commercial company?

In addition to these 'review' appointments at the general practitioner practice, he has outpatient appointments with specialists at the hospital every now and then, for his mental health and arthritis, but each doctor he sees pays attention only to their own specific area of expertise. The psychiatrist John sees never seems to know what blood tests his doctor has done recently for his diabetes, which is not well controlled at the moment, and says that their computer systems 'don't talk to each other'. Nobody seems to be able to help him prioritise one appointment above another if they clash and he cannot make it to both; attending all of them is a great deal of work [3], sometimes rather like a full-time job. When he missed an appointment once, he was discharged from a clinic and his general practitioner had to re-refer him. He no longer works, but he does not think he would be able to anyway, as all this 'self-management' takes so much time.

It sometimes feels to John as though nobody is actually interested in finding out what is worrying *him* about his health in the midst of all this frenetic yet increasingly fragmented 'provider' activity. He muddles through somehow. His daughter is worried about him, but she is not sure which doctor is the right person to tell and neither is John.

The Consequences of Specialisation and Fragmentation

There is nothing unusual about John's story. In some countries his story would even be more complex as he might also have to become involved in discussion with insurance companies about the cost of his care. John has access to more scientifically informed healthcare than at any period in the past. Yet the expansion in specialist information which has been generated has come without an improvement in our ability to integrate this knowledge optimally to meet John's personal needs. The World Health Organisation (WHO) [4] has drawn attention to this characteristic trend that is shaping health systems today:

- A disproportionate focus on specialist, tertiary care, or 'hospital centrism': in member countries of the Organisation of

Table 1. The consequences of fragmentation inefficiency: the most fragmented healthcare systems in the world are also the most expensive (adapted from Stange [6])

Ineffectiveness	spending more on the parts, such as through narrowly focussed pay-for-performance schemes does not improve the whole
Inequality	in a fragmented healthcare system people fall between a patchwork of 'safety nets' and specific barriers to access (e.g. for ethnic minority groups) are not addressed
Commoditisation	disease management programmes support narrow evidence-based care rather than integrated care; patients become 'customers' and doctors become 'providers'
Commercialisation	healthcare becomes 'market driven'
De-professionalisation	professionals become technicians delivering a narrow slice of care
De-personalisation and dissatisfaction	both patients and professionals are unhappy with their experience of the system

Economic Cooperation and Development (OECD), the 35% growth in the number of doctors between 1990 and 2005 was driven by a nearly 50% increase in specialists compared with a 20% rise in general practitioners [5]

- Fragmentation as a result of the multiplication of specialist programmes and projects built around 'priority programmes' focussed on single-disease control
- The pervasive commercialisation of healthcare in unregulated healthcare systems

In an editorial article in *Annals of Family Medicine*, Kurt Stange [6] highlighted the consequences of our increasingly specialised and fragmented healthcare systems (table 1). For the person with multimorbidity, the primary care professional, doctor or nurse, is a key person in helping them to navigate an increasingly complex landscape [7].

The Importance of Primary Care

The Alma Ata Declaration [8] defined primary care thus: 'the role of primary health care as the local, universally available, essential, first point of contact with the health system, based on practical, scientifically sound and socially acceptable methods and technology at a cost the community and country can afford'.

Numerous studies from multiple countries have shown that when systems are organised around primary care, outcomes are better with improved equity and lower costs. For example, when people have a primary care doctor as opposed to a specialist as their personal physician, their mortality risk drops by nearly 20% and their costs are about one third less [7].

The WHO views the development of primary healthcare as one of the key challenges for health system reform [4]. More than 30 years after the Alma Ata Declaration, the vision of primary care for all has yet to be achieved, but according to Gunn et al. [9] the generalist holds the key to providing truly personalised care (p. 111):

A fundamental role of the generalist is to balance the biotechnical with the biographical. The generalist must know and understand how each life story and social context are constantly influencing and being influenced by physical and emotional health. To achieve the balance between the biotechnical and biographical aspects of each interaction, the generalist must have the skills to reach a mutual understanding of the priorities and challenges that individual patients face when managing their health.

This very personal model of care is nevertheless greatly challenged by the forces such as those described above [1], which seek to fragment the process and provision of care in the belief that this will lead to improved quality of care [10]. Innovations such as the Quality and Outcomes Framework in the UK focus on single diseases rather than multimorbidity, and solely on disease-centred outcomes rather than also taking into consideration the patient's goals. This is particularly problematic when managing people with complex comorbid and multimorbid conditions [1].

Across the world, providers of primary care include not only doctors who have received specific vocational training in family medicine (including general internal medicine and general paediatrics in some countries such as the USA), but also non-physician primary care providers (such as nurses and physician assistants). Non-primary care physicians, in particular gynaecologists but also other specialists including psychiatrists, may also provide patient care services that are usually delivered by primary care physicians. These may focus on particular needs related to care such as prevention or chronic care, but they do not provide these services in the context of comprehensive, first contact and continuing care which is what characterises family medicine. Nevertheless, it is crucial that such specialists have a basic understanding of the diseases that are comorbid with those in which they specialise; for example, the need for psychiatrists to understand the role played by cardiovascular disease in the excess mortality and morbidity of people with a diagnosis of severe and enduring mental illness [11].

However, a crucial challenge faced by those seeking to develop services for comorbid physical and mental health problems is that patients themselves vary in how much they want to share their emotional problems with those caring for their physical health problems. Mental health problems still carry significant stigma, and additionally a person may feel that, in wanting to raise 'personal' issues, there is a sense that the professional is trying to dismiss the severity of physical symptoms or talk about issues which do not seem to the patient to be relevant to the problem they present. This is something we have particularly observed when patients present with what seem to the doctor to be 'medically unexplained symptoms' [12]; however, in a recent study of the implementation of a new model of care for depression and cardiovascular disease, uncertainty was also raised by some patients (and professionals) about how much they wanted physical and mental healthcare to be more integrated [13]. We have also noted that both primary care doctors, ostensibly providing holistic care for the person, and patients with long-term conditions may collude to avoid discussing emotional problems, preferring instead to keep to the 'safer ground' of physical health and 'normalising' the distress associated with conditions, such as diabetes and cardiovascular disease, rather than daring to try and raise the possibility that this might be 'depression' [14]. These form significant barriers to both detecting and managing emotional problems in the setting of long-term conditions and mean that professionals need to work hard to engage people sensitively in talking about their emotional problems (see below).

Similar barriers occur in the detection and management of physical illness in people with long-term mental health problems. Many people with severe and enduring mental illness do not feel stigmatised when receiving treatment in the setting of primary care [15], but some undoubtedly do [16]. In the UK, a significant minority do not attend their general practitioner for the routine physical health checks for which general practitioners are now financially rewarded. The degree to which people with severe mental illness receive equivalent physical healthcare to the general population from either primary care [17] or alternatively within mental health services [18] remains debatable.

Table 2. Elements of collaborative care (adapted from Gunn et al. [30])

Multiprofessional approach to patient care provided by a case manager working with the family doctor under weekly supervision from specialist mental health medical and psychological therapies clinicians
A structured management plan of medication support and brief psychological therapy
Scheduled patient follow-ups
Enhanced interprofessional communication of patient-specific written feedback to family doctors via electronic records and personal contact

Developing Novel Models of Care for Comorbidity and Multimorbidity

In recent years, numerous disease-management programs, incorporating clinician interventions (education, feedback, reminders) and/or patient interventions (education, reminders, financial incentives), to improve quality of care and outcomes for people with long-term conditions have been described in the literature. These programs, the best known of which is the Chronic Care Model developed by Wagner et al. [19] in Seattle, have been developed and extensively evaluated for single conditions, but less commonly for diseases in combination. A recent systematic review of complex interventions for patients with multimorbidity identified 10 randomised controlled trials, of which only 3 provided data on mental health outcomes [20].

However, there is now a growing body of literature on interventions for comorbid diabetes and depression. The Chronic Care Model informed the development of collaborative care (table 2) which has been extensively evaluated for the management of depression [21, 22].

A recent meta-analysis of 14 randomised controlled trials of interventions for depression in the setting of diabetes with a total of 1,724 patients [22] showed that treatment was effective in terms of reduction of depressive symptoms, but the effect on glycaemic control was substantially smaller. Collaborative care (utilising the components described below), which provided a stepped care

intervention with a choice of starting with psychotherapy or pharmacotherapy, to a primary care population yielded an effect size of −0.292 (95% CI: −0.429 to −0.155, n = 1,133) for depression outcomes. This is a moderate effect size, but the studies were based on community samples with few exclusion criteria (unlike studies of psychotherapies based in specialist settings), indicating this effect size could potentially be attained on a population scale. The authors concluded by saying, 'improvement of the general medical condition including glycemic control is likely to require simultaneous attention to both conditions.'

Reviewing the literature on the content of these complex interventions, Piette et al. [23] suggested an effective organisational management strategy for diabetes and depression should include all the following elements: (1) systematic identification of patients with diabetes and depression and quality-of-care reviews, (2) proactive patient monitoring between outpatient encounters, (3) intensive efforts to co-ordinate treatment across clinicians, (4) increased access to cognitive-behavioural or related therapies addressing patients' depressive symptoms *and* diabetes self-care, and (5) an emphasis on promoting physical activity to address both depressive symptoms and physiologic dysregulation.

Katon et al. in the TEAMcare study [24] have now both successfully addressed multimorbidity and improved physical and mental health outcomes. A specially trained and supported case manager was employed to 'treat to target' both

Table 3. Key skills for managing people with comorbid physical and mental health problems

Sensitively engaging the patient in discussing their worries and concerns
Finding out about the patient's problems
Exploring the impact of physical and mental health problems on the patient (and on each other)
Eliciting health beliefs
Clarifying and negotiating the patient's goals (and how these relate to their healthcare including self-management of chronic illness)
Motivating the patient to achieve their goals
Developing a therapeutic plan with the patient through shared decision-making
Employing simple psychological strategies (e.g. behavioural activation and problem solving) to help the person to achieve their goals

depression and other chronic disease-related outcomes in the primary care setting, achieving significant improvements in both. The TEAMcare nurse was integrated into primary care and supervised weekly by a psychiatrist and primary care physician. The intervention improved glycaemic control, lipid profile, systolic blood pressure and depression symptoms compared to usual primary care.

Implementing collaborative care into routine practice poses challenges. In the USA, the IMPACT model for depression care in older people with comorbid physical health problems has been implemented in a range of healthcare systems across the country [25], and this has also been highly influential internationally. Major changes (including re-allocation of resources) are needed to implement disease management and collaborative care models, and investment in clinical electronic information systems is essential [26]. Re-designed systems and care pathways must implement more frequent follow-up and routine monitoring of outcomes by case managers, promote integration of specialists into primary care to provide supervision and support, and develop self-management systems for patients and professionals. There are also problems in delivering such complex interventions in healthcare

systems where the general practitioner works alone without any additional person who might take the role of the 'case manager'. In these settings a more traditional approach to 'collaborative care' of developing the skills of the general practitioner in systematically following-up people with common chronic conditions with the support and supervision of specialists may still be the way forward [27].

In the USA the concept of the 'patient-centred medical home' is a delivery system and re-imbursement reform that aims to reduce care fragmentation and other inefficiencies associated with chronic disease management. Its supporters describe four 'cornerstones' that serve as the conceptual foundation for a successful medical home: (1) engaging patients actively in medical decision-making and enhancing their access, (2) incorporating evidence-based processes of care into practice, (3) adopting new payment structures that reimburse care activities occurring outside the traditional office visit and (4) enhanced primary care [28]. There is increasing recognition of the crucial role that primary care has in providing both mental healthcare for people with chronic illness and physical healthcare for people with severe mental illness in the 'medical home' [29].

Developing the Skills of Professionals

Finally, from our knowledge of the potential barriers to effective management, it is clear that at a micro-level the attitudes of professionals towards changing practices need to be challenged and knowledge needs to be acquired about common comorbidities they are likely to see in practice. For example, a psychiatrist may not be actively involved in managing a patient's diabetic care, but they should be able to recognise it and be able to work collaboratively with a physician in arranging care. Specific skills will need to be acquired by health professionals across the spectrum (including those who work in mental healthcare who cannot be assumed will possess all of these skills) to optimise the care for people who present with comorbid emotional and physical health problems (table 3). Acquisition of these skills will need to become embedded early in professional training if we are to meet the challenge successfully of developing more patient-centred services for comorbidity in the future.

References

1 Bower P, Macdonald W, Harkness E, Gask L, Kendrick T, Valderas JM, Sibbald B: Multimorbidity, service organization and clinical decision making in primary care: a qualitative study. Fam Pract 2011;28:579–587.

2 Chew-Graham CA, Hunter C, Langer S, Stenhoff A, Drinkwater J, Guthrie EA, Salmon P: How QOF is shaping primary care review consultations: a longitudinal qualitative study. BMC Fam Pract 2013; 14:103.

3 Vassilev I, Rogers A, Blickem C, Brooks H, Kapadia D, Kennedy A, Sanders C, Kirk S, Reeves D: Social networks, the 'work' and work force of chronic illness self-management: a survey analysis of personal communities. PLoS One 2013; 8:e59723.

4 World Health Report 2008: Primary Care – Now More than Ever. Geneva, WHO, 2008.

5 OECD health data; in: World Health Report 2008: Primary Care – Now More than Ever. Geneva, WHO, 2008, p 10.

6 Stange K: The problem of fragmentation and need for integrative solutions. Ann Fam Med 2009;7:100–103.

7 Ford D: Optimizing outcomes for patients with depression and chronic medical illnesses. Am J Med 2008;121:S38–S44.

8 Primary Health Care Report of the International Conference on Primary Health Care, Alma Ata, 6–12 September 1978. Geneva, World Health Organization, 1978.

9 Gunn JM, Palmer VJ, Naccarella L, Kokanovic R, Pope CJ, Lathlean J, Stange KC: The promise and pitfalls of generalism in achieving the Alma-Ata vision of health for all. Med J Aust 2008;189:110–112.

10 Mangin D, Toop L: The Quality and Outcomes Framework: what have you done to yourselves? Br J Gen Pract 2007; 57:435.

11 De Hert M, Dekker JM, Wood D, Kahl KG, Holt RI, Möller HJ: Cardiovascular disease and diabetes in people with severe mental illness position statement from the European Psychiatric Association (EPA), supported by the European Association for the Study of Diabetes (EASD) and the European Society of Cardiology (ESC). Eur Psychiatry 2009; 24:412–424.

12 Peters S, Rogers A, Salmon P, Gask L, Dowrick C, Towey M, Clifford R, Morriss R: What do patients choose to tell their doctors? Qualitative analysis of potential barriers to reattributing medically unexplained symptoms. J Gen Intern Med 2009;24:443–449.

13 Knowles SE, Chew-Graham C, Coupe N, Adeyemi I, Keyworth C, Thampy H, Coventry PA: Better together? A naturalistic qualitative study of inter-professional working in collaborative care for co-morbid depression and physical health problems. Implement Sci 2013;8: 110.

14 Coventry PA, Hays R, Dickens C, Bundy C, Garrett C, Cherrington A, Chew-Graham C: Talking about depression: a qualitative study of barriers to managing depression in people with long term conditions in primary care. BMC Fam Pract 2011;12:10.

15 Lester H, Tritter JQ, Sorohan H: Patients' and health professionals' views on primary care for people with serious mental illness: focus group study. BMJ 2005;330:1122.

16 Schizophrenia Commission. The Abandoned Illness: A Report from the Schizophrenia Commission. London, Rethink Mental Illness, 2012.

17 Osborn DP, Baio G, Walters K, Petersen I, Limburg H, Raine R, Nazareth I: Inequalities in the provision of cardiovascular screening to people with severe mental illnesses in primary care: cohort study in the United Kingdom THIN Primary Care Database 2000–2007. Schizophr Res 2011;129:104–110.

18 Lawrence D, Kisely S: Inequalities in healthcare provision for people with severe mental illness. J Psychopharmacol 2010;24(4 suppl):61–68.

19 Wagner EH, Austin BT, Von Korff M: Organizing care for patients with chronic illness. Milbank Q 1996;74:511–544.

20 Smith SM, Soubhi H, Fortin M, Hudon C, O'Dowd T: Managing patients with multimorbidity: systematic review of interventions in primary care and community settings. BMJ 2012;345:e5025.

21 Archer J, Bower P, Gilbody S, Lovell K, Richards D, Gask L, Coventry P: Collaborative care for depression and anxiety problems. Cochrane Database Syst Rev 2012;10:CD006525.

22 van der Feltz-Cornelis CM, van der Nuyen J, Stoop CH, Chan J, Jacobsen AM, Katon W, Snoek F, Sartorius N: Effect of interventions for major depressive disorder and significant depressive symptoms in patients with diabetes mellitus: a systematic review and meta-analysis. Gen Hosp Psychiatry 2010;32:380–395.

23 Piette JD, Richardson C, Valenstein M: Addressing the needs of patients with multiple chronic illnesses: the case of diabetes and depression. Am J Manag Care 2004;10:152–162.

24 Katon WJ, Lin EH, Von Korff M, Ciechanowski P, Ludman EJ, Young B, McCulloch D: Collaborative care for patients with depression and chronic illnesses. N Engl J Med 2010;363:2611–2620.

25 Unützer J, Powers D, Katon W, Langston C: From establishing an evidence-based practice to implementation in real-world settings: IMPACT as a case study. Psychiatr Clin North Am 2005;28:1079–1092.

26 Gunn J, Palmer V, Dowrick C, Herrman H, Griffiths F, Kokanovic R, Blashki G, Hegarty K, Johnson C, Potiriadis M, May C: Embedding effective depression care: using theory for primary care organizational and systems change. Implement Sci 2012;5:62.

27 Menchetti M, Sighinolfi C, Di Michele V, Peloso P, Nespeca C, Bandieri PV, Berardi D: Effectiveness of collaborative care for depression in Italy. A randomized controlled trial. Gen Hosp Psychiatry 2013;35:579–586.

28 Croghan TW, Brown JD: Integrating Mental Health Treatment into the Patient Centered Medical Home. Rockville, Agency for Healthcare Research and Quality, 2010.

29 Croghan TW, Brown JD: Integrating Mental Health Treatment Into the Patient Centered Medical Home. (Prepared by Mathematica Policy Research under Contract No. HHSA290200900019I TO2.) AHRQ Publication No. 10-0084-EF. Rockville, Agency for Healthcare Research and Quality, 2010.

30 Gunn J, Diggens J, Hegarty K, Blashki G: A systematic review of complex system interventions designed to increase recovery from depression in primary care. BMC Health Serv Res 2006;6:88.

Linda Gask, PhD, FRCPsych
Centre for Primary Care, Institute of Population Health
5th Floor Williamson Building, University of Manchester
Oxford Road, Manchester M13 9PL (UK)
E-Mail Linda.Gask@manchester.ac.uk

Sartorius N, Holt RIG, Maj M (eds): Comorbidity of Mental and Physical Disorders.
Key Issues Ment Health. Basel, Karger, 2015, vol 179, pp 165–177 (DOI: 10.1159/000365601)

Prevention of Comorbid Mental and Physical Disorders

Clemens Hosman

Emeritus Professor of Mental Health Promotion and Prevention, Maastricht University, Maastricht, and
Radboud University Nijmegen, Nijmegen, The Netherlands

Abstract

This chapter aims to explore the possibilities of preventing comorbid mental and physical disorders. It presents a framework of optional preventive strategies based on four explanatory models of comorbidity and six strategic dimensions. Addressing common early risk factors is discussed as one of these preventive strategies. Some examples of evidence-based prevention programs are presented that might contribute to prevention of comorbidity, needs for further research are discussed, and recommendations are presented for policy makers and practitioners to improve the perspectives for preventing mental and physical comorbidity. So far, preventing mental disorders and preventing physical disorders have been highly separated fields. It is recommended that both fields should broaden the range of baseline and outcome indicators and include longitudinal designs to understand the long-term broad-spectrum outcomes of preventive interventions better. Future policy plans and practices in physical and mental health should be more focused at preventing comorbidity, and enhance related expertise among policy-makers and practitioners. Finally, it is argued that the preventive approach of comorbidity should be broadened to 'smart clusters' of highly related mental, physical and social problems, with the last possibly referring to important common risk factors.

© 2015 S. Karger AG, Basel

As is extensively discussed and evidenced in this book, comorbidity of mental and physical disorders is a common phenomenon among patients in physical and mental healthcare, as well as in populations. Comorbidity with physical illnesses, particularly chronic physical illnesses, is reported especially for depression and anxiety disorders. This is in line with conclusions from the WHO World Mental Health Surveys in 18 countries, the results of which are presented in *Global Perspectives on Mental-Physical Comorbidity in the WHO World Mental Health Surveys* (2009) [1]. This international cross-sectional study measured the prevalence of mental and physical comorbidity during the year preceding data collection. Pooled across 18 surveys in developed and developing countries, odds ratios (ORs) between 1.8 and 3.3 were found for depression and dysthymia, and for different anxiety disorders in people with chronic pain conditions (arthritis, spinal pain, headache); among those with a heart disease, the ORs fell in the range of 1.9–2.7 [2]. Averaged across countries, the WHO study found that 36.9% of those with a depressive or anxiety disorder also suffered from a physical disorder. Prospective studies have shown that mental disorders could precede the onset of chronic physical disorders, but also that chronic physical disorders could precede the onset of mental disorders [3]. Mental and physical comorbidity represents a high burden to societies, as is illustrated by a recent Australian report on comorbidity. In 2007, almost 12% of Australians aged 16–85 had a mental disorder and a physical condition at the same time [4].

Comorbidity of mental disorders with physical disorders and comorbidity in general portends a poorer outcome for the patients and higher economic costs [2]. This includes poorer clinical course, higher risk of chronicity, disability, additive work-loss, poorer quality of life and mortality, as well as more healthcare utilization, poorer treatment adherence and reduced treatment success [5–7]. All of these outcomes stress the need to invest in prevention of comorbid disorders. If effective prevention strategies were implemented, such an investment could result in a tremendous reduction in human suffering, utilization of treatment services and huge cost savings in healthcare and social security.

Although the bulk of studies on comorbidity date from after 2000, there were studies on mental and physical comorbidity in the 1980s and 1990s [8–11]. By the 19th and 20th centuries, most mental hospitals had wards devoted to the treatment of physical illness of patients admitted because of mental illness. From the 1970s, a DSM-based assessment on the link between mental and physical diseases became an essential part of clinical diagnosis. Given this history, it is striking that there are very few publications on the prevention of comorbidity. Most of the current literature is almost exclusively focused on improving treatment for patients who already suffer from comorbid mental and physical illness.

This chapter aims to explore the possibility of preventing comorbid mental and physical disorders. It presents a theory-based framework of optional preventive strategies, describes examples of evidence-based prevention programs that might contribute to prevention of comorbidity, identifies further research needs and presents recommendations for policy makers and practitioners to improve the perspectives for preventing comorbidity.

Developments in Preventing Mental Disorders

Although the idea of preventing mental illness was introduced more than 100 years ago, science-based prevention has a history of around 30–40 years. Over the last decades, much progress has been made in understanding the risk and protective factors for mental disorders, which has been translated into a wide range of prevention programs. Prevention and health promotion, also in the mental health domain, have emerged internationally as a significant multidisciplinary field of science and practice, with a range of peer-reviewed scientific journals and specialized university departments and research centers in most continents. Currently, a wide range of science- and practice-based prevention programs are available. Thousands of controlled studies and a large range of systematic reviews and meta-analytic studies have been published showing that prevention programs targeting mental health can generate a wide range of positive outcomes [12–15]. These include strengthening protective factors (e.g. social-emotional skills, parenting competence, early parent-child interaction, coping with parental death and loss) and reducing the number of risk factors (e.g. child maltreatment, insecure attachment, early externalizing problems, bullying, substance use). There is also cumulative evidence of reductions in the onset of depression [16], anxiety symptoms and disorders [17, 18], eating disorders [19], externalizing problems and conduct disorders [20–22], and substance use problems [23]. Some randomized longitudinal studies have found significant effects even up to 15 and 40 years later. A growing number of economic evaluations of such programs have also provided evidence of their potential cost-effectiveness, especially early childhood programs [24].

To date, evidence-based prevention programs are internationally exchanged, disseminated and implemented, and supported by online international and national databases that are freely accessible to policymakers and practitioners. Given the steadily growing availability of effective prevention programs and the awareness of the enormous human and economic burden of mental disorders, it is likely that investments in preventing and treating mental disorders will become more balanced during this century.

In spite of these promising developments, major challenges exist in preventing mental disorders and promoting mental health. First, reviews and meta-analyses have shown that on average the effect sizes of prevention programs are small to moderate albeit significant, mostly ranging between 0.15 and 0.40. Meta-analyses have also shown large differences in effect sizes between programs, ranging from highly effective to showing no effect and in some cases even negative effects. This emphasizes the urgent need for program improvement and knowledge on the moderators and principles of effectiveness. Secondly, owing to the use of labor-intensive methods in many programs, low levels of implementation and poor resources and infrastructure for prevention, the population reach of these preventive interventions is still marginal. This contrasts with the much wider implementation and public reach of programs aimed at reducing the risk of chronic physical diseases such as those on reducing risk behaviors (e.g. smoking, substance use, consuming unhealthy food, risky driving) and environmental risk factors (e.g. air pollution, safe cars and roads, quality of food).

Finally, although Kessler and Price [25] already in 1993 advocated for investment in the prevention of comorbidity in psychiatric disorders, prevention research has only marginally addressed this issue. The fields of physical diseases and mental disorders prevention are highly separated. Even in cases where risk factors are addressed with a potential broad-spectrum outcome, testing their impact on the onset of both mental and physical illnesses is exceptional. Most disorder prevention programs in mental health are targeted at preventing a single disorder (e.g. depression).

To understand how to prevent physical and mental comorbidity and to measure if interventions are effective in preventing comorbidity, we first need to understand what comorbidity means, how we can differentiate between types of comorbidity and what the causal processes are underlying comorbidity.

Types of Comorbidity

Comorbidity can be defined at an *individual level* and at a *population level,* paralleling a clinical and a public health approach. This is a relevant distinction as prevention encompasses both preventive treatment and public health actions. Clinicians in physical and mental healthcare are challenged to identify the risk of comorbidity in individual patients and to act accordingly to prevent comorbidity. This requires widening clinical assessment and treatment to address the risk of multiple disorders in the physical and mental health domains, and, if needed, to involve other clinical disciplines.

Preventing comorbidity at the population level requires a public health way of thinking [26]. This includes population-based assessment, finding groups at high risk of comorbidity, identifying risk and protective factors, taking policy measures, initiating intervention programs to reduce the risk of disorders and comorbidity, and rigorously testing their efficacy and effectiveness. As discussed in the next section, interventions could range across a wide spectrum of optional preventive strategies that could start before the onset of a primary disorder and even before birth.

A distinction is commonly made between concurrent comorbidity and sequential comorbidity. *Concurrent comorbidity* refers to a situation in which a person has two or more disorders at the same time or at least during the same period. In such cases, taking timely action to prevent the onset of both disorders would be the most desirable approach. This is only possible when both disorders have evidence-based common risk or protective factors that are measurable and malleable during the antecedent period. For instance, growing empirical support exists for serious childhood adversities as a risk factor for both mental disorders and chronic physical diseases [1, 27]. Serious motor vehicle accidents with life-threatening experiences represent another example, as they could result in both serious physical injuries and a posttraumatic stress disorder among survivors. The many successful measures that have been adopted in recent decades to reduce serious traffic accidents have likely prevented many physical diseases or disability as well as comorbid posttraumatic stress disorders.

Sequential comorbidity refers to the onset of a secondary disease that is significantly associated with or influenced by an already existing primary disease. A well-known example of sequential comorbidity within the mental health domain is the relation between child anxiety disorders and adolescent major depression. In their longitudinal community study, Wittchen et al. [28] found that in the case of comorbidity, anxiety disorders mainly precede the onset of major depression. The ORs for later onset of depression ranged from 2.5 for specific phobia to 3.7 and 3.8 for panic disorder and agoraphobia. The time delay between the onset of the two related disorders could be short (e.g. a month or a year) or might even extend over one or more decades. The development of sequential comorbidity could encompass longitudinal pathways from the start of life into late adulthood [28]. It should be stressed, however, that anxiety symptoms might be an expression of child depression, which means that the ex-

ample might not reflect the sequential onset of two comorbid disorders, but age-related manifestations of a similar underlying long-term depressive disorder.

The distinction between concurrent and sequential comorbidity is less transparent than it looks at first sight. Concurrent refers to the co-occurrence of two disorders during a specific period of measurement, which could be the preceding week, month or year. In the case of a chronic physical disease, the onset of a reactive depression might follow months after the onset of a chronic heart disease. When their illness periods (prevalence) overlap, they could be considered as concurrent diseases, but as sequential comorbidity when we use onset as the criterion. As primary prevention aims to reduce onset of diseases, the onset criterion is of more strategic value as it offers more information on possible causal sequences and timing of preventive interventions and their outcomes. The onset of a primary disease could then be used as a trigger for interventions to prevent the onset of a related secondary disease. Further, when the secondary disorder is likely to start during the episode of the primary disorder, it is most practical that clinicians integrate efforts to prevent a secondary disorder in their treatment of the primary disorder. Finally, even when sequential comorbidity is established, how disorders are related remains an important question. Theory-based prospective studies are needed to establish if the onset of the second disorder is mediated by the features and outcomes of the primary disorder, or a delayed result from a common risk factor.

Four Explanatory Models

Most research on comorbidity is targeted at increasing the knowledge on prevalence and consequences of comorbidity, and on early detection and appropriate treatment. The causes of comorbidity are studied much less [7]. For prevention policies and programs, the latter type of studies are crucial, as preventive interventions typically aim to influence causes of diseases to lower the risk of onset. Designing an effective prevention approach to mental and physical comorbidity is only possible when we have insight into the underlying causal mechanisms. For this reason, this section is focused on understanding how multiple diseases could be related and how risk and protective factors might contribute to comorbidity. Next, we present a comprehensive framework of optional preventive strategies to reduce comorbidity.

To describe how and why disorders could be related, we differentiate between four models: (1) common antecedent model, (2) sequential comorbidity model, (3) bidirectional comorbidity model and (4) accidental comorbidity model.

The *common antecedent model* assumes that common, broad-spectrum factors influence the onset of multiple disorders, irrespective of whether the onset and prevalence of these disorders is co-occurring or separated over time. For childhood adversities (e.g. child abuse and neglect, parental mental illness, parental death and divorce), especially in the case of an accumulation of childhood adversities, extensive evidence exists for a wide range of long-term negative outcomes such as increased risk of depression, conduct disorders, drug and alcohol abuse, low self-esteem, poor emotional competence, risky sexual behavior, suicidal behavior, and adult-onset asthma, obesity and hypertension [1, 3].

The *sequential comorbidity model* presumes that features and outcomes of a primary disorder or its treatment increase the onset of a secondary disorder. Examples of factors that mediate the causal relationship between both disorders are serious stress experiences resulting from the primary disorder (e.g. pain, psychotrauma, physical disability, dependency, unemployment, social isolation), harmful coping behaviors (e.g. smoking, alcohol use, inactivity), negative social reactions (e.g. social stigma) or negative side effects of

medication. Preventive interventions could aim to reduce or compensate for these mediating outcomes. In the *bidirectional model,* two disorders and their outcomes are assumed to reinforce each other's development and chronic course. In this case, preventive interventions could address mediating outcomes of both disorders. Finally, in the *accidental comorbidity model* comorbid disorders are considered to be a random phenomenon, with no evidence of mutual influence or common causes. Each disorder is assumed to have an independent causal trajectory. The prevention of both disorders would require the implementation of separate primary preventive interventions, each addressing a different disorder.

Strategies to Prevent Comorbidity

To prevent comorbid mental and physical illness, one could choose from different intervention scenarios. Each strategy is defined by the combination of choices on a range of target- and strategy-related dimensions that roughly represent the 'what-who-why-when framework'. This framework of choices is composed of six dimensions:

(1) *Target.* This dimension concerns choices such as 'Which combination of comorbid disorders is targeted?', 'Which of them should be prevented?' and 'The mental disorder, physical disorder, or both?'.

(2) *Target population.* Should the target population be chosen through universal, selective or indicated prevention? This refers to a choice about the width and level of risk of the targeted population. Universal prevention targets whole populations, selective prevention targets groups at risk and indicated prevention targets persons or groups at high risk when they show subclinical symptoms that might grow into a diagnosable disorder. Targeted persons or groups could be at risk of the primary disorder, the secondary disorder or both. Identifying persons at high risk re-

quires the use of risk assessment tools that are still poorly developed in psychiatry.

(3) *Factors*. Which evidence-based risk or protective factors are targeted? This concerns especially the choice between addressing common causal factors or disorder-specific factors. Common factors are shared by multiple disorders, also called broad-spectrum factors. Disorder-specific factors could be related to either a physical disorder or a comorbid mental disorder. Risk factors for depression include, for instance, a parental mental illness, negative cognitive style, serious loss experiences, physical illnesses (e.g. diabetes, stroke, cardiac disease, loss of hearing), poverty and exposure to childhood traumas, while parental care, secure attachment, coping skills, social-emotional competence and social support are considered to protect against depression. Several of these factors (e.g. poverty, childhood maltreatment, secure attachment, social support) can also be considered as broad-spectrum factors. There is growing evidence that high risk is not just defined by single risk factors, but by the number of accumulating risk factors [28–30]; reducing this number by targeting the most malleable factors might be a cost-effective strategy to prevent disorders.

(4) *Timing*. This refers to choices concerning *when* to intervene. In the case of sequential comorbidity, the options are to provide a preventive intervention prior to, during or after a primary disorder, or prior to the secondary disorder. For instance, some studies suggest that depression in children, adolescents and young adults increases the risk of adult obesity [31, 32]. To lower the risk of secondary obesity, one could aim to prevent depression in adolescents, treat first episodes of depression effectively, prevent relapses, educate people with depression about healthy lifestyles, or detect and treat early eating problems among those with chronic depression. When common factors are targeted, a choice needs to be made about when to intervene along the life span. This will depend on

when a common risk or protective factor emerges and the most sensitive period during which such a factor could be influenced. For instance, research outcomes suggest that maternal depression, anxiety and chronic stress during pregnancy and early child maltreatment may result in a disturbed emotional brain and stress-response system (HPA axis) in childhood that is associated with long-term vulnerability to mental disorders and weakened immunity against chronic diseases. This points to the need to start preventive interventions as early as during pregnancy and infancy.

(5) *Provider*. Who will provide the preventive intervention and from which setting? This could be general practitioners, public nurses, mental health professionals, medical specialists in hospitals, public health professionals, health educators, or peers and experts-by-experience. It is highly desirable to integrate prevention in the work of all of these disciplines. Related to this is the choice between providing preventive support integrated in the treatment process (e.g. following a stepped care model) or by a referral to separately provided prevention programs.

(6) *Method*. This concerns the choice of intervention methods and theories and principles of change. Evidence-based prevention programs use a wide variety of intervention methods, such as home-visiting, parenting education, school-based programs, group-based courses, internet-based interventions, self-help books, support groups, individual counseling and preventive medication. These methods make use of different mechanisms of change to influence causal factors, such as providing information, feedback, modeling, competence training, emotional support and biological agents, as well as through environmental changes.

Figure 1 offers an overview of six alternative prevention strategies (PS) that could contribute to the prevention of comorbidity-based on combinations of choices at the target, target population, factor and timing dimensions. Preventive inter-

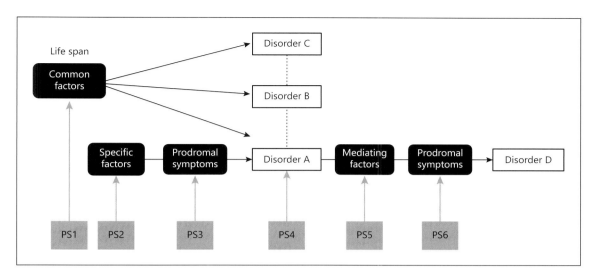

Fig. 1. Model of strategies to prevent comorbidity across the developmental trajectory and targeted at common or disorder-specific factors.

ventions could start during pregnancy and infancy to influence the development of common risk and protective factors early in life or during childhood and adolescence (PS1). Other interventions are targeted at disorder-specific risk factors (PS2) and prodromal or subclinical symptoms preceding the primary disorder (PS3), at effective treatment of the primary disorder (PS4), reducing negative outcomes of the primary disorder or its treatment (PS5), and addressing specific risk factors and subclinical symptoms of secondary disorders (PS6).

Promising Evidence-Based Preventive Programs

Following the strategic framework, many available evidence-based prevention programs might be useful as components of an integral approach to reduce comorbidity, although they were not developed originally for this purpose. We do not have the opportunity here to review all prevention programs that might be useful to

reduce comorbidity, but some examples will show that effective preventive actions might be possible.

Preventing Child Abuse and Neglect
The first example concerns the prevention of early child abuse and neglect, earlier identified as a broad-spectrum risk factor for both mental disorders and chronic physical diseases. In their *Lancet* review on interventions to prevent child maltreatment in 2009, Macmillan et al. [33] concluded that some home-visit programs have shown significant results in controlled trials. Effective programs include among others the Nurse-Family Partnership program that was evaluated in three randomized controlled trials across different US regions [34]. The program uses trained nurses that visit low-income first-time mothers during pregnancy and infancy, many of whom are single mothers or who have to cope with other life stressors. The nurses offer parent education, promote a healthy lifestyle, help the mothers to develop supportive relationships, and link them to appropriate health and

social services. The studies showed a wide variety of positive outcomes, including healthier maternal diets and less smoking, 75% fewer preterm deliveries, less irritable and fussy babies, a large drop in cases of child maltreatment, fewer emergency visits and less injury requiring medical examination, higher IQ among children of smoking mothers, and shorter periods of maternal dependency on social welfare. Fifteen years later, children from the intervention group showed dramatically less exposure to child abuse over this period, and lower levels of adolescent substance abuse, arrests and convictions than children from the control condition. Several other home-visit programs were not successful in reducing child maltreatment. Likely conditions for successful programs are a theory base, use of trained professionals (nurses) and safeguarding program fidelity during implementation. Also starting home-visiting during pregnancy might have significantly contributed to the success of the Nurse-Family Partnership program.

Two other types of programs have shown significant benefits in randomized trials, as reported by Macmillan et al. [33]. In the Safe Environment for Every Kid (SEEK) program, pediatric residents were trained to identify family problems and to link families to a social worker if needed. Families served by these trained residents showed fewer child-protection service reports, fewer instances of medical neglect, and less harsh punishment reported by parents, although the results were only marginally significant. Triple P is an Australian multicomponent program on positive parenting that addresses both universal and targeted populations of parents, using a wide variety of educational methods (e.g. group work, mass media, books, lectures). The results across 48 controlled studies showed significant reductions in ineffective parenting and depression among parents and less behavioral problems among their children, and in one large randomized trial across 18 US counties around 1 in 5 less cases of regis-

tered child abuse and less child maltreatment injuries [35, 36]. The program is currently implemented in a wide range of countries around the world.

Selected and Indicated Prevention of Depression
Most intervention programs that aim to prevent the onset of depression make use of cognitive-behavioral treatment principles to educate at-risk individuals to challenge negative beliefs, enhance positive thinking, and strengthen their problem solving and social skills. A wide variety of such programs have been standardized for adolescents, adults and elderly. The best known are the Coping with Depression Course and the Penn Resilience Program. These types of programs are provided in different formats such as group-based courses, self-help books in combination with telephone support and as internet-based programs. Each of these formats can easily be provided by physical and mental health services or by national institutes or nongovernmental organizations in the case of internet-based programs. Several reviews and meta-analyses across a large range of controlled trials have shown that these programs are effective in reducing depression-prone risk factors and depressive symptoms in different age groups, including older adults [37, 38]. Face-to-face, internet-based and self-help formats were all found to be effective. A meta-analysis of 19 randomized controlled trials that tested the impact of selected and indicated depression prevention programs found an average 22% reduction in the onset of depressive episodes as a result of participation in comparison to the incidence in the control groups [17]. One randomized controlled trial tested the integration of preventive interventions in a stepped care mental health service model for elderly with an elevated level of depressive symptoms [39]. Implementation of this prevention-oriented stepped care model resulted in a 50% reduction in incident depression or anxiety among elderly people aged 75 years or older, which was sustained over 24 months.

Healthy Lifestyle Programs

While chronic physical illnesses increase the risk of secondary mental disorders, such as depression and anxiety disorders, one might expect that public health efforts to prevent physical illnesses might also result in a lower incidence of secondary mental disorders. For instance, meta-analyses and systematic reviews have shown that the risk of type 2 diabetes and cardiovascular disease can be reduced through behavioral counseling to promote physical activity and a healthy diet [40–42]. No insight exists, however, on the impact of such programs at the onset of secondary depression among those at risk.

Challenges for Research

This exploratory paper has revealed a range of weaknesses in current knowledge and challenges for future prevention research. These challenges concern both the development of basic knowledge on the causal mechanisms of comorbidity, and the need to understand what works and how to prevent comorbidity.

The first challenge is to better understand what common risk and protective factors and shared developmental trajectories are in the etiology of mental disorders and chronic physical diseases. The science of developmental psychopathology could serve as a great source for such knowledge as this field is typically multidisciplinary in nature and studies complex and long-term etiological trajectories. The aim is to understand the spectrum of long-term mental and physical outcomes of common early risk factors (multifinality) as well as the different etiological paths toward a similar disorder (equifinality). Its multidisciplinary nature facilitates the integration of knowledge from genetic and epigenetic, biological, neurological, psychological and social research. This cross-fertilization of research approaches offers great opportunities to understand the interplay of biological, behavioral and social forces along the life span, and how the development of mental and somatic disorders is intertwined.

The growing knowledge on the narrow relationships between mental and physical disorders challenges the current practice in prevention research of treating the mental and physical disease domains as completely separated fields. As a consequence, in current prevention studies in the physical and mental health domains, major opportunities are missed to understand possible broad-spectrum effects of prevention programs that surpass the originally targeted domain. It is likely that both programs could contribute to outcomes in the other domain – outcomes that have remained undetected so far. Breaking through the borders between both domains could also open research on innovative approaches where prevention programs from both domains could be combined to create a higher level of 'collective impact'. For instance, under what conditions could lifestyle programs contribute to the prevention of depression and anxiety? How can depression prevention and mental health promotion programs be combined with lifestyle education in order to reduce smoking and obesity more effectively?

To understand the relationship between mental and physical processes and disorders better, it is necessary to broaden the range of baseline and outcome indicators in prevention studies. In prevention studies primarily targeting common mental disorders, more physical health indicators should be added, and likewise, mental health indicators should be added to studies primarily targeting physical disorders. Currently, it is common practice in trials targeted at the prevention of a specific disorder to measure at baseline only the presence of that disorder to exclude those with the disorder from participation in the trial. It is, however, likely that many included subjects had other disorders in the preceding year or at baseline that remained unnoticed. Including a

Table 1. Policy- and practice-based strategies to prevent comorbidity of mental and physical disorders

Policy-based
    Addressing comorbidity issues in health and mental health policies as well as in prevention and health promotion policies, and enhancing integrated approaches that address 'smart clusters' of multiple health and social problems
    Special focus on prevention and health promotion policies at reducing common early risk factors (e.g. childhood adversities) and strengthening protective factors (e.g. emotional resilience)
    Reducing the barriers between health and mental health policies, and between healthcare and mental healthcare
    Define quality standards in care for addressing prevention of comorbidity
    Making evidence-based preventive interventions more accessible through international and national databases
    Safeguarding professional and financial resources for prevention of comorbidity
    Investing in research and development of effective interventions to prevent comorbidity
Practice-based
    Adoption of risk assessment practices in primary health services and pediatric care for early identification of common risk factors
    Training practitioners in risk assessment and interventions to prevent comorbidity in different stages of the life span
    Enhancing integrated practices that address related health, mental health and social problems

wider set of health and mental health indicators could offer more insight into the impact of prevention trials on comorbidity, as well as in the impact of comorbid disorders on the outcomes of prevention trials.

Lastly, it would be desirable to combine the use of a wider spectrum of outcome indicators with longitudinal research designs in prevention studies. Many prevention and mental health promotion programs address early risk and protective factors (e.g. child maltreatment, parenting, social and emotional resilience) that might be related to a broad spectrum of mediating or long-term health outcomes. Studies that measure only short-term outcomes will likely undervalue the potential spectrum of effects of a prevention program.

In conclusion, a major issue for the future research agenda is to study what the potential of current evidence-based programs in the mental health domain is to prevent comorbidity, to improve both physical and mental health, and to learn how physical and mental health are related along the lifespan.

Challenges for Policy and Practice

The analysis and findings presented in this chapter show that a wide range of policy- and practice-based strategies are possible to prevent comorbidity, as illustrated in table 1. This should have implications for the work of individual physical and mental health practitioners, as well as for national and local public health and prevention policies.

Recognizing the interrelatedness of mental disorders with chronic physical diseases, and the role of common risk and protective factors, future policy plans should be more focused at integrated approaches, addressing mental and physical outcomes simultaneously. Currently, prevention of mental disorders still occupies a marginal and undervalued position in public health policies and health budgets worldwide. Finding opportunities for shared preventative and health promotion approaches might open new perspectives for preventing mental disorders. It will offer better opportunities to expand the reach in the population. It will also offer opportunities to increase the resources and professional capacity to implement prevention for mental health. This will be more likely when evidence shows that preventive interventions in the mental health domain are successfully targeting risk and protective factors that also have an impact on the development of chronic physical diseases. Given the growing knowledge of the impact of stress and depression on the functioning of the immune system, such a perspective is not imaginary.

To make practitioners and local health and mental health services more willing and capable to address the prevention of comorbidity, their expertise in preventative strategies and interventions needs to be expanded. This initially requires making prevention and comorbidity a standard element in the training of general practitioners, nurses, psychiatrists, psychologists and social workers. Secondly, the knowledge and accessibility of available evidence-based preventative interventions need to be increased. This could be facilitated by easily accessible databases of effective prevention programs as these are already available in some countries, such as the USA, the Netherlands, Norway and Germany. By establishing an international network of such databases, international exchange of new evidence-based programs and best practices could be improved.

Finally, this book is devoted to the relationship between mental and physical disorders. There are good reasons, however, to assume that the relationship between both types of problems is caused or at least reinforced by existing social problems, such as poverty, unemployment, discrimination, domestic violence, war-related traumas, housing problems, poor social networks, social isolation and social stigma. Such social circumstances could be considered as common risk factors or even as the 'root of the roots'. For this reason, the message of this book is that the single disorder approach to address mental-physical comorbidity should be expanded to focus on social-mental-physical comorbidity. The public health and prevention approaches in the future should not be targeted at single disorders one by one, but at so-called 'smart clusters' of highly related social, mental and physical problems, especially those clusters that concentrate in low-income countries, problem areas, disadvantaged communities or populations at high risk for an accumulation of problems. This challenges health and public health managers, health promoters, nongovernmental organizations, community leaders, citizen groups, private companies, policy makers and politicians to sit together and communicate about an effective integral preventive approach to such clusters of problems. In such a comprehensive approach, multiple social measures and preventive interventions could be combined in a complementary way, where the collective impact is larger and has a broader spectrum than could be achieved by stand-alone interventions and programs. Such a smart cluster and integral approach could be concentrated at crucial stages of the life span, such as a 'healthy start in life' to facilitate children growing up in healthy, safe and caring environments that enhance their physical, mental and social resilience, and immune systems, and will contribute to less mental, physical and social problems during their adolescence and adulthood. Integrating a focus on the social determinants in a mental health approach is in line with the core messages of the recent WHO Comprehensive Mental Health Action Plan 2013–2020 [43].

In conclusion, the field of mental health and physical health should become more integrated, which would make working on the prevention of comorbidity a normal phenomenon instead of an exception. In the end it will be the well-being of the person that will gain most from it.

References

1 Von Korff MR, Scott KM, Gureje O: Global Perspectives on Mental-Physical Comorbidity in the WHO World Mental Health Surveys. New York, Cambridge University Press, 2009.

2 Gureje O: The pattern and nature of mental-physical comorbidity: specific or general?; in Von Korff MR, Scott KM, Gureje O (eds): Global Perspectives on Mental-Physical Comorbidity in the WHO World Mental Health Surveys. New York, Cambridge University Press, 2009, pp 51–83.

3 Gilbert R, Spatz Widom C, Browne K, Fergusson D, Webb E, Janson S: Burden and consequences of child maltreatment in high-income countries. Lancet 2009; 373:68–81.

4 Australian Institute of Health and Welfare: Comorbidity of Mental Disorders and Physical Conditions 2007. Cat. No. PHE 155. Canberra, AIHW, 2011.

5 Buist-Bouwman MA, de Graaf R, Vollebergh WA, Ormel J: Comorbidity of physical and mental disorders and the effect on work-loss days. Acta Psychiatr Scand 2005;111:436–443.

6 Fried LP, Ferrucci L, Darer J, Williamson JD, Anderson G: Untangling the concepts of disability, frailty, and comorbidity: implications for improved targeting and care. J Gerontol A Biol Sci Med Sci 2004;59:255–263.

7 Gijsen R, Hoeymans N, Schellevis FG, Ruwaard D, Satariano WA, van den Bos GA: Causes and consequences of comorbidity: a review. J Clin Epidem 2001;54: 661–674.

8 Romano J, Turner J: Chronic pain and depression: does the evidence support a relationship? Psychol Bull 1985;97:18–34.

9 Turner R, Noh S: Physical disability and depression: a longitudinal analysis. J Health Soc Behav 1988;29:23–37.

10 Eaton WW, Armenian H, Gallo J, Pratt L, Ford DE: Depression and risk for onset of type II diabetes. A prospective population-based study. Diabetes Care 1996;19:1097–1102.

11 Penninx BW, Beekman AT, Ormel J, Kriegsman DM, Boeke AJ, Eijk JT, Deeg DJ: Psychological status among elderly people with chronic diseases: does type of disease play a part? J Psychosom Res 1996;40:521–534.

12 Hosman CM, Jane-Llopis E, Saxena S (eds): Prevention of Mental Disorders: Effective Interventions and Policy Options. WHO Summary Report 2004. Geneva, World Health Organization, 2004.

13 Saxena S, Jane-Llopis E, Hosman C: Prevention of mental and behavioral disorders: implications for policy and practice. World Psychiatry 2006;5:5–14.

14 Institute of Medicine and National Research Council: Preventing Mental, Emotional, and Behavioral Disorders among Young People: Progress and Possibilities. Committee on Prevention of Mental Disorders and Substance Abuse among Children, Youth and Young People. Washington, National Academic Press, 2009.

15 Anderson P, Jane-Llopis E, Hosman C: Reducing the silent burden of impaired mental health. Health Prom Int 2011; 26(suppl 1):i4–i9.

16 Cuijpers P, Van Straten A, Smit F, Mihalopoulos C, Beekman A: Preventing the onset of depressive disorders: a meta-analytic review of psychological interventions. Am J Psychiatry 2008;165: 1272–1280.

17 Fisak BJ Jr, Richard D, Mann A: The prevention of child and adolescent anxiety: a meta-analytic review. Prev Sci 2011;12:255–268.

18 Teubert D, Pinquart M: A meta-analytic review on the prevention of symptoms of anxiety in children and adolescents. J Anxiety Disord 2011;25:1046–1059.

19 Taylor CB, Bryson S, Luce KH, Cunning D, Doyle AC: Prevention of eating disorders in at-risk college-age women. Arch Gen Psychiatry 2006;63:881–888.

20 Bierman KL, Coie JD, Dodge KA, et al: The effects of the Fast Track Program on serious problem outcomes at the end of elementary school. J Clin Child Adolesc Psychol 2004;33:650–661.

21 Grove AG, Evans SW, Pastor DA, Mack SD: A meta-analytic examination of follow-up studies of programs designed to prevent the primary symptoms of oppositional defiant and conduct disorders. Aggress Violent Behav 2008;13:169–184.

22 Wilson WJ, Lipsey MW: School-based interventions for aggressive and disruptive behavior: update of a meta-analysis. Am J Prev Med 2007;33(2 suppl):S130–S143.

23 Jackson C, Geddes R, Haw S, Frank J: Interventions to prevent substance use and risky sexual behavior in young people: a systematic review. Addiction 2011; 107:733–747.

24 Aos S, Lieb R, Mayfield J, Miller M, Pennucci A: Benefits and Costs of Prevention and Early Intervention Programs for Youth. Olympia, Washington State Institute for Public Policy, 2004.

25 Kessler R, Price R: Primary prevention of secondary disorders: a proposal and agenda. Am J Community Psychol 1993; 21:607–633.

26 Oldenburg B, O'Neil A, Cocker F: Public health perspectives on the co-occurence of non-communicable diseases and common mental disorders; in Sartorius N, Holt RIG, Maj M (eds): Comorbidity of Mental and Physical Disorders. Key Issues Ment Health. Basel, Karger, 2015, vol 179, pp 15–22.

27 Scott KM: The development of mental-physical comorbidity; in Von Korff MR, Scott KM, Gureje O (eds): Global Perspectives on Mental-Physical Comorbidity in the WHO World Mental Health Surveys. New York, Cambridge University Press, 2009, pp 97–107.

28 Wittchen HH, Kessler RC, Pfister H, Lieb M: Why do people with anxiety disorders become depressed? A prospective longitudinal community study. Acta Psychiatr Scand Suppl 2000;406:14–23.

29 Appleyard K, Byron E, Van Dulmen MH, Sroufe LA: When more is not better: the role of cumulative risk in child behavior outcomes. J Child Psychol Psychiatry 2005;46:235–245.

30 Rutter M, Quinton D: Parental psychiatric disorder: effects on children. Psychol Med 1984;14:853–880.

31 Hassler G, Pine DS, Gamma A, Milos G, Ajdacic V, Eich D, Rössler W, Angst J: The associations between psychopathology and overweight: a 20-year prospective study. Psychol Med 2004;34:1047–1057.

32 Kawada T, Inagaki H, Wakayama Y, Katsumata M, Li Q, Li Q, Otsuka T: Depressive state and subsequent weight gain in workers: a 4-year follow up study. Work 2011;38:123–127.

33 Macmillan HL, Wathen CN, Barlow J, Fergusson DM, Leventhal JM, Taussig HN: Interventions to prevent child maltreatment and associated impairment. Lancet 2009;373:250–266.

34 Olds DL: The nurse-family partnership: an evidence-based preventive intervention. Infant Ment Health J 2006;27:5–25.

35 De Graaf I, Speetjens P, Smit F, de Wolff M, Tavecchio L: Effectiveness of the Triple P Positive Parenting Program on parenting: a meta-analysis. Fam Relat 2008;57:553–566.

36 Prinz RJ, Sanders MR, Shapiro CJ, Whitaker DJ, Lutzker JR: Population-based prevention of child maltreatment: the US Triple P system population trial. Prev Sci 2009;10:1–12.

37 Forsman AK, Schierenbeck I, Wahlbeck K: Psychosocial interventions for the prevention of depression in older adults: systematic review and meta-analysis. J Aging Health 2011;23:387–416.

38 Calear AL, Christensen H: Systematic review of school-based prevention and early intervention programs for depression. J Adolesc 2010;33:429–438.

39 van't Veer-Tazelaar PJ, van Marwijk HW, van Oppen P, van der Horst HE, Smit F, Cuijpers P, Beekman AT: Prevention of late-life anxiety and depression has sustained effects over 24 months: a pragmatic randomized trial. Am J Geriatr Psychiatry 2011;19:230–239.

40 Esposito K, Kastorini CM, Panagiotakos DB, Giugliano D: Prevention of type 2 diabetes by dietary patterns: a systematic review of prospective studies and meta-analysis. Metab Syndr Relat Disord 2010;8:471–476.

41 Lin JS, O'Connor E, Whitlock EP, Beil TL: Behavioral counseling to promote physical activity and a healthful diet to prevent cardiovascular disease in adults: a systematic review for the U.S. Preventive Services Task Force. Ann Intern Med 2010;153:736–750.

42 Rawal LB, Tapp RJ, Williams ED, Chan C, Yasin S, Oldenburg B: Prevention of type 2 diabetes and its complications in developing countries: a review. Int J Behav Med 2012;19:121–133.

43 World Health Organization: Comprehensive Mental Health Action Plan 2013–2020. Geneva, WHO, 2013.

Prof. Dr. Clemens Hosman, PhD
Hosman Prevention Consultancy and Innovation
Knapheidepad 6
NL–6562 DW Groesbeek (The Netherlands)
E-Mail Hosman@psych.ru.nl

Sartorius N, Holt RIG, Maj M (eds): Comorbidity of Mental and Physical Disorders.
Key Issues Ment Health. Basel, Karger, 2015, vol 179, pp 178–181 (DOI: 10.1159/000365606)

Conclusions and Outlook

Norman Sartorius[a] · Richard I.G. Holt[b] · Mario Maj[c]

[a]Association for the Improvement of Mental Health Programmes, Geneva, Switzerland;
[b]Human Development and Health Academic Unit, Faculty of Medicine, University of Southampton,
University Hospital Southampton NHS Foundation Trust, Southampton, UK; [c]Department of Psychiatry,
University of Naples, Naples, Italy

Abstract

The reviews of evidence presented in the chapters of this volume lead to several conclusions and four recommendations. The prevalence and incidence of comorbidity of mental and physical disorders are high and likely to grow. The problems of comorbidity are not the simple addition of problems related to the diseases involved, as they worsen the prognosis of all diseases involved to a significantly greater extent. At present there is no clear strategy of action concerning comorbidity at the primary, secondary or tertiary levels of healthcare or in the local, provincial, national or international decision-making systems. The evidence presented in the book also allows the formulation of recommendations concerning the training of healthcare staff and the organization of healthcare. To support the changes proposed and to evaluate their effects it will be necessary to strengthen research concerning comorbidity and seek ways of sharing experience obtained by the use of different models of care catering to the needs of people with comorbid illnesses.

Several conclusions emerge from the chapters that have been included in this volume. First, comorbidity between mental and physical disorders is frequent in the population and its prevalence grows with age and with successes of medicine saving lives (but not curing diseases) [Rosenblat et al., pp. 42–53; Holt, pp. 54–65; Monteleone and Brambilla, pp. 66–80; Kariuki-Nyuthe and Stein, pp. 81–87; Lawrence et al., pp. 88–98; Müller, pp. 99–113; Gordon et al., pp. 114–128]. Second, comorbidity does not simply add problems related to one disease to those of the other: by and large the simultaneous presence of several diseases makes the prognosis of all the diseases involved worse, their complications more frequent and their treatment more complicated [Fisher et al., pp. 1–14; Oldenburg et al., pp. 15–22]. Third, no medical discipline has a clear strategy of action required when a disease that does not belong to its special field of interest accompanies one that is within the domain of their specialty. Fourth, the current trend of super-specialization and fragmentation of medicine may make matters worse unless appropriate action is taken promptly [Fisher et al., pp. 1–14]. Fifth, primary healthcare professionals (e.g. general practitioners or family physicians) are aware of the problems related to comorbidity because they encounter them even more frequently than other medical specialists;

however, most have not received specific training in the use of skills that might be central in dealing with comorbidity [Boeckxstaens et al., pp. 129–136; Cushing and Evans, pp. 137–147; Gask, pp. 157–164].

The material presented also indicates directions of future work at different levels. First, it is clear that changes in the delivery of education of healthcare personnel are urgently needed [Cushing and Evans, pp. 137–147; Millar et al., pp. 148–156; Gask, pp. 157–164]. This is true for all categories of healthcare professionals including nurses, medical assistants, general practitioners and specialists, at both undergraduate and postgraduate levels. Problem-based learning was seen as an educational method that would lead to a better understanding of the problems and solutions and that would be in harmony with the environment in which the patient lives and the service operates. Unfortunately, the training materials that were produced by specialists, who were to lead problem-based learning as well as the implementation of the training, have neglected, to a large degree, the comorbidity of mental and physical disorders. The education of healthcare personnel in institutions which are usually uneasy federations of specialized departments did not help in developing an attitude of dealing with illnesses fully aware of the person who suffers from that illness and possibly from various other ills and problems. Teachers of the disciplines are usually specialists knowledgeable in their own field and somewhat distant or even possibly disdainful of other specialists and matters with which they deal. In many parts of the world, family physicians are rarely invited to train medical students and other students of health professions. By contrast, in the UK general practitioners are invited to teach increasingly often and it is to be hoped that this will soon happen elsewhere. Carers who often have a vast array of experiences in dealing with comorbid chronic mental and physical diseases are only excep-

tionally invited to serve as teachers of health professional students.

The distinction of psychological reactions to being ill and mental disorders in a strict sense is also a problem. Many of those surrounding the patient – professional and nonprofessional carers – are ready to dismiss the notion that the patient they have before them has a depressive illness that requires specific treatment, preferring to explain the symptoms in 'logical' terms as the reaction of patients who were told that they have a serious illness and that they have to live with it. Occasionally both the patient and the doctor realize that a mental disorder as well as a physical illness is present, but they are united in a tacit collusion about the presence of the mental illness which they hope will vanish once the treatment of the physical illness has been successfully completed and therefore focus on the treatment of the physical illness only. This way of proceeding is also seen and emulated by the medical students who in later years of their training often learn by imitating the behavior of more experienced general practitioners or other specialists.

A second line of recommendations that could be made concerns in-service training of doctors and other health personnel. The two examples given in the chapters by Cushing and Evans [pp. 137–147] and Millar et al. [pp. 148–156] concern the in-service training of nurses and general practitioners. In the chapter by Cushing and Evans, which describes the training of senior nurses and nurse trainers in African countries, the participants are cited as saying they found it useful to discuss how to organize their service in a manner that would facilitate the management of problems arising for people with comorbid depression and diabetes because they have not been trained in ways in which this should be done. Bearing in mind that in the countries from which the nurses attending the course came, and where nurses are the backbone of health service, it is clear that the training of nurses about the ways in which their service should be organized is a neglected priority in the effort to provide appropriate care to people who have the misfortune of suffering from more than one illness at the same time [Beran, pp. 33–41; Millar et al., pp. 148–156]. Family physicians seem to be clear about the need to see the patients in their totality and to pay attention to all of their ills; there is, however, no consensus about the ways in which this type of approach to the patients they see can best be supported by referral and feedback arrangement within the health system as a whole [Boeckxstaens et al., pp. 129–136].

A third recommendation that could be formulated concerns funding. At present a considerable proportion of research funding is channeled through institutions which deal with a single disease or a group of diseases. This is the principle on which the National Institutes of Health in the USA as well as many funding agencies in other countries have been constructed. Some of the major foundations fund various types of research, but even there a major part of the funding follows a call for proposals on a single disease or disease group. There are very few calls for proposals on comorbidity and even fewer that would specifically invite applications for research on comorbid mental and physical disorders [Hosman, pp. 165–177]. Universities, which should, if true to their mission, fund research on topics of major public health importance and could therefore be expected to fund research on comorbidity, are increasingly adopting the strategy of making a good part of their living from overhead charges to projects which have been funded by someone else and only rarely provide their researchers funds for projects that would express the universities' public health mission. It might therefore be recommended that universities take it upon themselves to fund research and other work related to comorbidity at least until it dawns on the other agencies that comorbidity should be at the center of their interest rather than being seen as a confounding factor. Wheth-

er the universities will be in a position to play the role of being leaders in research which is of public health importance will to a large extent depend on the support of their governments – which unfortunately in recent times they have refused to provide.

Finally, in addition to the recommendations on funding of research and reorientation of training, a fourth recommendation could be directed to the search for opportunities to study and test the most appropriate models of service for people with comorbid mental and physical disorders. In the 19th century, mental hospitals were obliged to have wards for inpatients who in addition to their mental disorder also had a physical illness. These wards were usually run by specialists in internal medicine who in the course of time acquired considerable experience and knowledge about mental disorders. In the early 20th century a new category of super-specialists came into existence – the liaison psychiatrists who often, in addition to their postgraduate education in psychiatry, also had attended postgraduate courses in internal medicine. To an extent, the existence of this group is a sad admission of the fact that the vast majority of psychiatrists was not willing or able to deal with physical illness in their patients. This refusal to perform all that undergraduate and postgraduate education gave to these doctors has not been typical for other specialties; for example, there are no liaison surgeons, liaison dermatologists or liaison ophthalmologists although these specialists, among others, often deal with patients who have a mental disorder as well as a dermatological illness or problems with their eyes. Liaison psychiatry and 'general hospital psychiatry' are clearly not the best way to a solution of the comorbidity problem and therefore there is an urgent need to develop service models that will be better suited to meet the needs of people with comorbid illnesses and to provide training in ways of doing it.

Recommended Reading

Glassman A, Maj M, Sartorius N: Depression and Heart Disease. Hoboken, Wiley-Blackwell, 2010.

Gordon AJ: Physical Illness and Drugs of Abuse: A Review of the Evidence. Cambridge, Cambridge University Press, 2010.

Katon W, Maj M, Sartorius N: Depression and Diabetes. Hoboken, Wiley-Blackwell, 2010.

Kissane DW, Maj M, Sartorius N: Depression and Cancer. Hoboken, Wiley-Blackwell, 2011.

Kurrle S, Brodaty H, Hogarth R: Physical Comorbidities of Dementia. Cambridge, Cambridge University Press, 2012.

Leucht S, Burkard T, Henderson JH, Maj M, Sartorius N: Physical Illness and Schizophrenia: A Review of the Evidence. Cambridge, Cambridge University Press, 2007.

O'Hara J, McCarthy J, Bouras N: Intellectual Disability and Ill Health: A Review of the Evidence. Cambridge, Cambridge University Press, 2010.

Prof. Norman Sartorius, MA, MD, PhD, FRCPsych
President, Association for the Improvement of Mental Health Programmes
14, Chemin Colladon
CH–1209 Geneva (Switzerland)
E-Mail sartorius@normansartorius.com

Author Index

Subject Index

Low-income countries
    definition 33
    health system limitations 36–39
    local immunity involvement 39
    multimorbidity overview 34, 35
Luteinizing hormone, eating disorder effects 74

Marijuana
    cancer risks 116
    cardiovascular disease risks 117, 118
    ear, nose and throat disorders 118
    female reproductive system effects 120, 121
    gastrointestinal disorders 119
    hematopoietic disorders 116, 117
    immune system effects 115
    infection risks 116
    metabolic, nutritional and endocrine
        disorders 120
    neurological disorders 121, 122
    overview of effects 123, 124
    renal and male urogenital disorders 120
    respiratory dysfunction 119
Medical school, see Training, medical students about
    comorbidity
Multimorbidity
    concept 130
    evidence base 131–133
    general practitioner role in management 134,
        135
    goal-oriented care 132, 134
    implications for health system 133
    low-income countries 34, 35

Obesity
    antipsychotic medication effects 57
    cardiovascular disease
        management 61, 62
        risk in severe mental illness 56
Obsessive-compulsive disorder, see Anxiety disorders
Opioids
    cardiovascular disease risks 118
    ear, nose and throat disorders 118
    immune system effects 115
    infection risks 116
    neurological disorders 122
    overview of effects 123, 124
    pregnancy effects 121
    renal and male urogenital disorders 120
    respiratory dysfunction 119

PANDAS 108
Panic disorder, see Anxiety disorders
Patient-centered care
    care model development for comorbidity and
        multimorbidity 161, 163
    collaborative care elements 161
    fragmentation of healthcare 157, 158
    physician training 140, 141, 163
Phobia, see Anxiety disorders
PREDIMED trial 18
Pregnancy, substance abuse effects 120, 121
Primary care
    fragmentation of healthcare
        consequences of specialization and
            fragmentation 158, 159
        overview 157, 158
    general practitioner role in multimorbidity
        management 134, 135
    goal-oriented care 132, 134
    importance 159, 160
    overview 131
    patient-centered care, see Patient-centered care
Prolactin, eating disorder effects 75
Public health intervention
    comorbid non-communicable diseases and mental
        disorders
        control in high-risk populations 18, 19
        economic impact 20, 21
        implementation and scale-up of programs
            context 19
            cost and responsibility 19, 20
        prevention 17, 18
        prospects 21
    definition 17

Respiratory disease
    global burden of chronic disease 15, 34
    smoking, see Smoking
    substance abuse and dysfunction 119

Schizophrenia
    cardiovascular disease comorbidity
        antipsychotic medication effects on physical
            disease 57–59
        epidemiology of cardiovascular disease
            comorbidity 55
        etiology of cardiovascular disease comorbidity
            diabetes 56, 57
            dyslipidemia 56